Clinical Pharmacy

Clinical Pharmacy

Editor: Winter Hayes

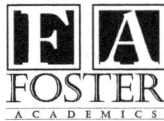

FA FOSTER
ACADEMICS

www.fosteracademics.com

www.fosteracademics.com

FOSTER
ACADEMICS

Cataloging-in-Publication Data

Clinical pharmacy / edited by Winter Hayes.
    p. cm.
Includes bibliographical references and index.
ISBN 978-1-63242-826-4
1. Pharmacy. 2. Clinical pharmacology. 3. Clinical medicine. I. Hayes, Winter.
RS153 .C55 2019
615--dc23

© Foster Academics, 2019

Foster Academics,
118-35 Queens Blvd., Suite 400,
Forest Hills, NY 11375, USA

ISBN 978-1-63242-826-4 (Hardback)

Contents

Preface

The purpose of the book is to provide a glimpse into the dynamics and to present opinions and studies of some of the scientists engaged in the development of new ideas in the field from very different standpoints. This book will prove useful to students and researchers owing to its high content quality.

Clinical pharmacy is a sub-field of pharmacy. It is concerned with providing direct care to the patients by optimizing the use of medication and promoting health and wellness. A specialist in this field is called a clinical pharmacist. The main task of clinical pharmacists involves the care of patients in all health care settings. In order to carry out their tasks in a smooth and effective manner, they are often required to collaborate with nurses, physicians and other healthcare professionals. They play a significant role in the health care system by providing information regarding the safe and cost-effective uses of medications. This book unfolds the innovative aspects of clinical pharmacy, which will be crucial for the progress of this field in the future. It studies, analyzes and upholds the pillars of clinical pharmacy and its utmost significance in modern times. Students, researchers, experts and all associated with clinical pharmacy will benefit alike from this book.

At the end, I would like to appreciate all the efforts made by the authors in completing their chapters professionally. I express my deepest gratitude to all of them for contributing to this book by sharing their valuable works. A special thanks to my family and friends for their constant support in this journey.

Editor

A Comparison of Competences for Healthcare Professions in Europe

Antonio Sánchez-Pozo

Department of Biochemistry, Faculty of Pharmacy, University of Granada, Campus Cartuja s/n, Granada 18071, Spain; sanchezpster@gmail.com

Academic Editor: Jeffrey Atkinson

Abstract: In Europe and elsewhere, there is increasing interest in competence-based education (CBE) and training for professional practice in healthcare. This review presents competences for pharmacy practice in Europe and compares them with those for medicine and dentistry. Comparisons amongst competence frameworks were made by matching the European Directive for Professional Qualifications in sectoral professions such as healthcare (EU directive) with the frameworks of competences elaborated by European consortia in pharmacy (PHAR-QA), medicine (MEDINE), and dentistry (ADEE). The results show that the recommendations of the EU directive for all three professions are similar. There is also widespread similarity in the formulation of competences for all healthcare professions. Furthermore, for medicine and pharmacy, the rankings by practitioners of the vast majority of competences are similar. These results lay the foundations for the design of more interdisciplinary educational programs for healthcare professionals, and for the development of team-based care.

Keywords: competences; education; pharmacy; healthcare professions

1. Introduction

In Europe, and elsewhere in the world, there is an increasing shift from content-based to competence-based education (CBE) and practice. In healthcare sciences, this process started in medicine [1] and is now developing in pharmacy. This shift can bring many advantages. Competences for practice are better understood by the society at large, and thus provide a clearer public statement of the role of the healthcare practitioner. Competences are useful in the mutual recognition of qualifications amongst institutions and government bodies, especially at an international level as amongst European member states. CBE promotes greater comparability and compatibility in educational programs, thus facilitating student and practitioner mobility. The CBE approach also stimulates the development of advanced practice. In European pharmacy, CBE is at present limited; student [2] and practitioner mobility is low [3], and advanced practice, although developing, is still not recognized by the EU [4].

Competence frameworks for pharmacy education have emerged during the last years both at national, European, and worldwide levels. These have been promoted by professional chambers and associations, and academia [5–15]. European frameworks have been proposed for other healthcare sciences such as medicine (MEDINE: Medical education in Europe) [16] and dentistry (ADEE: Association for Dental Education in Europe) [17].

In this paper, we compared the CBE framework for EU pharmacies developed by the PHAR-QA (Quality assurance in European pharmacy education and training) [13] consortium (a follow-up to the PHARMINE (Pharmacy education in Europe) [14] project) with those for medicine (MEDINE [16]) and dentistry (ADEE [17]).

The comparison was carried out in three parts:

1.   The recommendations for the minimum requirements of the EU directive [4].
2.   The formulations of the academic proposals for CBE in healthcare sciences.
3.   The perception by practitioners of the framework proposals for pharmacy and medicine. (This step has not to our knowledge been undertaken in dentistry).

EU Directives of the European Parliament and of the Council on the recognition of professional qualifications have consolidated a system of mutual recognition. It provides for automatic recognition for a limited number of professions based on harmonized minimum training requirements (sectoral professions), a general system for the recognition of evidence of training and automatic recognition of professional experience. The directives have also established a new system of the free provision of services.

Evaluation of the perception of practitioners is an essential step in building a framework. To do this, practitioners rank the competences proposed according to their own development needs, after reflection on the competences required for their particular professional practice. Faculties and other academic institutions have collaborated in the establishment of a framework of competences based on the scientific advances and new methodologies in education. Examples of this collaboration include the PHARMINE and MEDINE. However, the academic knowledge of the problems have to be tested in the working places. This dual approach—an academic proposal followed by ranking by practitioners—is an integral part of the production of a viable framework.

2. Results and Discussion

2.1. The Recommendations for Minimum Requirements of the European Directive

The 2013 EU directive on the recognition of professional qualifications [4], an amendment of the 2005 EU directive [18], deals mainly with structural management issues, such as length of degree course and the attributes of training, rather than competences. It does, however, set out a series of minimum requirements for the healthcare sciences (Table 1).

Table 1. The minimum requirements for healthcare professions as given in the 2005 EU directive [4].

Requirement	Pharmacy	Medicine	Dentistry
The sciences upon which practice is based	X	X	X
The scientific methods including the principles of measurement	X	X	X
Evaluation of scientific data	X	X	X
Structure, function and behavior of healthy and sick persons	X	X	X
Traineeship in a community or hospital setting	X	X	X
Clinical disciplines and practices		X	X

As shown in Table 1, the requirements of the EU directive for the sectoral professions of pharmacy, medicine (general practice), and dentistry have many things in common. Education and training for all three types of practitioner require basic science, human physiopathology, and clinical experience.

Only the requirements for medicine and dentistry, however, emphasize clinical disciplines in which the professional is in direct contact with healthy or sick individuals. However, there has been an evolution in pharmacy from the EU directive in its 2005 version [18] to its 2013 version [4] (Table 2), with the installation of a more "clinical" role for pharmacists as far as patient centered care and public health is concerned. Others professions such as nurses and midwives have also had changes in their requirements, whereas medicine and dentistry remain unchanged.

Table 2. Description of the roles of pharmacist given in the 2005 and 2013 EU directives. Differences in EU directives concerning patient care and public health issues are given in bold.

EU Directive 2005 [18]	EU Directive 2013 [4]
Preparation of the pharmaceutical form of medicinal products; manufacture and testing of medicinal products; testing of medicinal products in a laboratory for the testing of medicinal products; storage, preservation and distribution of medicinal products at the wholesale stage	Same as 2005
Preparation, testing, storage and supply of medicinal products in pharmacies open to the public	Ordering, manufacture, testing, storage and dispensing of safe, high quality medicinal products in public pharmacies
Preparation, testing, storage and dispensing of medicinal products in hospitals	Same as 2005
Provision of information and advice on medicinal products	Medication management and provision of information and advice about medicinal products and **general health information**
	Provision of advice and support to patients in connection with the use of non-prescription medicines and self-medication
	Contributions to public health and information campaigns

It should be noted that the elements given in Tables 1 and 2 are not competences. They describe knowledge or activities. For instance, the requirement "the sciences upon which practice is based" corresponds to the levels ("knows" and "knows how") of Miller's triangle [19]; or the "Provision of information and advice on medicinal products" corresponds to the levels ("shows how" and "does"). However, the EU directive still lacks detail on "competences for practice" and this is one of the reasons why the PHAR-QA, MEDINE, and ADEE academic consortia produced their detailed frameworks for pharmacy, medicine, and dentistry, respectively.

2.2. The Formulations of the Academic Proposals for CBE in Healthcare Sciences

A comparison was made of the competence frameworks proposed by academia for pharmacy (PHAR-QA), medicine (MEDINE), and dentistry (ADEE). The major competences were divided into domains as shown in Table 3. We grouped the competences in clusters of related competences: first in groups of very close competences that we called major competences, and then in domains of related major competences. For example, the major competence "professional attributes" includes competences such as probity, honesty, commitment to maintaining good practice, concern for quality, critical and self-critical abilities, reflective practice, and empathy, and the domain "professionalism" includes professional attributes, professional work, and ability to apply ethical and legal principles. This grouping facilitates comparisons, as the individual definitions of competences by the three consortia concerned are not always identical, even though they are talking about the same concept.

The following domains are common to all three professions: professionalism, interpersonal competences, communication and social skills, knowledge base, information and information literacy, clinical information gathering, diagnosis and treatment planning, therapy, establishing and maintaining health, and prevention and health.

The major competences included in the domains of Table 3 account for more than 95% of the major competences described in the frameworks. They can thus be considered as representative of the frameworks proposed.

Table 3. Domains and major competences in frameworks of competences for the pharmacist (PHAR-QA), general medical practitioner (MEDINE) and dentist (ADEE).

Domain	Major Competences		
	PHAR-QA	MEDINE	ADEE
1. Professionalism	Personal competences: values.	Professional attributes	Professional attitude and behavior
	Personal competences: learning and knowledge.	Professional working	
	Personal competences: values.	Apply ethical and legal principles	Ethics and jurisprudence
2. Interpersonal, communication and social skills	Personal competences: communication and organizational skills.	Communicate effectively in a medical context	Communication
3. Knowledge base, information and information literacy	Personal competences: learning and knowledge.	Apply the principles, skills and knowledge of evidence-based medicine	Application of basic biological, medical, technical and clinical sciences
	Personal competences: learning and knowledge.	Use information and information technology effectively in a medical context	Acquiring and using information
4. Clinical information gathering	Patient care competences: patient consultation and assessment.	Carry out a consultation with a patient	Obtaining and recording a complete history of the patient's medical, oral and dental state
		Assess psychological and social aspects of a patient's illness'	
5. Diagnosis and Treatment planning	Patient care competences: need for drug treatment.	Assess clinical presentations, order investigations, make differential diagnoses and negotiate a management plan	Decision-making, clinical reasoning and judgment
	Patient care competences: drug interactions.	Provide immediate care of medical emergencies, including First Aid and resuscitation'	
	Patient care competences: drug dose and formulation.		
	Patient care competences: provision of information and service.		
6. Therapy, establishing and maintaining health	Patient care competences: monitoring of drug therapy.	Carry out practical procedures	Establishing and maintaining oral health
		Prescribe drugs	
7. Prevention and health promotion	Patient care competences: patient education.	Promote health, engage with population health issues and work effectively in a health care system	Improving oral health of individuals, families and groups in the community

For each domain, peer major competences appear on the same line, whereas non-equivalent major competences appear on different lines (Table 3). There are gaps in the table (perhaps) representing major competences that (one or more) professions consider implicit.

The first three domains relate to personal competences and are very similar in all healthcare professions. A specific attitude and behavior to patients, together with an ethical commitment, are common aspects of these healthcare professions. Communication and social skills are clearly needed for the information and education of patients. As in many other professions, the use of information technology and the ability to solve problems is a common denominator.

The last four domains (4–7) comprise the specific competences related to patient care. Patient care requires (1) clinical judgment based on competences for gathering information included in the domain "Clinical information gathering"; (2) assessment and treatment planning, included in the domain "Diagnosis and Treatment planning"; and (3) monitoring the results, included in the domain "Therapy, establishing and maintaining health." These latter domains are present in all three healthcare professions. We suggest that the decisions about the need for a drug, the selection, dosage, the adverse effects, etc., typically performed by the pharmacist, follow the same principles as other clinical disciplines and thus require the same competences. This is reflected in the increasing role of pharmacists in patient care as recognized by the EU (see above).

2.3. The Perception by the Practitioners of the Framework Proposals for Pharmacy and Medicine

In the PHAR-QA [14] and MEDINE [16] projects the competences were ranked by practitioners in each profession.

Figure 1 shows that all competences were considered "necessary" (rank > 2/4), although with a considerable degree of variability. Globally, ranking scores for pharmacists and general practitioners were similar, although there were some differences. Knowledge of a second language and research skills were ranked higher by pharmacists; competences such as the ability to work autonomously and to recognize limits were ranked higher by general practitioners.

All patient care competences were considered "necessary" (rank >2/4) (Figure 2). The spread for patient care competences (2.9–3.8) was higher than for personal competences (2–3.8), suggesting that all practitioners rank patient care competences as more important. Rankings were similar for pharmacy and medicine with the global rank being lower for pharmacy than for medicine (delta = −0.5).

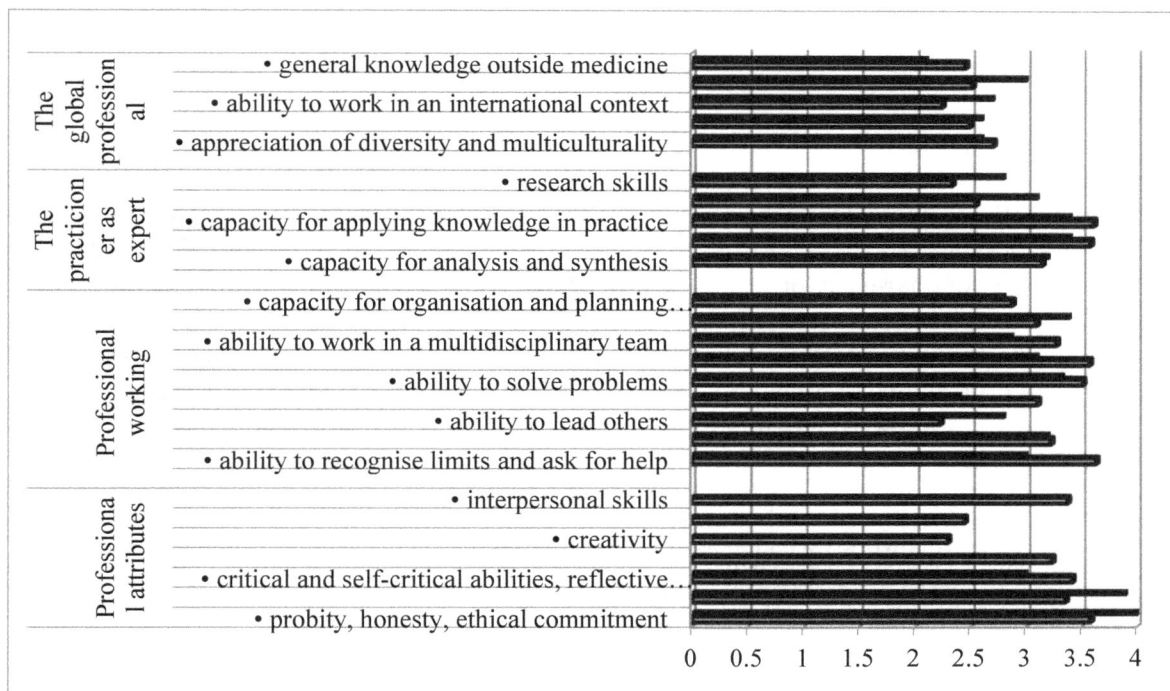

Figure 1. Ranking of personal competences by pharmacy (full columns) and medicine (open columns) practitioners. Ranking was on a 4-point scale (1 = least and 4 = most important). Pharmacy data are from PHAR-QA [19–22], and for medicine MEDINE [16].

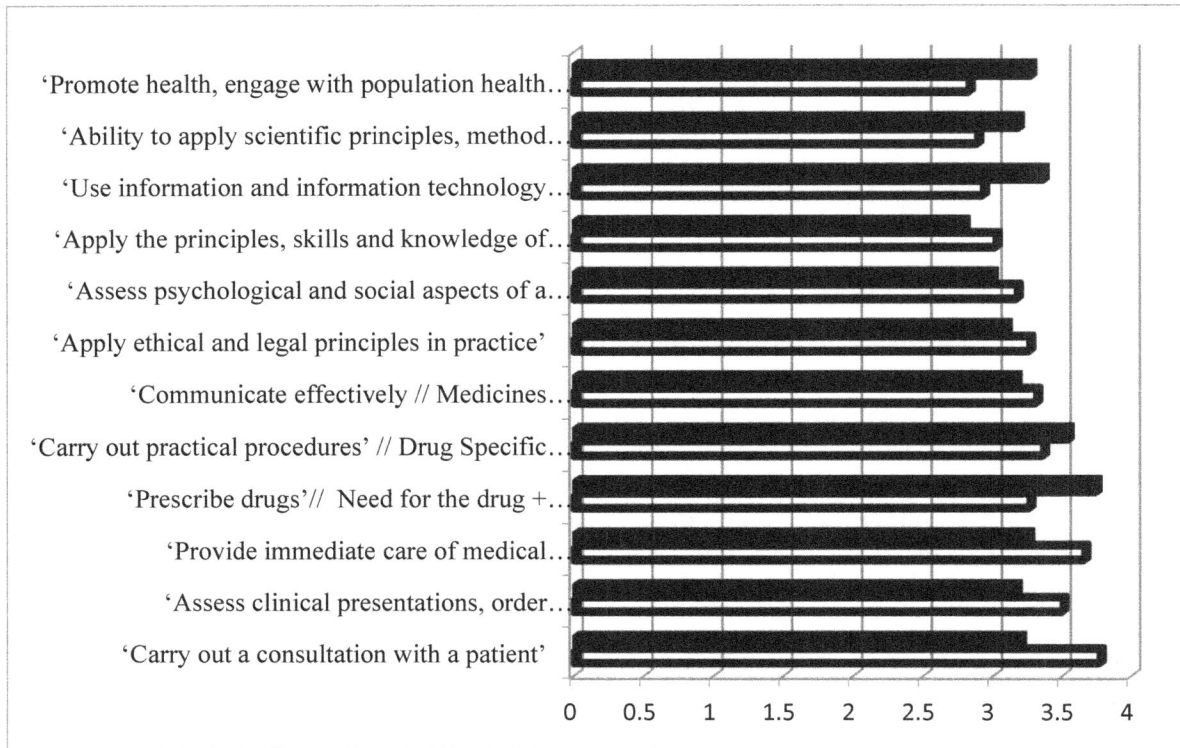

Figure 2. Ranking of patient care competences by pharmacy (full columns) and medicine (open columns) practitioners. Ranking was on a 4-point scale (1 = least and 4 = most important). Pharmacy data are from PHAR-QA [19–22], and for medicine MEDINE [16].

3. Conclusions

The results show that there is much similarity in competences for practice amongst all healthcare professions. This is seen in the recommendations for practice in the EU directive. It is also seen in the formulation of the competences by the different EU academic consortia that have proposed competence frameworks for pharmacy (PHAR-QA, medicine (MEDINE) and dentistry (ADEE)). Finally, it is seen in the perception of pharmaceutical and medical practitioners through their relative ranking of the proposals for competences.

The identification of a large number of competences that are similar in healthcare professions opens up the possibilities of a new design in educational programs with the installation of CBE, of more interaction in the different healthcare disciplines regarding education and practice, and, globally, of programs that are more adequate to an era of team-based healthcare.

Acknowledgments: I wish to thank J. Atkinson for his continuous help and support and for the revision of the manuscript. This work was supported by the Lifelong Learning program of the European Union: 527194-LLP-1-2012-1-BE-ERASMUS-EMCR.

References

1. Frank, J.R.; Snell, L.S.; Cate, T.O.; Holmboe, E.S.; Carraccio, C.; Swing, S.R.; Harris, P.; Glasgow, N.J.; Campbell, C.; Dath, D.; et al. Competency-based medical education: Theory to practice. *Med. Teach.* **2010**, *32*, 638–645. [CrossRef] [PubMed]
2. Data on Intra-EU Student Mobility: Strengths and Diversity of European Student Mobility—Agence Erasmus. Available online: https://www.agence-erasmus.fr/docs/2115_soleoscope-10-en.pdf (accessed on 13 January 2017).

3. Wismar, M.; Maier, C.B.; Glinos, I.A.; Dussault, G.; Figueras, J. (Eds.) *Health Professional Mobility and Health Systems: Evidence from 17 European Countries*; Observatory Studies Series 23; WHO Regional Office for Europe on Behalf of the European Observatory on Health Systems and Policies: Copenhagen, Denmark, 2011. Available online: http://www.healthpolicyjrnl.com/article/S0168-8510(15)00214-6/fulltext#bibl0005 (accessed on 13 January 2017).

4. Directive 2013/55/EU of the European Parliament and of the Council of 20 November 2013 Amending Directive 2005/36/EC on the Recognition of Professional Qualifications and Regulation (EU) No 1024/2012 on Administrative Cooperation through the Internal Market Information System ('the IMI Regulation'). Available online: http://eur-lex.europa.eu/legal-content/EN/ALL/?uri=celex%3A32013L0055 (accessed on 13 January 2017).

5. General Level Framework. A Framework for Pharmacists Development in General Pharmacy Practice. Available online: http://www.codeg.org/fileadmin/codeg/pdf/glf/GLF_October_2007_Edition.pdf (accessed on 13 January 2017).

6. Core Competency Framework for Pharmacists. The Pharmaceutical Society of Ireland. Available online: http://www.thepsi.ie/gns/pharmacy-practice/core-competency-framework.aspx (accessed on 13 January 2017).

7. Competencias del Farmacéutico Para Desarrollar Los Servicios Farmacéuticos (SF) Basados en Atención Primaria de Salud (APS) y las Buenas Prácticas en Farmacia (BPF). Available online: http://forofarmaceuticodelasamericas.org/wp-content/uploads/2015/04/Competencias-del-farmacéutico-para-desarrollar-los-SF-basados-en-APS-y-BPF.pdf (accessed on 13 January 2017).

8. The American College of Clinical Pharmacy (ACCP). White Paper Clinical Pharmacist Competencies: The American College of Clinical Pharmacy. *Pharmacotherapy* **2008**, *28*, 806–815.

9. Medina, M.S.; Plaza, C.M.; Stowe, C.D.; Robinson, E.T.; DeLander, G.; Beck, D.E.; Melchert, R.B.; Supernaw, R.B.; Roche, V.F.; Gleason, B.L.; et al. Center for the Advancement of Pharmacy Education 2013 Educational Outcomes. *Am. J. Pharm. Educ.* **2013**, *77*, 162. [CrossRef] [PubMed]

10. Competency Framework for the Pharmacy Profession. Pharmacy Council of New Zealand, 2009. Available online: http://www.pharmacycouncil.org.nz/cms_show_download.php?id=201 (accessed on 13 January 2017).

11. NAPRA. Professional Competencies for Canadian Pharmacists at Entry to Practice. 2007. Available online: http://napra.ca/content_files/files/comp_for_cdn_pharmacists_at_entrytopractice_march2014_b.pdf (accessed on 13 January 2017).

12. National Competency Standards Framework for Pharmacists in Australia. Pharmaceutical Society of Australia, 2010. Available online: https://www.psa.org.au/downloads/standards/competency-standards-complete.pdf (accessed on 13 January 2017).

13. PHAR-QA (Quality Assurance in European Pharmacy Education and Training). 2016. Available online: http://www.phar-qa.eu/ (accessed on 13 January 2017).

14. The PHARMINE (Pharmacy Education in Europe) Consortium. Work Programme 3: Final Report. Identifying and Defining Competences for Pharmacists. Available online: http://www.pharmine.org/wp-content/uploads/2014/05/PHARMINE-WP3-Final-ReportDEF_LO.pdf (accessed on 13 January 2017).

15. A Global Competency Framework. FIP Pharmacy Education Taskforce, 2012. Available online: https://www.fip.org/files/fip/PharmacyEducation/GbCF_v1.pdf (accessed on 13 January 2017).

16. Learning Outcomes/Competences for Undergraduate Medical Education in Europe (MEDINE) the Tuning Project (Medicine). Available online: http://tuningacademy.org/medine-medicine/?lang=en (accessed on 13 January 2017).

17. Cowpe, J.; Plasschaert, A.; Harzer, W.; Vinkka-Puhakka, H.; Walmsley, A.D. Profile and Competences for the Graduating European Dentist—Update 2009. *Eur. J. Dent. Educ.* **2010**, *14*, 193–202. [CrossRef] [PubMed]

18. Directive 2005/36/EC of the European Parliament and of the Council of 7 September 2005 on the Recognition of Professional Qualifications. Available online: http://eur-lex.europa.eu/legal-content/EN/TXT/?uri=celex:32005L0036 (accessed on 15 February 2017).

19. Miller, G.E. The assessment of clinical skills/competences/performance. *Acad. Med.* **1990**, *65*, 63–67. [CrossRef]

20. Atkinson, J.; de Paepe, K.; Sánchez Pozo, A.; Rekkas, D.; Volmer, D.; Hirvonen, J.; Bozic, B.; Skowron, A.; Mircioiu, C.; Marcincal, A.; et al. How do European pharmacy students rank competences for practice? *Pharmacy* **2016**, *4*, 8. [CrossRef]

21. Atkinson, J.; de Paepe, K.; Sánchez Pozo, A.; Rekkas, D.; Volmer, D.; Hirvonen, J.; Bozic, B.; Skowron, A.; Mircioiu, C.; Marcincal, A.; et al. What is a pharmacist: Opinions of pharmacy department academics and community pharmacists on competences required for pharmacy practice. *Pharmacy* **2016**, *4*, 12. [CrossRef]

22. Atkinson, J.; Sánchez Pozo, A.; Rekkas, D.; Volmer, D.; Hirvonen, J.; Bozic, B.; Skowron, A.; Mircioiu, C.; Sandulovici, R.; Marcincal, A.; et al. Hospital and Community Pharmacists' Perceptions of Which Competences Are Important for Their Practice. *Pharmacy* **2016**, *4*, 21. [CrossRef]

Pharmacy Practice and Education in Romania

Roxana Sandulovici [1]**, Constantin Mircioiu** [2]**, Cristina Rais** [2] **and Jeffrey Atkinson** [3,*]

[1]   Faculty of Pharmacy, Titu Maiorescu University, 22, Dâmbovnicului, Sector 4, 040441 Bucharest, Romania; roxana.sandulovici@yahoo.com or farmacie@univ.utm.ro

[2]   Faculty of Pharmacy, University of Medicine and Pharmacy "Carol Davila", 6th Traian Vuia, Sector 2, 020956 Bucharest, Romania; constantin.mircioiu@yahoo.com (C.M.); cristina_rais@yahoo.com (C.R.)

[3]   Pharmacolor Consultants Nancy, 12 rue de Versigny, 54600 Villers, France

*   Correspondence: jeffrey.atkinson@univ-lorraine.fr

Abstract: The PHARMINE (*"Pharmacy Education in Europe"*) project examined the organisation of pharmacy practice and education in the European Union (EU). An electronic survey was sent out to representatives of different sectors (community, hospital, industrial pharmacists, university staff, and students) in each individual EU member state. This paper presents the results of the PHARMINE survey on pharmacy practice and education in Romania. In the light of this data we examine to what extent harmonisation of practice and education with EU norms has occurred, whether this has promoted mobility of pharmacy professionals, academics and students, and what impact it has had on healthcare in Romania. The survey reveals the substantial changes in Romanian pharmacy practice and education since the 1989 change in government and Romania joining the EU in 2007. Romania remains, however, a poor country with expenditure on healthcare less than one-third of the EU average. This factor also impacts pharmacy practice. Although practice seems aligned with EU norms, this masks the substantial imbalance between the situation in the richer capital, Bucharest, and that of the poorer countryside. Harmonisation to EU norms in pharmacy education has not promoted student exchange and mobility but, rather, a brain drain in pharmaceutical graduates to other EU countries. Specialisation in industrial practice has been lost since 1989 with pharmacists being replaced by chemists. In hospitals the hospital pharmacist is being replaced by the clinical pharmacist.

Keywords: pharmacy; education; practice; Romania; European Union

1. Introduction

The PHARMINE (*"Pharmacy Education in Europe"*) consortium surveyed the state of pharmacy practice and education in the member states of the EU, including Romania, between 2008 and 2011, with an update in 2017. The methodology used and the principal results obtained have already been published [1].

PHARMINE gathered information on general (community) practice and specialisation in hospital and industrial practice. PHARMINE also dealt with assistant pharmacists—their education, training, and responsibilities were surveyed.

PHARMINE studied the administrative context of practice and education in the EU. In the EU pharmacy practice and education fall under two jurisdictions: national and European. The latter involves a confederal approach to decision-making. Freedom of movement, of residence, and of the right to work anywhere in the EU, is the cornerstone of the EU. In the case of pharmacy and other sectoral professions (nurses, midwives, doctors, dentists, architects, and veterinary surgeons) this is regulated by a system of automatic recognition of professional qualifications. To work in another EU member state, pharmacists apply to the relevant authority, providing proof of their qualifications. For sectoral professions, the EU issues directives which are ordinances laying down the broad imperatives [2]. An EU directive requires member states to achieve a particular result (in this case harmonisation of practice and education) without dictating the exact means of achieving that result. Directives leave the different member states with leeway to organise systems that are more or less harmonised with the EU paradigm. Thus member states may introduce national legislation relating to specialisation in practice and education, to ownership and management of pharmacies, etc.

In parallel to the EU directive, pharmacy education and training in Europe is also impacted by the Bologna agreement on the harmonization of degree courses and student and staff exchange [3]. The Bologna agreement, signed by the education ministers of the governments of the European Higher Education Area (48 members including the 28 EU member states), proposed several recommendations. In contrast to the EU directive Bologna recommendations are not legally binding. They include a degree structure for all university degrees with a bachelor (three years) followed by a master (two years). As with the EU directive, the idea behind the Bologna recommendations is to improve student mobility. However, the Bologna agreement and the EU directive do differ. The latter requires a five-year, "tunnel" degree structure for pharmacy, i.e., a degree course that offers no possibility for intermediate mobility after accomplishment of a three-year bachelor period.

Mobility is also behind other aspects of the Bologna process: firstly, the development of tools to promote student exchange programmes, such as the European Credit Transfer and Accumulation System (ECTS). This provides credits to students for defined learning outcomes and their associated workload. Secondly, ECTS are coupled to a Diploma Supplement that describes the nature, level, context, content, and status of the studies that were successfully completed by the student at a given university. This system allows students to validate studies carried out at the host university by their home university.

This paper looks at how the Bologna process has developed in Romanian universities. It is particularly interesting to examine how this affects pharmacy practice and education in a country that recently joined the EU in its fifth enlargement in 2007, following the 1989 revolution and the introduction of a multi-party, democratic government and free market measures.

In order to place pharmacy within the general health context in Romania compared to the EU, it can be noted that in Romania life expectancy at birth (Table 1) is lower than (males) or equal to (females) the EU average of 79 years. Healthy life expectancy (EU average 70 years) is much lower. Furthermore, expenditure on health is less than one-third of the EU average ($3611 per capita).

Table 1. Health statistics for Romania [4,5].

Total Population	19,511,000
Life expectancy at birth m/f (years)	71/79
Healthy life expectancy at birth m/f (years)	59/59
Total expenditure on health per capita	$1074

2. Design

Information was obtained from Romanian experts who replied to a questionnaire on:

- Pharmacy practice

  - Community, hospital, and industry
  - Organisation
  - Legislation
  - Education and training

- The adoption of the EU sectoral directive 2013/55/EU [2] in pharmacy practice and education
- The impact of the Bologna declaration [3]:

  - Organisation of the degree course with the existence or not of a bachelor/master structure,

○   Implementation of ECTS and the Erasmus programme on student and staff exchange [6].

The information is presented in the form of tables in order to facilitate legibility. This form of presentation was developed in association with this journal's editorial board of directors and has been described in detail in a previous publication [7]. This presentation is aimed at easing the comparison of different EU countries as all country profiles are presented in the same tabular form.

3. Evaluation and Assessment

3.1. Organisation of the Activities of Pharmacists, Professional Bodies

Table 2 provides details of the numbers and activities of community pharmacists and pharmacies in Romania. Items are expounded in the "comments" column also include opinions and trends for the future.

Table 2. Numbers and activities of community pharmacists and pharmacies in Romania.

Item	Numbers	Comments
Pharmacists	*Circa* 13,600	3533 work in Bucharest and 10,067 elsewhere 1435 inhabitants/community pharmacist (Bucharest 525 inhabitants/community pharmacist) EU average: 2145 [1]
Pharmacies	5938	Inhabitants/pharmacy: 3286. EU average: 4407 [1] Pharmacists/pharmacy: 2.3. EU average: 2.1 [1]
Competences and roles of community pharmacists		The competencies of community pharmacists are: a. Supplying prescription medicines b. Managing medicines for some ailments c. Giving advice on medicines d. creening, diagnostic services
Is ownership of a community pharmacy limited to pharmacists?	No	The community pharmacies are private institutions. Their owners need not be pharmacists as long as they hire a pharmacist as the manager.
Rules on geographical distribution of pharmacies?	Yes	Demographic criteria only [8,9]. • Bucharest: one pharmacy per 3000 inhabitants • cities that are capital of their respective district: one pharmacy per 3500 inhabitants • other cities: one pharmacy per 4000 inhabitants Exceptions from these provisions are the community pharmacies found in railway stations, airports, and in large surface commercial centres.
Are drugs and health care products available to the general public by channels other than pharmacies?	Yes	Through stores that sell plants or medicines from plants and OTC (*Plafar*) only. Recently e-pharmacies have appeared, but their legal status is not yet clearly established. Despite the fact that present legislation imposes a series of conditions for the way pharmacies work and how they sell drugs, these do not directly restrict marketing them online. According to a draft normative act, online marketing for OTC drugs will be allowed for authorised pharmacies only, with the goal to reduce the risks to which the online buyers are exposed at present.

Compared to the EU linear regression estimation (for definition and calculation see [1]), the ratio of the actual number of community pharmacists in Romania (per population) = 0.90. Thus, the number of pharmacists per population is slightly lower than the EU norm. The same comparison for community pharmacies produces a ratio of 0.90, again slightly below the EU norm. The activities and occupations of pharmacists in Romania are similar to those of community pharmacists in other EU member states.

Globally, as far as pharmacy practice is concerned, Romania is close to EU norms and in line with the EU directive 2013/55/EU, thus, pharmacy practice is harmonised with that in other member states. However, behind the mean data there are highly non-homogeneous distributions. Thus, in Bucharest there are too many pharmacists and (almost) all small localities no longer have a pharmacy. There are various reasons behind this situation, but it is primarily connected to the low quality—especially economic—of life in villages. Furthermore, following the widespread emigration of young people to urban areas, only small numbers of old, poor people remain in the countryside so, economically, a pharmacy is no longer profitable.

Table 3 provides details of the numbers and activities of persons other than pharmacists working in pharmacies in Romania.

Table 3. Numbers and activities of other personnel working in pharmacies in Romania.

Item	Numbers	Comments
Are persons other than pharmacists involved in community practice?	Yes	There are two types of assistants working in pharmacies: - pharmacy assistants have three years' education in a postsecondary school (technical college). This represents the pre-1989 education system survived and is still predominant. - medical assistants for pharmacy follow a three-year course in a university faculty of pharmacy [10]. This second category was introduced in 2004 in order to assure recognition in Europe. In Romanian pharmacy practice no difference is made between the two categories and both are also called "pharmacy assistants". They perform dispensing and counselling of drug products, under the guidance of a pharmacist.
Their numbers and status	>120,000	
Organisations providing and validating education and training of the 3-year courses		The curricula of postsecondary schools was up-graded and extended by university pharmacy faculties for the education of medical assistants for pharmacy starting from 2004 onwards, and validated by Romanian Agency for Quality of University Education (ARACIS) [11]. In a second phase the Ministry of Education and the Ministry of Health imposed the same curricula on post-secondary schools. Thus practically the structure is essentially similar with some quantitative differences. Entrance exams and final evaluations are similar, but they receive a different diploma [12].
Subject areas		Fundamental disciplines: • human anatomy, physiology, physiopathology, microbiology, clinical pathology, • cellular and molecular biology, • general and inorganic chemistry, organic chemistry, • mathematics, computer sciences, Applied disciplines: • chemical bases of the drug (inorganic and organic chemistry), • physical-chemical bases of drug formulation, • medicinal plants, • descriptive and metabolic biochemistry, • instrumental analysis techniques, • medical semiology/clinical pathology, • first-aid, • pharmaceutical and medical terminology, • elements in nutrition, • bioethics and ethics,

Table 3. *Cont.*

Item	Numbers	Comments
Subject areas		Specialty disciplines: <ul><li>drug analysis,</li><li>the bases of pharmaceutical techniques,</li><li>therapeutic chemistry,</li><li>communication in pharmacy,</li><li>elements of industrial pharmaceutical technology,</li><li>elements of toxicology, pharmacology, phyto-therapy,</li><li>notions of pharmacovigilance,</li><li>cosmetic products,</li><li>para-pharmaceutical and medical products,</li><li>vegetal products, dietary supplements),</li></ul> Complementary disciplines: <ul><li>medical information technology,</li><li>modern languages,</li><li>scientific research methodology,</li><li>elements of pharmaceutical management and marketing.</li></ul>
Competences and roles		Dispensing and counselling of: Medical assistants: OTC medicines and plant products Pharmacy assistants: drug products

The legal opportunity for pharmacy assistants to complete their education in order to become medical assistants for pharmacy is to be examined starting in 2017. Legislation in Romania tried to ensure compatibility of medical assistants for pharmacy with their European counterparts, but the practical consequences concerning the possibility of Romanian medical assistants for pharmacy to work elsewhere in the EU are unclear. As seen below, one aspect of harmonisation with the EU that is somewhat specific to Romania is the possibility that such harmonisation allows for Romanian pharmacy professionals to work elsewhere in the EU.

Table 4 provides details of the numbers and activities of hospital pharmacists in Romania.

Table 4. Numbers and activities of hospital pharmacists in Romania.

Item	Numbers	Comments
Does such a function exist?	Yes	
Number of hospital pharmacists	692	One hundred and twenty in Bucharest (17%) and 572 in the rest of the country. Hospital pharmacies are small with 1–2 pharmacists and 2–3 medical assistants. The number of specialists is insufficient to cope with the demands of the numerous patients hospitalized. Therefore it is necessary to increase the numbers of staff for the development of patient care. The lack of specialist staff is also due to the low salaries in hospitals.
Number of hospital pharmacies	564	One hundred and twenty in Bucharest (21%) and 444 in the rest of the country.
Competences and roles of hospital pharmacists		These are similar to those in other EU member states [1].

In previous generations hospital pharmacy was connected to industrial pharmacy with the preparation, for example, of perfusions for hospital wards and many semisolid formulations. This type of hospital pharmacist is changing due to the low salary incentives in the national health service and the development of "clinical pharmacists". These undergo specialisation in a 3-year internship *"rezidentiate"*. They are able to participate with the clinical team in the individualization of treatment of patients in a hospital. They act as clinical pharmacologists". Thus in the future hospital pharmacists will become more clinical pharmacists.

Table 5 provides details of the numbers and activities of industrial pharmacists and pharmacists in other sectors in Romania.

Table 5. Numbers and activities of industrial pharmacists and pharmacists in other sectors in Romania.

Item	Numbers	Comments
Industrial Pharmacy and Pharmacists		
Number of pharmacists working in industry	Around 120	
Competences and roles		• Synthesis and production of chemical entities and drugs • Research and development, including formulation and control of drug systems, evaluation of bioavailability of active substances • Cooperation in preclinical drug evaluation (safety and efficacy) • Cooperation in clinical trials (safety and efficacy) • Quality assurance of production • Registration of drugs • Marketing • Distribution
Pharmacists working in other sectors		
	100–200	
Sectors in which pharmacists are employed		Clinical Trials, Armed Forces, National Medicinal Agency

Industrial pharmacists in Romania have similar practices and duties to those in other EU countries [1]. As accurate numbers of industrial pharmacists were not available for most European countries, a comparison with the EU average is not possible.

Pre-1989, specialists in industry were pharmacists. The same was true in clinical laboratories in hospitals ("biochemistry laboratories"). After the liberalisation of community pharmacy practice, pharmacists migrated toward community pharmacies, where it was possible to obtain higher salaries. They were replaced by chemists in industry and by medical doctors in hospitals.

Pharmacists from the public laboratories for drug control (ICSMCF—Institute for State Control of Drugs and Pharmaceutical Research) disappeared following the disappearance of industrial and hospital laboratories in a purported harmonization with EU models. This had a negative impact on public control of the quality of drugs.

Table 6 provides information on professional associations for pharmacists in Romania.

Table 6. Professional associations for pharmacists in Romania.

Item		Comments
Registration of pharmacists	Yes	The National College of Pharmacists has colleges in each district, including Bucharest [13]. All the branches are active in registration of pharmacists. After graduation, in order to work as a pharmacist, the candidate must obtain the Pharmacists' Membership Certificate from the National Pharmacy College. Further continuous educational training is required—pharmacists have to accumulate 40 continuous education credit points/year in order to carry on with their pharmacy practice.

Table 6. *Cont.*

Item		Comments
Creation of pharmacies and control of territorial distribution	Yes	A dossier has to be presented in order to open a new community pharmacy. This contains information on: The registration number from the Trade Register of the new commercial society created The personal employed (professional qualification, number) The work programme The proof of ownership The proof of the demographic criteria. This must be sent to the Ministry of Health, Department of Strategies and Medicine Politics. After verification of legal criteria, inspections are performed, by the Ministry of Health and the College of Pharmacists, in order to release the authorisation to function.
Ethical and other aspects of professional conduct	Yes	Romania has a Code of Ethics for pharmacists approved by the General Assembly of Pharmacists in 2009 [13].
Quality assurance and validation of university courses	Yes	

3.2. Pharmacy Faculties, Students, and Courses

Table 7 provides details of pharmacy higher education institutions (HEIs), staff and students in Romania.

Table 7. Pharmacy higher education institutions (HEIs), staff, and students in Romania.

Item	Number	Comments
Number of pharmacy HEIs in Romania	11	1. West University *Vasile Goldis* Arad, http://www.uvvg.ro/site/; http://www.4icu.org/reviews/12323.htm 2. University of Medicine and Pharmacy *Carol Davila*, Bucharest, http://www.ceebd.co.uk/ceeed/un/rom/ro003.htm 3. University of Medicine and Pharmacy Cluj Napoca, http://www.ceebd.co.uk/ceeed/un/rom/ro020.htm; http://www.umfcluj.ro/ 4. Ovidius University, Constanta, http://www.euroeducation.net/euro/ro025.htm; http://www.univ-ovidius.ro/ 5. University of Medicine and Pharmacy Craiova, http://www.umfcv.ro/en/index.html 6. University of Medicine and Pharmacy Iassy, https://www.medicaldoctor-studies.com/study-medicine-abroad/study-medicine-in-romania/university-of-medicine-pharmacy-in-iasi/ 7. Oradea University, http://www.uoradea.ro/ 8. University of Medicine and Pharmacy Targu Mures, http://www.euroeducation.net/euro/ro048.htm; http://www.umftgm.ro/ 9. University of Medicine and Pharmacy Timisoara, http://www.umft.ro/ 10. University Lower Danube, Faculty of Medicine and Pharmacy, Galati, http://www.ugal.ro/ 11. Titu Maiorescu University, Faculty of Pharmacy, Bucharest, http://www.utm.ro/en/
Public pharmacy HEIs	2	1. West University *Vasile Goldis* Arad 2. Titu Maiorescu University, Faculty of Pharmacy, Bucharest

Table 7. *Cont.*

Item	Number	Comments
Independent faculty	Part of "Medicine & Pharmacy" HEIs	1. University of Medicine and Pharmacy *Carol Davila*, Bucharest 2. University of Medicine and Pharmacy Cluj Napoca 3. University Ovidius, Constanta 4. University of Medicine and Pharmacy Craiova 5. University of Medicine and Pharmacy Iassy 6. University Oradea, 7. University of Medicine and Pharmacy Targu Mures 8. University of Medicine and Pharmacy Timisoara
Faculty attachment	Attached to a medical faculty	1. Faculty of Medicine, Dentistry and Pharmacy, at the "University Vasile Goldis" Arad 2. Faculty of Medicine and Pharmacy, Galati 3. Faculty of Pharmacy, Titu Maiorescu University, Bucharest
Do HEIs offer B and M degrees?	No	All pharmacy schools have a five-year integrated system. There is no split between the first years 1–3 and years 4–5, and there is no "diploma" that gives the right to work after completing the first three years.
		Teaching staff
Staff	Around 100 at each HEI = *circa* 1000 in all	There is no national database of teaching staff in pharmacy.
Professionals from outside the HEIs, involved in E&T	Around 3% of staff	The professionals from outside the HEI's involved in education and training are community pharmacists in charge of the traineeship period, researchers from hospitals or research units.
		Students
Number of places on entry following secondary school	Around 50–250 per HEI	Around 50–200 students for smaller faculties, and 250 for Bucharest and Cluj, together with 50–100 places for training in English or French languages.
Number of applicants for each entry place	100–400 per HEI	Around two applicants per place, but the number of candidates diminishes in time following massive emigration of the young population to other countries.
International students (EU)	2%	Students from Greece, Bulgaria.
International students (non EU)	20%	Students from: Albania, Jordan, Iraq, Iran, Israel, Lebanon, Macedonia, Moldavia, Mongolia, Morocco, Nigeria, Palestine, Syria, Tunisia.
Specific pharmacy-related entrance examination.	Yes	Botany or anatomy and organic chemistry—subjects with potential application in pharmacy.
Other form of entry requirement at a national level	Yes	Graduates who already have a degree from other faculties (medicine, chemistry, biology) and want to obtain a pharmacy degree can start on advanced entry, 2nd or the 3rd year based on ECTS.
Graduates that become registered pharmacists.		Difficult to establish given drop-out rate.
		Advanced entry
Entrance after a first bachelor year.	no	
		Fees per year
For home and EU students	9000 RON (*circa* €2000)	
For non-EU students	€6000	

Compared to the EU average (for definition and calculation see [1]); the ratio for staff is 1.8 and, for students, 2.0. The student/staff ratio is around 2. It should be noted that a university post is not economically attractive compared to one in a community pharmacy. Furthermore, the number of students is decreasing and academic staff risk becoming jobless in the future. Tentative increases in student numbers include the French degree section at Cluj.

In Table 8 below are given the electives (courses open to choice) in the Romanian course.

Table 8. Specialisation electives in pharmacy HEIs in Romania.

Item		Comments
Do HEIs Provide Specialised Courses?	Yes	In order to work in industry or a hospital as an executive it is sufficient to be a graduate of the integrated five-year programme. One can become a "Qualified Person" after two years' activity in certified (Good Manufacturing Practice, Good Clinical Practice, Good Laboratory Practice) industrial units in the field of qualitative analysis of the medicines, quality control of active substances, or any other tests required to check the quality of medicines. The certification is validated by the National Medicines Agency after evaluation of the activity of the candidate. It is not mandatory to be a pharmacist in order to become a Qualified Person. In order to obtain a leading position in a hospital pharmacy it is necessary to become a "specialist" following two years' education in the framework of "*rezidentiate*" in a faculty of pharmacy and a final exam. Only a small number of hospitals have pharmacists specialized in clinical pharmacy. Most of them are "specialists" in community pharmacy.

Table 9 provides details of past and present changes in pharmacy education and training in Romania.

Table 9. Past and present changes in education and training in Romania pharmacy HEIs.

Item	Comments
Have there been any major changes since 1990?	The change in the governmental regime in 1989 and the preparation for joining the EU in 2007, promoted harmonisation with EU pharmacy practice and education. Other forces were at work. Privatization of pharmacies induced a substantial increase in the number of pharmacies leading to an increase in the number of faculties of pharmacy (from four to 11) and ten times the number of students. Following a drastic reduction in the preparation of medicines in the pharmacy, the preponderance of chemical sciences disciplines has diminished in favour of medical disciplines in the pharmacy degree.
Are any major changes envisaged before 2019?	Two factors: (1) the decrease in the number of young people in Romania, and (2) the increase in emigration of pharmacists to other EU countries, impose an in-depth analysis of the aims and methods of pharmacy education and training, based on the competences required by the labour market and future practice.

3.3. Teaching and Learning Methods

Table 10 provides details of hours by learning method (for further details on the definitions of the different methods see Reference [1]).

Table 10. Student hours by learning method.

Method	Year 1	Year 2	Year 3	Year 4	Year 5	Total	%
Lecture	308	336	350	350	238	**1582**	32.4
Tutorial + Practical	434	462	490	434	266	**2086**	42.8
Project	0	0	0	0	60	**60**	1.2
Traineeship (community or hospital pharmacy)	60	60	60	120	780	**1140**	22.1
Electives + Optional	14	14	14	14	14	**70**	1.4
Total	816	872	914	918	1358	**4878**	100

The degree is characterised by the substantial amount of hands-on training (65%).

3.4. Subject Areas

Table 11 provides details of student hours by subject area (for further details on the definitions of the subject areas see [1]). Student hours are presence hours, not student workload hours.

Table 11. Student hours by subject area.

Subject Area	Year 1	Year 2	Year 3	Year 4	Year 5	Total	%
CHEMSCI	238	238	238	168	0	882	20.1
PHYSMATH	238	0	0	56	0	294	6.7
BIOLSCI	154	14	336	14	14	532	12.1
PHARMTECH	28	14	84	140	210	476	10.8
MEDISCI	0	182	98	392	168	840	19.1
LAWSOC	14	14	0	42	56	126	2.9
GENERIC + TRAINEESHIP	172	172	60	60	780	1244	28.3
Total	844	634	816	872	1228	4394	100

CHEMSOC: chemical sciences; PHYSMATH: physical and mathematical sciences; BIOLSCI: biological sciences; PHARMTECH: pharmaceutical technology; MEDISCI: medicinal sciences; LAWSOC: law and social sciences; GENERIC: generic competences.

Taking the MEDISCI/CHEMSCI ratio, medicinal sciences are still less than chemical sciences but, in the last 20 years, the proportion of medicinal sciences has increased continuously. It should also be noted that basic subjects (CHEMSCI, PHYSMATH, BIOLSCI) are concentrated in the early years, whereas more applied subjects (MEDISIC, PHARMTECH) in the later years. Traineeship is in the 5th year. Such chronological harmonisation is similar to that observed in other EU member states and should facilitate student exchange programmes.

3.5. Impact of the Bologna Recommendations [3]

Table 12 provides details the various ways in which the Bologna Declaration impacts on the pharmacy HEIs of Romania.

Table 12. Ways in which the Bologna Declaration impacts on Romanian pharmacy HEIs.

Item	Comments
"Comparable degrees with diploma supplement"	The degree structure is comparable to that observed in other EU member states (see above). A diploma supplement is delivered according to European directives (it is both in Romanian and English).
"Two main cycles (B and M) with entry and exit at B level"	There is a five-year integrated course with no possibility of graduation after three years
"European Credit Transfer System (ECTS) system of credits with links to life-long learning (LLL)"	Theoretically, this system was accepted and formally adopted in 1998. Practically, it was applied step-by-step. The transfer of credits was accepted between faculties of pharmacy and later between faculties of pharmacy, medicine and chemistry, all inside Romania. The acceptance of credits from foreign universities is discussed case-by-case.
"Addressing obstacles to mobility"	Both language barriers and lack of financial support. Only incoming students receive language tuition.
European/international quality assurance of courses	Maybe in the near future. Pharmacy courses and traineeship are validated by the Ministry of Education and the Romanian Agency for Quality Assurance in Higher Education (ARACIS [11]).
European dimension	Our staff was involved in European Projects: Cooperation in Science and Technology (COST) Joint Research Center (JRC) Ispra PHAR-QA the follow-on from PHARMINE
ERASMUS staff exchange to Romania from elsewhere	Rare

Table 12. *Cont.*

Item	Comments
ERASMUS staff exchange from Romania to other HEIs	Not frequently
ERASMUS student exchange to Romania from elsewhere	Less than 5 students/year
ERASMUS student exchange from Romania to other HEIS	Number of student months: 3–6 2 students in 2008, 3 students in 2009, all to Italy

The application of the Bologna recommendations was subject to a long debate by the Council of Deans of the Faculties of Pharmacy of Romania in the 2004–2008 period. One argument was that young people have to enter earlier in their professional activity. A second argument was that in community pharmacy practice there is no longer a need for such detailed studies in chemistry, physics, and other fundamental sciences. This was evident in the PHAR-QA results [14]. The opinion of EU community pharmacists was that, for example, physics and analytical chemistry are no more than "quite important". Furthermore, in the Romanian countryside, many pharmacies have only assistants with pharmacists dropping in from time to time. On this basis it could be argued that a three-year degree may be sufficient. The main argument against this is the specific nature of drug dispensation and the primordial element of patient safety.

Romania is in a somewhat unique situation relating to the harmonisation of pharmacy education and practice with other European countries in that harmonisation has led to emigration rather than exchange. In the last 10 years many young pharmacists from Romania left to work as pharmacists in several EU countries. Their numbers are increasing and approximately 3–4% of graduates currently leave Romania to work abroad. The phenomenon is still under control. This is different from the case of medical doctors who emigrated in large numbers such that Romania has, at the moment, an acute lack of medical personal.

3.6. Impact of EU Directive 2013/55/EC [2]

Table 13 provides details the various ways in which the EC directive impacts on pharmacy education and training in Romania.

Table 13. Ways in which the elements of the EC directive (left column) impact on Romanian pharmacy HEIs.

Item	Comments
"Evidence of formal qualifications as a pharmacist shall attest to training of at least five years' duration, … "	This applies.
" … four years of full-time theoretical and practical training at a university or at a higher institute of a level recognised as equivalent, or under the supervision of a university."	Yes, applied ad literam (4.5 years of full time theoretical and practical training and six months traineeship in a hospital or community pharmacy). Professors from the pharmaceutical technology department validate the traineeship through an oral/written examination in which the student must solve a problem in pharmaceutical technology (e.g., a pharmaceutical preparation). At the end of this period, the student must also present a notebook with his/her activity in the practice period and be able to answer questions regarding pharmaceutical practice.
" … six-month traineeship in a pharmacy which is open to the public or in a hospital, under the supervision of that hospital's pharmaceutical department."	Industrial traineeship is allowed in a community or hospital traineeship, but for only one of the six compulsory months

Romania mainly conforms to the different aspects of the EU directive with, notably, a tunnel degree. It should be noted that the directive clearly orients pharmacists toward community pharmacy practice reducing the possibilities for the development of pharmacy practice in clinical trials, industry, regulatory affairs, hospital pharmacy, etc.

4. Discussion and Conclusions

In essence, the survey reveals substantial changes in Romanian pharmacy practice and education since the 1989 change in government and Romania joining the EU in 2007. Some elements of the previous regime remain, such as the education of pharmacy assistants. Progress has been made towards harmonisation with the EU. Romania remains, however, a poor country with expenditure on healthcare at less than one-third of the EU average. This factor thwarts the impact of harmonisation on pharmacy practice. Thus, although practice seems aligned with EU norms, this masks substantial imbalance between the situation in the richer capital, Bucharest, and that of the poorer countryside. Harmonisation to EU norms in pharmacy education has not promoted student exchange and mobility but, rather, a brain drain in pharmaceutical graduates to other EU countries. Although this has not yet had the very serious consequences of emigration of medical general practitioners, the situation calls for remediate measures. Specialisation in industrial practice has been lost since 1989 with pharmacists being replaced by chemists. In hospitals the hospital pharmacist has been replaced by the clinical pharmacist.

The question arises as to whether harmonization could lead to an improvement in the Romanian health system and, more generally, what can do pharmacists in this respect? As seen above, harmonisation with EU norms is not always positive in that this can lead to pharmacy professionals emigrating to other countries. Another aspect of this concerns the prescription of generic drugs. This accounts for 88% of all prescriptions in the USA and approximately 20% in Romania [15]. Several causes are involved here including not only government economic policy but also the diminution in the competences of industrial pharmacists in areas such as bio-pharmacy and pharmacokinetics, good manufacturing practice, good clinical practice, and quality assurance systems, etc.—essential information for a clear understanding that bioequivalence implies therapeutic equivalence.

Finally the general context is that Romania is a poor country, with worse health conditions in comparison with other European countries. This situation is generated by many causes but one of these is clearly connected with education in the medical and pharmaceutical domain. Given this situation harmonization with EU norms was considered as a way for improving the actual situation. Harmonization started with the EU directives, first of all with curricula and, particularly, with the ratio between theoretical and practical education. The most important consequence of this legislative harmonization was the recognition of diplomas obtained from Romanian faculties of pharmacy and opportunity for pharmacists to work practically in all European countries. Unfortunately, this did not have the expected impact on student and staff exchange in other EU member states. Another negative effect was the alignment of EU directives with the most basic levels of knowledge and education. This promoted ignorance of new disciplines, such as information technology, bio-pharmacy, advanced pharmacokinetics, clinical pharmacy, etc., thus proving a bad model for Romania.

The final conclusion is that harmonization with EU norms is a long, ever-evolving process which is to be pursued in parallel with in-depth analysis, starting from local traditions and institutions, of all possible consequences.

Acknowledgments: With the support of the Lifelong Learning Programme of the European Union (142078-LLP-1-2008-BE-ERASMUS-ECDSP).

Author Contributions: Constantin Mircioiu, Roxana Sandulovici, and Cristina Rais provided data and information, and helped with the revisions of the manuscript; Constantin Mircioiu and Jeffrey Atkinson wrote the manuscript; and Jeffrey Atkinson coordinated the revisions.

References

1. Atkinson, J.; Rombaut, B. The 2011 PHARMINE report on pharmacy and pharmacy education in the European Union. *Pharm. Pract.* **2011**, *9*, 169–187. [CrossRef]
2. The European Commission Directive 2013/55/EU on Education and Training for Sectoral Practice Such as That of Pharmacy. Available online: http://eur-lex.europa.eu/legal-content/FR/TXT/?uri=celex:32013L0055 (accessed on 5 October 2017).
3. The European Higher Education Area (EHEA)—Bologna Agreement of Harmonisation of European University Degree Courses. Available online: http://www.ehea.info/ (accessed on 9 November 2017).
4. WHO World Health Organisation, Health statistics 2017. Available online: http://www.who.int/countries/rou/en/ (accessed on 9 November 2017).
5. Health Care Systems in Transition: Romania, European Observatory on Health Care Systems, WHO Regional Office for Europe, 2015. Available online: http://ec.europa.eu/health/ph_information/dissemination/hsis/hsis_13_nhs_en.htm (accessed on 9 November 2017).
6. Erasmus Plus Programme for Student and Staff Exchange in the EU. Available online: https://info.erasmusplus.fr/ (accessed on 9 November 2017).
7. Atkinson, J. The Country Profiles of the PHARMINE Survey of European Higher Educational Institutions Delivering Pharmacy Education and Training. *Pharmacy* **2017**, *3*, 34. [CrossRef] [PubMed]
8. Law of Pharmacy 2015. Legea nr. 266/2008—Legea Farmaciei, Republicata in 2 Februarie 2015, Publicată în Monitorul Oficial al României, Partea I, Nr. 85/02.II.2015. Available online: https://www.avocatnet.ro/articol_39799/Legea-farmaciei-nr-266-2008-republicata-in-2-februarie-2015.html (accessed on 9 November 2017).
9. Order from the Minister of Health for Approving the Establishment, Organisation and the Operation of Pharmacies and Drugstores, with Subsequent Amendments. Ordinul Ministrului Sanatatii nr 962/2009 Pentru Aprobarea Normelor Privind Infiintarea, Organizarea si Functionarea Farmaciilor si Drogheriilor, cu Modificarile si Completarile Ulterioare, MOf al Romaniei, Partea I nr 538/3.08.2009. Available online: http://www.colegfarm.ro/images/pdf/mo_0538.pdf and http://www.ms.ro/2017/08/21/ordin-pentru-modificarea-ordinului-nr-9622009-pentru-aprobarea-normelor-privind-infiintarea-organizarea-si-functionarea-farmaciilor-si-drogheriilor-cu-modificarile-si-completarile-ulterioare/ (accessed on 9 November 2017).
10. The Practice of the Medical Assistant, the Midwife and the Organization and the Function of the Order of Medical Assistants and Midwifes in Romania. Legea nr. 307/2004 privind exercitarea profesiei de asistent medical si a profesiei de moasa, precum si organizarea si functionarea Ordinului Asistentilor Medicali si Moaselor din Romania. Monitorul Oficial, Partea I nr. 578 din 30/06/2004. Available online: http://www.oamr.ro/legislatie/nationala/LEGEA_NR_307.pdf (accessed on 9 November 2017).
11. The Agency for Quality Assurance in University Training (ARACIS). Available online: http://www.aracis.ro/fileadmin/ARACIS/Comunicate_Media/2016/Standarde_specifice_consultare/Standardelor_specifice_7_OCTOMBRIE_2016_MED2.pdf (accessed on 9 November 2017).
12. An Example of a Postsecondary school Organization and Curricula Can Be Found at: "*Scoala postliceală Carol Davila*". Available online: http://www.scoalacdavila.ro (accessed on 9 November 2017).
13. The Romanian National College of Pharmacists. Available online: www.colegfarm.ro (accessed on 9 November 2017).
14. Atkinson, J.; De Paepe, K.; Sánchez Pozo, A.; Rekkas, D.; Volmer, D.; Hirvonen, J.; Bozic, B.; Skowron, A.; Mircioiu, C.; Marcincal, A.; et al. PHAR-QA Results. The PHAR-QA Project: Competence Framework for Pharmacy Practice—First Steps. The Results of the European Network Delphi Round 1. *Pharmacy* **2015**, *3*, 307–329. [CrossRef] [PubMed]
15. Romania-Insider. Manufacturers: Romanian Market Could Lose over 1,000 Generic Drugs. Available online: https://www.romania-insider.com/manufacturers-romanian-market-could-lose-generic-drugs/ (accessed on 9 November 2017).

3

Assessment of Drug Information Service in Public and Private Sector Tertiary Care Hospitals

Sawsan Abdullah Alamri [1], **Raniah Ali Al Jaizani** [2], **Atta Abbas Naqvi** [2] (ID)
and **Mastour Safer Al Ghamdi** [1,*]

[1] College of Clinical Pharmacy, Imam Abdulrahman Bin Faisal University (University of Dammam),
     Dammam 31441, Saudi Arabia; sawsan.ama94@gmail.com
[2] Department of Pharmacy Practice, College of Clinical Pharmacy, Imam Abdulrahman Bin Faisal University
     (University of Dammam), Dammam 31441, Saudi Arabia; raaljaizani@uod.edu.sa (R.A.A.J.);
     bg33bd@student.sunderland.ac.uk (A.A.N.)
*   Correspondence: msalghamdi@uod.edu.sa

Abstract: Drug information service is a dedicated and specialized service provided by pharmacists to enhance knowledge of medicines use, promote rational prescribing among prescribers, and reduce medication errors. Saudi Arabia has a National Drug and Poison Information Center (NDPIC) responsible for answering drug queries. There is a lack of literature that reports the current scenario of drug information services in the country, especially the Eastern Province. This study reported the current status of drug information services being provided among tertiary care hospitals of the Eastern Province of Saudi Arabia. All hospitals provided drug information services. The qualification of personnel was mostly bachelor's level (46.2%) and without proper training (54.8%). The most common queries received in a day were related to drug alternatives, dosage, and administration, as well as the availability of drugs. Physicians were the main users of the service. The most common health resources employed for the service was Lexi-Comp (76.9%) and Micromedex (69.2%). The use of Saudi National Formulary was not reported by any hospital, which highlights a potential research gap to address i.e., to investigate the lack of use of SNF by practitioners.

Keywords: drug information service; pharmacists; Saudi Arabia

1. Introduction

Drug information service is a specialized service provided by pharmacists to enhance drug knowledge, empower rational prescribing, and reduce medication errors [1]. This service is provided in response to the queries sought by allied health professionals in addressing medication-related problems pertaining to pharmacotherapy and medicine management issues of patients [2,3]. One of the most important aspects of drug information is to be unbiased in its contents [4]. Thus, the unbiased nature of information is of paramount importance to enhance patient outcomes and reduce adverse drug reactions (ADRs) [5].

Saudi Arabia has a National Drug and Poison Information Center (NDPIC) responsible for answering drug queries. The center has a total of 31 hospitals with established drug information centers. It is distributed in the following manner: the Central region has 11 established drug information centers, while there are nine in the Eastern region, three in the South, five centers in the West and two drug information centers in the Northwestern region of the country [6]. The country's health authority has a policy on the minimum standards required for drug information services that includes organizational and clinical objectives [7]. However, there is a dearth of research literature reported in Saudi Arabia on the quality parameters of this service, especially in the Eastern region with regard to the work operations of drug information services provided in tertiary care hospitals.

2. Methods

This descriptive study, which was five months in duration (January 2017 to May 2017), was conducted in five cities including Dammam, Dhahran, Al Hufuf, Khobar, and Qateef, located in the Eastern Province of Saudi Arabia. The study incorporated tertiary care hospitals across five cities of the Eastern Province of Saudi Arabia i.e., seven hospitals in Dammam (53.8%), two hospitals (15.4%) each in Dhahran and Al Hufuf, and one hospital each (7.7%) in Khobar and the city of Qateef. This amounted to a total of 13 healthcare facilities to assess drug information services. The data source or target population was the pharmacy department of the hospital, particularly the head of the pharmacy department or pharmacy manager. The study used a structured, closed-ended survey questionnaire to assess the service parameters, which was exclusively developed by reviewing the literature. The survey questionnaire contained a total of 10 questions. It included questions related to the demographic information of the drug information personnel, quality assessment information such as mode of delivery, frequency of information sought, type of drug information sought, and the persons seeking such information, lag time, etc., as well as the use of resources to obtain such information. Prior permission was sought from the hospitals before the commencement of the study. The survey was conducted among the hospital pharmacy managers by dropping off the questionnaire and collecting it again at their time of choosing. The study was noninvasive in nature and the participants were briefed about the objectives before completing the questionnaire. The study was exempted from review, however, a letter addressed to the concerned hospital was produced on request.

3. Results

Most of the hospitals were in the public sector ($N = 10$, 76.9%) while some were in the private sector ($N = 3$, 23.1%). All hospitals ($N = 13$, 100%) confirmed that they provide drug information services. Moreover, almost half of the hospitals ($N = 7$, 53.8%) had a dedicated drug information office followed by a third proportion ($N = 4$, 30.8%) that provided the service through a clinical pharmacy department. One hospital utilized an on-duty pharmacist and another hospital reported that anyone, whether pharmacist, pharmacy manager, or a technician present on the telephone line in the pharmacy department provided the service.

Furthermore, the qualification of the personnel was mostly bachelor's level i.e., Bachelors in Pharmacy (B.Pharm) ($N = 6$, 46.2%) and Doctor of Pharmacy (Pharm.D) ($N = 2$, 15.4%), followed by few hospitals ($N = 4$, 30.8%) which declined to mention the qualification of the staff responsible for the service. One hospital had a pharmacist with Master's qualification. Additionally, almost half of the hospitals ($N = 6$, 46.2%) had previously trained staff for the said purpose followed by a third ($N = 4$, 30.8%) that did not mention the details, and almost a quarter ($N = 3$, 23.1%) that did not have such training. The mode of inquiry was mainly direct access and via telephone ($N = 5$, 38.5%), followed by emails ($N = 4$, 30.8%) and direct access alone ($N = 2$, 15.4%). One hospital provided drug information service by telephone only and another by all modes.

Additionally, information relating to the quality assurance (QA) of the service was also sought from the hospitals. In this context, we found out that the majority of the hospitals provided immediate response to the drug information queries received, but only half of them kept a record for quality assurance purposes. The response was mostly verbal. Moreover, only two hospitals assimilated that information to produce newsletters. This hospital focused on continuous education programs for the patients as well as healthcare professionals. The data pertaining to the quality of service is tabulated in Table 1.

Table 1. Details of drug information service.

Information (N = 13)	Sample (N)	Percentage (%)
Keeping Record of Received Queries		
Yes	7	53.8
No	6	46.2
Average Response Time		
Immediately	10	76.9
Within 24 h	3	23.1
Most Common Mode of Response		
Verbal	4	30.8
Verbal and written	4	30.8
Verbal and written and mail	2	15.3
Mail	1	7.7
Verbal and printed literature	1	7.7
Printed literature	1	7.7
Participate in Patient Education Programs		
Yes	12	92.3
No	1	7.7
Report Adverse Drug Reactions (ADRs)		
Yes	8	61.5
No	5	38.5
Provide Educational Program for Healthcare Professionals		
Yes	9	69.2
No	4	30.8
Produce Newsletter		
Yes	2	15.4
No	11	84.6

With regard to the resources used for answering queries, we found that most of the hospitals used Lexi-Comp's Drug Information Handbook ($N = 10$, 76.9%) and Micromedex ($N = 9$, 69.2%). The data is presented in Table 2.

Table 2. Resources used in hospitals.

	Resources Used (Online Included)	Type of Hospitals (N = 13)		
		Public Yes (No)	Private Yes (No)	Total Yes (%)/No (%)
1	Lexi-Comp's Drug Information Handbook	7 (3)	3 (0)	10 (76.9)/3 (23.1)
2	Micromedex	7 (3)	2 (1)	9 (69.2)/4 (30.8)
3	Iowa Drug Information Service	1 (9)	0 (3)	1 (7.7)/12 (92.3)
4	Uptodate	6 (4)	1 (2)	7 (53.8)/6 (46.2)
5	Meyler's Side Effects on Drugs	1 (9)	1 (2)	2 (15.4)/11 (84.6)
6	Martindale's Extra Pharmacopoeia	2 (8)	1 (2)	3 (23.1)/10 (76.9)
7	American Hospital Formulary Service (AHFS) Drug Information	1 (9)	0 (3)	1 (7.7)/12 (92.3)
8	Pharmacotherapy: A Pathophysiologic Approach	3 (7)	1 (2)	4 (30.8)/9 (69.2)
9	Applied Therapeutics: The Clinical Use of Drugs	4 (6)	2 (1)	6 (46.2)/7 (53.8)
10	Pediatric Dosage Handbook	3 (7)	1 (2)	4 (30.8)/9 (69.2)
11	Drugs in Pregnancy and Lactation	4 (6)	3 (0)	7 (53.8)/6 (46.2)
12	British National Formulary (BNF)	5 (5)	2 (1)	7 (53.8)/6 (46.2)
13	Australian Medicine Handbook	1 (9)	0 (3)	1 (7.7)/12 (92.3)

Furthermore, the frequency of different types of drug information queries received at the pharmacy was also sought from the hospitals. The most common queries were related to seeking drug alternatives, administration and dosage, compatibility and safety issues, contraindications and availability of drugs in the pharmacy. Queries regarding adverse drug reactions (ADRs), pregnancy and lactation issues, as well as drug interactions were sought occasionally. Information regarding the toxicological parameters of drugs was rarely sought. The summary of these results is tabulated in Table 3.

Table 3. Frequency of different queries sought from drug information services.

Nature of Query	Hospital	Frequency of Drug Queries			
		Never	Rarely	Sometimes	Commonly
Adverse Drug Reactions	Government	1	4	4	1
	Private	1	0	1	1
	Total	2	4	5	2
Drug Alternatives	Government	0	0	2	8
	Private	0	0	1	2
	Total	0	0	3	10
Administration and Dosage	Government	0	0	2	8
	Private	0	0	0	3
	Total	0	0	2	11
Drug Interactions	Government	0	3	3	4
	Private	0	0	2	1
	Total	0	3	5	5
Drug Compatibility and Stability	Government	0	1	4	5
	Private	0	2	0	1
	Total	0	3	4	6
Drug Safety and Contraindications	Government	2	2	3	3
	Private	0	1	0	2
	Total	2	3	3	5
Availability of Drug in Pharmacy	Government	0	0	1	9
	Private	0	0	2	1
	Total	0	0	3	10
Drug Pharmacokinetics	Government	5	2	2	1
	Private	2	1	0	0
	Total	7	3	2	1
Drug Toxicity	Government	1	4	4	1
	Private	0	1	1	1
	Total	1	5	5	2
Pregnancy and Lactation	Government	0	4	4	2
	Private	0	0	1	2
	Total	0	4	5	4

The frequency of queries received per day from allied healthcare professionals and patients was also documented. Most commonly, the queries were received from physicians and pharmacists followed by nurses. The drug information service sometimes received queries from patients and interns. The summary of these results is presented in Table 4.

Table 4. Frequency of drug queries received from different persons.

Nature of Query	Hospital	Frequency of Drug Queries			
		Never	Rarely	Sometimes	Commonly
Physicians	Government	0	0	1	9
	Private	0	0	0	3
	Total	0	0	1	12
Nurses	Government	0	1	2	7
	Private	1	0	2	0
	Total	1	1	4	7
Pharmacists	Government	0	0	1	9
	Private	0	1	0	2
	Total	0	1	1	11
Patients	Government	1	1	6	2
	Private	0	0	1	2
	Total	1	1	7	4
Interns	Government	1	2	5	2
	Private	1	2	0	0
	Total	2	4	5	2

4. Discussion

Our study revealed that drug information service is now provided in all major tertiary care hospitals across five cities in the Eastern Province. Though all hospitals provide the service, most of the pharmacists providing the information had bachelor's qualification and only half of them had specialized training. This is not in accordance with the standards normally assumed for the service. While all pharmacists can provide drug information to consumers and healthcare professionals to some extent, the quality of the service is believed to improve if the pharmacist has had formal training or supervision of a drug information specialist [8]. This will offer greater support in combating medication errors, as expert pharmacists will be more poised and experienced in countering such problems. Hence, incorporating qualified and trained pharmacists may be more beneficial for achieving positive patient outcomes. The study also reported that the most common health resources employed for the service was Lexi-Comp and Micromedex. A similar study conducted among pharmacy students and faculty at a university in the USA also reported the high preference for Lexi-Comp for seeking information [9]. Secondly, the increased use of Micromedex was also reported from hospitals across the globe [1,10].

Our study also found that most of the queries were received from physicians. Studies conducted in other parts of the world also observed physicians being the most common enquirers of drug information [1,11]. The information related to the type of query was also sought from drug information personnel. We found that most the queries received in a day were related to drug alternatives, dosage and administration, as well as the availability of drugs. This finding was unusual, as it reported a high frequency of queries related to dosage and administration which was previously reported in studies conducted in different locations. However, it also observed that queries related to ADRs were reported rarely. This observation is contradictory to previous findings, as studies conducted in a hospital in India reported that a quarter of the total queries received were of such a nature [1]. Furthermore, the study observed that the other most common queries were the availability of the drug in the pharmacy and the drug alternatives. This highlights the growing use of online resources by physicians to seek ADRs and toxicology profiles of drugs to prescribe. Hence, physicians only sought information pertaining to the logistical constraints.

Since the common resources used did not contain information about the local availability and alternatives available in Saudi Arabia, perhaps a better solution to this problem may be the use of the Saudi National Formulary (SNF), as it can serve as a better alternative to other resources in such situations. The Saudi National Formulary contains drug information tailored for use in the country with related information [12]. However, the formulary needs to be updated more frequently to incorporate the latest information and must be freely available to all practicing healthcare professionals in Saudi healthcare settings. Further investigation is needed to find out the reasons that led to the decreased or lack of use of the SNF among healthcare practitioners in Saudi Arabia. The service should also field calls pertaining to the questions related to non-emergent cases and must promote direct interactions with the patients. This practice may increase the patient-pharmacist interaction, invest patient trust in pharmacists, and have the potential to achieve positive patient outcomes. One of the minimum standards pertaining to drug information services in Saudi Arabia is to monitor and report medication errors [7]. This standard has been mentioned in the official directives, however, it still needs to be put in practice.

Overall, it is believed that the drug information service may be improved by an upgrade of personnel i.e., pharmacists with higher qualification, training in drug information service, and appropriate experience should be hired, followed by updating the Saudi National Formulary (SNF) and establishing a mechanism for medication error identification and reporting.

5. Conclusions

Drug information service was provided in all major healthcare settings. Pharmacists working as a drug information specialist mostly held a bachelor's degree in pharmacy, with most of them not having any specialized training in the domain. This issue needs to be addressed for the future as it may be considered as a shortcoming and may require upgradation. Physicians benefitted the most from the drug information service, however, their queries were mostly related to the logistical constraints of drug availability and alternatives. Overall, the service is adequate. The use of the Saudi National Formulary was not reported by any hospital, which highlights a potential research gap to address i.e., to investigate the decreased use of the SNF by practitioners. This study will help understand the potential areas for improvement of the service and the ways in which drug information service in the country can contribute to positive patient outcomes.

Acknowledgments: This manuscript is based on undergraduate research thesis submitted by Sawsan Alamri (ID 2130006235) student of Pharm.D 5th Year for partial fulfillment of the degree of Doctor of Pharmacy (Pharm.D) at College of Clinical Pharmacy, Imam Abdulrahman Bin Faisal University (previous University of Dammam), Dammam 31441, Eastern Province, Saudi Arabia. The study was subjected to ethical approval by the ethics committee and was granted exemption from review. No funding was sought for the study.

Author Contributions: S.A., R.A.A.J. and M.S.A.G jointly conceived the idea. S.A. conducted the project. A.A.N. designed the methodology and wrote the manuscript. S.A., R.A.A.J and M.S.A.G. jointly designed and validated the questionnaire. A.A.N. revised and edited the manuscript in response to reviewers' comments. All authors read and approved the final draft of the manuscript.

References

1. George, B.; Rao, P.G. Assessment and evaluation of drug information services provided in a South Indian teaching hospital. *Indian. J. Pharmacol.* **2005**, *37*, 315–318.

2. Shah, A.; Naqvi, A.A.; Ahmad, R. The need for providing pharmaceutical care in geriatrics: A case study of diagnostic errors leading to medication-related problems in a patient treatment plan. *Arch. Pharm. Pract.* **2016**, *7*, 87–94.

3. Naqvi, A.A.; Shah, A.; Ahmad, R.; Ahmad, N. Developing an integrated treatment pathway for a post coronary artery bypass grafting (CABG) geriatric patient with comorbid hypertension (HTN) and type 1 diabetes mellitus (DM) for treating acute hypoglycemia and electrolyte imbalance. *J. Pharm. Bioallied Sci.* **2017**, in press.

4. Khan, N.; Naqvi, A.A.; Ahmad, R.; Ahmed, F.R.; McGarry, K.; Fazlani, R.Y.; Ahsan, M. Perceptions and Attitudes of Medical Sales Representatives (MSRs) and Prescribers Regarding Pharmaceutical Sales Promotion and Prescribing Practices in Pakistan. *J. Young Pharm.* **2016**, *8*, 244–250. [CrossRef]

5. Ali, A.A.; Yusoff, S.M.; Joffry, S.M.; Wahab, M.A. Drug information service awareness program and its impact on characteristics of inquiries at DIS unit in Malaysian public hospital. *Arch. Pharm. Pract.* **2013**, *4*, 9–14. [CrossRef]

6. Drug Information Centers in Saudi Arabia. Available online: http://webcache.googleusercontent.com/search?q=cache:mwykMjiP1VsJ:faculty.ksu.edu.sa/hisham/Documents/My_Books_pdf/DI/14-_1%2B%2B.pdf+&cd=5&hl=en&ct=clnk&gl=sa (accessed on 27 June 2017).

7. Ministry of Health, KSA. Minimum Standard of Drug Information Centre at MOH. Available online: http://www.moh.gov.sa/depts/Pharmacy/Documents/MINIMUM%20STANDARD%20OF%20DRUG%20INFORMATION%20CENTERS%20AT%20KSA.pdf (accessed on 27 June 2017).

8. Brand, K.A.; Kraus, M.L. Drug Information Specialists. *Am. J. Health Syst. Pharm.* **2006**, *63*, 712–714. [CrossRef] [PubMed]

9. Hanrahan, C.T.; Cole, S.W. Assessment of drug information resource preferences of pharmacy students and faculty. *J. Med. Libr. Assoc.* **2014**, *102*, 117–121. [CrossRef] [PubMed]

10. Moorman, K.L.; MacDonald, E.A.; Trovato, A.; Tak, C.R. Assessment and use of drug information references in Utah pharmacies. *Pharm. Pract. (Graneda)* **2017**, *15*, 839. [CrossRef] [PubMed]

11. Strobach, D.; Gruber, A.C.; Möhler, N.C.; Vetter-Kerkhoff, C. Clinical impact of the hospital pharmacy drug information service: How does information on drug-drug interaction enquiries translate into clinical decisions? *Eur. J. Hosp. Pharm.* **2015**, *22*, 83–88. [CrossRef]

12. Al-Shaqha, W.M. *Saudi National Formulary (SNF)*, 4th ed.; Saudi Food & Drug Authority and Saudi Pharmaceutical Society: Riyadh, Saudi Arabia, 2009.

4

'I Can Step outside My Comfort Zone.'

Morag C. E. McFadyen * (iD) **and Lesley Diack**

School of Pharmacy and Life sciences, Robert Gordon University, Riverside East, Garthdee Road,
Aberdeen AB10 7GJ, UK; h.l.diack@rgu.ac.uk
* Correspondence: m.mcfadyen@rgu.ac.uk

Abstract: On embarking upon such a multifactorial, professional degree as Pharmacy, students often find it difficult to meld the scientific- and practice-based components of the course. In final year of the undergraduate Masters of Pharmacy degree (MPharm) within the School of Pharmacy and Life Sciences at Robert Gordon University (RGU), students undertake a research project within a specific area. The aims of this study were to explore the effectiveness of a novel practice based approach to a biomedical science project, to identify elements of difficulty in the process, and to explore students' perceptions and reflections. Final year students were assigned to perform a systematic literature review working within a defined area of pharmacovigilance. Students were given individual ownership of the research question and were able to choose a topic of interest. Following the successful completion of the assignment, students were invited to explore their attitudes and views of the project and reflect on the process through a focus group using a talking wall method. The findings clearly identified a shift in mindset from predominantly negative opinions initially to an overwhelming positive viewpoint.

Keywords: evidence-based medicine; undergraduate pharmacy; thematic analysis; science practice integration; systematic review

1. Introduction: Evidence Based Medicine and Pharmacy

This paper investigates the views and attitudes of final year pharmacy students to the substitution of a science based project to a systematic review of a science topic. The innovative project was developed to highlight the centrality of the pharmacist's role in evidence based practice and pharmacovigilance (otherwise known as 'drug safety', which involves monitoring adverse events associated with the use of pharmaceutical products). The responsibility for pharmacovigilance falls under the Medicines and Healthcare products Regulatory Agency (MHRA) [1]. MPharm students at RGU are introduced to the MHRA in the first year of the course. Within the United Kingdom (UK), the MHRA uses adverse drug event (ADE) data collected from patients and healthcare professionals such as the pharmacist (the 'yellow card scheme') in addition to clinical studies [2]. Using this information, the MHRA assesses whether the potential for benefit outweighs the potential for harm, which in turn leads to a decision being made on whether a particular product will be given a marketing authorization, knowledge and understanding of this process is vital for pharmacy students. Using a systematic approach to review scientific literature in their final year has highlighted this and how their understanding could be important in their professional practice.

In the UK, the General Pharmaceutical Council (GPhC) is the accrediting body for Pharmacy education in Great Britain and the statutory regulator for pharmacists. A GPhC-accredited Master of Pharmacy (MPharm) degree is part of the pathway from a first year MPharm student to registration as a pharmacist. Increasingly in the 21st century, the role of the pharmacist is that of a healthcare professional, expert in medicines, and with a strong grounding in the science that underpins their practice. As such, the GPhC has adopted Miller's Triangle (Figure 1) as the pedagogical model for the development of clinical competencies to ensure safe and effective practice, is established as early as possible within training programmes, including the undergraduate MPharm [3,4]. The introduction of this project in final year allows the student to progress from knows to does in Miller's triangle (Figure 1).

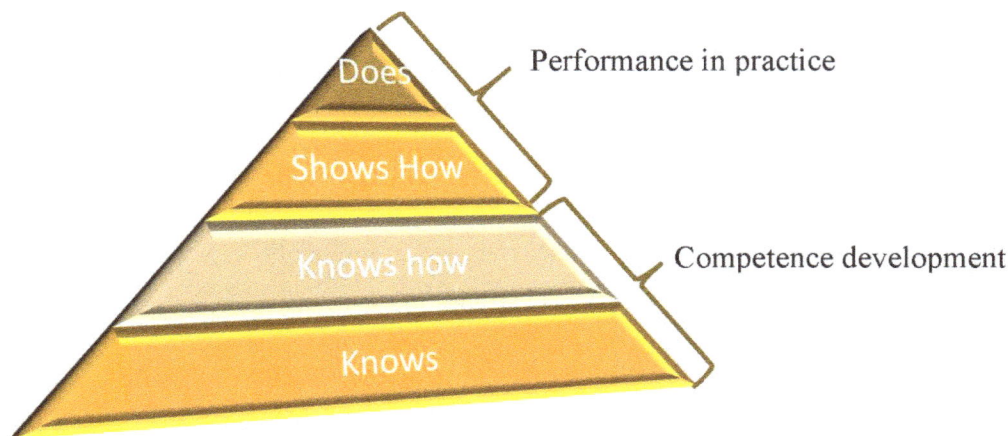

Figure 1. Miller's Triangle [3].

Standard 10 of the GPhC's 2011 education standards identifies the outcomes for the initial education and training of pharmacists [5]. An essential competency for the MPharm graduate is that they are expected to show how to 'assess and critically evaluate evidence to support safe, rational and cost effective use of medicines' (10.2.1b). They are also expected to be able to review the evidence base for current practice (10.2.1c). Several authors including Sackett (1979) [6] and Cochrane [7] advocated evidence-based practice (EBP) and called for "the conscientious use of current best evidence in making decisions about the care of individual patients or the delivery of health care services". Archibald Cochrane defined EBP as "current best evidence is up-to-date information from relevant, valid research about the different forms of health care" [7].

The curriculum of the school of Pharmacy and Life sciences at Robert Gordon University (RGU) is designed so that evidence-based medicine underpins all teaching within the MPharm. During the early stages of the course, students demonstrate that they know how to use the evidence to review current practice in written examinations. This project allows students to use the evidence base to review current practice in a final (fourth) year SQF level 10 five-week research project in biomedical sciences.

Student research projects within pharmacy have always been problematical, issues of finance, technical support, and laboratory space negatively impact not only on staff availability but also on the scope of the student's project being relevant and meaningful to their future practice.

Increasing complexity in pharmaceutical intervention and advancement in person centered care mean that pharmacy students often find it difficult to make sense of the wealth of data available and to appreciate the importance of this to scientific evidence-based practice. During the first three years of the course students are introduced to, and develop a knowledge and understanding of, problem based learning and evidence based practice. However, by the time students undertake their final year project it is often the application of their knowledge that is in question rather than the knowledge itself. The critical awareness and analysis as to whether the evidence they are provided with is valid or not is often overlooked within a busy curricula.

The aims of this evaluation study were to explore the effectiveness of a novel practice-based approach to a biomedical science project, identify elements of difficulty in the process, and to explore students' perceptions and reflections.

2. Methodology

This was a longitudinal qualitative case study research project conducted over four years with four or five students in each year. The research aim was to give a snapshot of the outcomes of the project to assess whether there was a need to adapt the project or the process. The project was split into three phases: mentoring, systematic review, and evaluation.

2.1. Phase 1: Mentoring

Students' expectations of a biomedical science project is that all five weeks of data collection will be within a laboratory setting. Nevertheless, prior to the research project data collection period MPharm students involved in this type of project were asked to undertake a modified systematic review of a scientific topic following Cochrane guidelines [7] entitled "Global perspectives of pharmacovigilance and adverse drug reactions: a cytochrome P450 case study".

During the third year of the MPharm, students undertake a narrative literature review in a related area to their fourth year project. Providing the opportunity to gather and interpret previous research in the area drawing a conclusion about the studies selected. Due to the students' limited knowledge and appreciation of the area, it rapidly became apparent that they would require considerable assistance and mentoring when it came to undertaking a successful systematic review. Unlike a narrative review, systematic reviews contain explicit rules for selecting the studies to be included in the review. These rules guide the reviewers to which findings they can and cannot include in the review, thereby lessening the probability that bias will influence the conclusions. A structured format is used for consistent presentation of information and data [7].

On commencing this project, it was essential to manage their expectations of the research project and to mentor and support them on their systematic review journey. Central to the review was the scientific premise that in humans six of the 57 different cytochrome P450's are the principal phase1 enzymes responsible for the metabolism of at least 60% of all drugs [8]. These P450s—namely CYP1A2, CYP2C9, CYP2C19, CYP2D6, CYP3A4, and CYP3A5—have polymorphic variants which affect their metabolic capacity [9]. As future pharmacists, it is important that the students are not only conversant with these particular enzymes but have the capacity to understand the importance of evidence based medicine relating to their role in drug metabolism.

Therefore, prior to the project start, weekly meetings were arranged to direct students to specific tasks building their knowledge, understanding, and confidence to successfully complete a systematic review. At the initial meeting, a student driven contract was instigated by which agreed milestones were set and achievements documented. Subsequent meetings provided the opportunity to identify challenges and concerns and to take action to resolve these in a timely manner, a brief synopsis of these is provided in Table 1.

Table 1. Pre-project milestones and student tasks.

Week	Topic	Milestone	Student's Task
1	Introduction	Research aim and objectives explained.	Identify paper for week 2 journal club (JC).
2	Journal club 1	Students presented at journal club. Discussion on evidence and critical appraisal tools.	Familiarise themselves with research area.
3	Research question	Initial discussion on research question Students provided with SIGN 50: a guideline developer's handbook	Decide area of interest (disease state) provide paper for next JC.
4	Journal club 2	Paper discussed, Methodology examined	Familiarise with bias.
5	Importance of bias	Understanding of research question; bias and confounding factors.	Identify a paper for week 6 JC.
6	Journal club	Development of search strategy	Develop search strategy for week 7.
7	Search strategy	Search strategy and plan how to undertake a systematic review.	Organise additional sessions on database searching and referencing with the librarian.

2.2. The Systematic Review Process

The first step to developing a systematic review involves defining the purpose of the review: The most common method used when creating a question is to use the PICO method. PICO is an acronym which describes a framework around which a question can be built—the question should include a description of: the participants (the patient group); intervention (action being taken to improve patient's health); comparison (a different intervention, to which the former intervention is being compared); and outcome (indicator of efficacy or harm resulting from intervention(s)). It should be noted that the comparison can in some cases be 'no intervention'. PICO can on occasion be expanded to PICOS where 'S' is representative of the setting of the studies [7].

As one of the purposes of a systematic review is to identify relevant research, it is important that the search is as thorough as possible; all relevant keywords and the appropriate databases must be identified and recorded for optimum coverage of the body of evidence pertaining to the particular clinical subject. While this can be achieved by maximising the number of databases used, this will prolong the search time as more time is spent tailoring search strategies to the individual databases; in addition to the fact that one spends more time screening a larger volume of duplicated articles. In addition to being time-consuming, selecting a large quantity of databases to search has also been proven to have only a modest benefit over using a select few of the most appropriate databases [10]. For this reason, it was important to select databases which have an extensive coverage of the area of interest for the purpose of the review; the databases should not be too similar in their coverage, as this would cause duplication of effort with few or no unique papers yielded—essentially making the process less efficient. With this in mind, following initial meetings with the supervisor, students were required to seek the assistance of a librarian. Following which they were required to discuss their databases and reasoning with their supervisor. Search strategy development was an iterative process—it involved defining keywords and synonyms to search for, and how to combine them when searching; the strategy often needed to be refined and adjusted according to the database being searched, which was why piloting of the strategy was also a part of the initial development process. Individual sessions with the supervisor ensured students were cognisant not only with other search methods (inverted commas for phrase searching, truncation, and wildcards) specific to each database and the use of Boolean operators, but with Cochrane's methodology and the necessity for the development and piloting of their search strategies [7].

After the search strategy had been developed and piloted, the next step was to assess results for relevance to the question. This involved confirming that inclusion and exclusion criteria were adequately defined, necessary to ensure only papers which specifically answered a student's research question were included in the review. Five to six databases were selected for the final search which involved individual searches of each of the PICOS component, then a combined search of all the PICOS terms. In addition to electronic databases, other methods were employed to identify studies including snowballing and 'grey literature'; literature which has not been peer-reviewed defined as "that which is produced on all levels of government, academics, business and industry in print and electronic formats, but which is not controlled by commercial publishers" [11]. At the end of the search process, all identified studies were uploaded to RefWorks, a reference management tool. The studies were assessed against the eligibility criteria in four stages:

- removing duplicates
- scoping assessment of titles
- assessing abstracts of the remaining studies
- reading of potentially eligible studies.

Once the relevant papers were identified they were analysed using data extraction tools. This was done systematically to improve validity of the review and extract necessary information about study characteristics and results from the included studies.

The data extraction proforma provided by the supervisor was initially developed from ones used by Mann et al. [12] and the North York Public Health Department, Ontario [13] amended to include statistical analysis. This was further adapted by the students to ensure relevance for their study, research question, inclusion/exclusion criteria, and articles. The students' data extraction form was used for their studies to provide consistency within the review, improve validity and reliability, and reduce bias. The form was piloted and validated by extracting data from an initial study and checked by the supervisor prior to the commencement of further data extraction.

Finally, a protocol based on the critical appraisal skills assessment (CASP) tools [14] (which the students were familiar with from their third year of study) was decided for critical appraisal of the papers; the protocol was essential to ensure that the papers were being critiqued in a systematic way, reducing bias. This allowed the reviewer to make a valid conclusion based on the data found from the identified papers.

Although all projects were focused upon the generic "Global perspectives of pharmacovigilance and adverse drug reactions: a cytochrome P450 case study", the titles were different and focused on such diverse topics as: an investigation into the adverse drug reactions and required pharmacokinetics associated with an increased dose of donepezil in Alzheimer's disease; impact of genetic polymorphisms in CYP2C9 on adverse drug reactions in patients administered with fluvastatin; gender specific responses to clopidigrel; comparison of P450 associated tardive dyskinesia in schizophrenics treated with atypical antipsychotics.

2.3. Evaluating the Process

After completion of this project the students were invited to take part in a 'talking wall' focus group on completion of the project. First described by Parsell, Gibbs, and Bligh in 1998 [15] to enhance interprofessional learning, 'talking walls' are a simple technique to collect data and enhance reflection by discussion with the other participants and was adapted from the commercial world. Our intention with this approach was to obtain student feedback to explore and analyse issues, opinions, and reflections and develop an action plan which could be fed forward to future years.

Student responses were analysed by grouping into themes and sub themes as summarised in Table 2 below.

Table 2. Themes identified from the students responses in their own words.

Question	Student Response/Themes	—ve/+ve
What did you feel when you were first given your research topic?	Disappointed, a dawdle (Scottish for easy), lost, mixed feelings, worried/dread /discomfort, staff intimidating	Predominantly negative
How would you describe the experience of undertaking a systematic review?	Time consuming/ demanding, rewarding/ steep-learning-curve, lots-of-work, tedious, more work than lab projects, progress slow at times, liked more as went on, chose area, understanding beyond systematic approach, changing viewpoints, new and demanding, really useful.	Negative to positive
How do you feel now having completed your project?	Achievement, greater understanding of evidence base, relief, it was tough, happy, staff so nice, prerequisite knowledge, importance of research methods,	More positive than negative
What impact do you think the project will have on your future career?	Knowledge of evidence base, systematic approach, critically appraise, confidence to question therapeutic intervention, project—area of research	All +ve

3. Discussion

This use of systematic reviews as an alternative to a lab based project allowed the students to develop appropriate and relevant skills and enhanced knowledge of biomedical research methodology and the underpinning theory. This fits with the GPhC competencies required of an MPharm graduate [5]. This project introduced a robust understanding of evidence-based medicine to the students and by the end of the research they were very aware of the impact of guidelines and the background to their development. Their confidence and understanding of the topics grew during the review process and many of the students contacted regulators and guideline developers to discuss their topic area [2]. This was particularly impactful for several students whose initial perception of a drug class and their efficacy changed with the development of the evidence base during their systematic reviews. By the end of the project, it had been reinforced to all students that their knowledge of drugs had to be based on evidence rather than on assumption that 'new' meant 'improved' or 'better' for the patient.

4. Impact

The 'sea change' observed from the students was unexpected, however the positive change in attitude and the findings have been fed-forward to develop this approach further to subsequent biomedical science practice based projects. Particularly reassuring to the authors was the change in attitude from a predominantly negative to more positive. Using systematic reviews to develop knowledge and understanding of biomedical research and methodology has been perceived as successful by the students involved and enabled them to utilise this newly acquired skill on the remainder of their fourth year modules to great effect. Anecdotally, the majority of students indicated that these skills were important ones to take into their pharmacy practice—a serendipitous outcome of the project. This was a robust project that allowed the students to develop their own topic and gave them ownership of their own research. It empowered, engaged, and educated them in the development of their own evidence based practice.

For the school, the impact created a more effective use of laboratory space, and minimised the financial burden that science-based projects often bring with them. For the university, it utilised the skills and knowledge base of the support services, especially the library, in an effective and efficient manner. For academic staff within the school, it provided the opportunity for continuous professional development and the further integration of science and practice within the MPharm curriculum.

At the end of the project, students agreed that they could step outside their comfort zone and learn about biomedical topics in a novel evidence-based way.

Acknowledgments: The authors wish to acknowledge all the students who have been involved in this project and who kindly shared their opinions and reflections on this novel practice-based approach to a biomedical sciences project.

Author Contributions: The authors contributed jointly to the research and writing of this manuscript.

References

1.   Medicines & Healthcare Products Regulatory Agency MHRA. Available online: https://www. gov.uk/government/organisations/medicines-and-healthcare-products-regulatory-agency (accessed on 4 September 2017).
2.   Yellow Card Scheme: Report a Problem with a Medicine or Medical Device. Available online: https://www.gov.uk/report-problem-medicine-medical-device (accessed on 4 September 2017).
3.   Miller, G.E. The assessment of clinical skills/competence/performance. *Acad. Med.* **1990**, *65*, S63–S67. [CrossRef] [PubMed]
4.   General Pharmaceutical Council GPhC: Millers Triangle. Available online: https://www. pharmacyregulation.org/content/millers-triangle (accessed on 4 September 2017).
5.   General Pharmaceutical Council. Standards for the Initial Education and Training of Pharmacists. 2011. Available online: http://www.pharmacyregulation.org/education/educationstandards (accessed on 4 September 2017).
6.   Sackett, D. Bias in analytic research. *J. Chronic Dis.* **1979**, *32*, 51–63. [CrossRef]
7.   Higgins, J.; Green, S. Cochrane Handbook for Systematic Reviews of Interventions. The Cochrane Collaboration, 2011. Available online: http://handbook.cochrane.org/ (accessed on 4 September 2017).

8. Zhou, S.; Liu, J.; Chowbay, B. Polymorphism of human cytochrome P450 enzymes and its clinical impact. *Drug Metab. Rev.* **2009**, *41*, 89–295. [CrossRef] [PubMed]

9. Pirmohamed, M. Cytochrome P450 enzyme polymorphisms and adverse drug reactions. *Toxicology* **2003**, *192*, 23–32. [CrossRef]

10. Shariff, S.Z.; Sontrop, J.M.; Iansavichus, A.V.; Haynes, R.B.; Weir, M.A.; Gandhim, S.; Cuerden, M.S.; Garg, A.X. Availability of renal literature in six bibliographic databases. *Clin. Kidney J.* **2012**, *5*, 610–617. [CrossRef] [PubMed]

11. Farace, D. GL'99 Conference Program. GreyNet, Grey Literature Network Service. In Proceedings of the 4th International Conference on Grey Literature, New Frontiers in Grey Literature, Washington, DC, USA, 4–5 October 1999.

12. Mann, V.; DeWolfe, J.; Hart, R.; Hollands, H.; LaFrance, R.; Lee, M.; Ying, J. *The Effectiveness of Food Safety Interventions (Report)*; Effective Public Health Practice Project (EPHPP): Hamilton, ON, Canada, 2001; Available online: https://www.healthevidence.org/view-article.aspx?a=effectiveness-food-safety-interventions-report-16155 (accessed on 4 September 2017).

13. North York Public Health Department. *Food Safety: Program Descriptions and Systematic Review of the Effectiveness of Documented Interventions*; Prepared for the Ontario Ministry of Health; North York Public Health Department: North York, ON, Canada, 1997.

14. Critical Appraisal Skills Programme (CASP). CASP Checklists. 2014. Available online: http://www.casp-uk.net/casp-tools-checklists (accessed on 4 September 2017).

15. Parsell, G.; Gibbs, T.; Bligh, J. Three visual techniques to enhance interprofessional learning. *Postgrad. Med. J.* **1998**, *74*, 387–390. [CrossRef] [PubMed]

5

Antipsychotic Polypharmacy among Children and Young Adults in Office-Based or Hospital Outpatient Department Settings

Minji Sohn [1,*]**, Meghan Burgess** [2] **and Mohamed Bazzi** [1]

[1] College of Pharmacy, Ferris State University, 220 Ferris Drive, Big Rapids, MI 49307, USA;
   bazzim5@ferris.edu

[2] College of Health Professions, Ferris State University, 200 Ferris Drive, Big Rapids, MI 49307, USA;
   burgem10@ferris.edu

* Correspondence: minjisohn@ferris.edu

Abstract: The purpose of the study was three-fold: (1) to estimate the national trends in antipsychotic (AP) polypharmacy among 6- to 24-year-old patients in the U.S.; (2) to identify frequently used AP agents and mental disorder diagnoses related to AP polypharmacy; and (3) to assess the strength of association between AP polypharmacy and patient/provider characteristics. We used publicly available ambulatory health care datasets to evaluate AP polypharmacy in office-based or hospital outpatient department settings to conduct a cross-sectional study. First, national visit rates between 2007 and 2011 were estimated using sampling weights. Second, common diagnoses and drugs used in AP polypharmacy were identified. Third, a multivariate logistic regression model was developed to assess the strength of association between AP polypharmacy and patient and provider characteristics. Between 2007 and 2011, approximately 2% of office-based or hospital outpatient department visits made by 6- to 24-year-old patients included one or more AP prescriptions. Of these visits, 5% were classified as AP polypharmacy. The most common combination of AP polypharmacy was to use two or more second-generation APs. Also, bipolar disorder and schizophrenia were the two most frequent primary mental disorder diagnoses among AP polypharmacy visits. The factors associated with AP polypharmacy were: older age (young adults), black, having one or more non-AP prescriptions, and having schizophrenia or ADHD.

Keywords: antipsychotics; polypharmacy; children; adolescents; young adults

1. Introduction

Over the last two and half decades, a wide variety of psychotropic medications have reinvented psychiatric therapy, especially for children and young adults. In particular, the profession of medicine has observed an increased frequency in the use of antipsychotic (AP) medication in the age group [1–4]. First-generation, typical APs were developed in the 1950s, and second-generation APs (i.e., also known as atypical APs) were developed in the 1990s. Second-generation APs boasted reduced extrapyramidal symptoms and other health problems caused by the use of first-generation APs [5,6]. As a result, the overall utilization of APs has increased significantly over time in patients of all ages, including children [7–16]. According to a study by Sieda et al., by 1996, APs were prescribed for 8.6 per 1000 children. By 2002, this statistic rose drastically to include as many as 39.4 per 1000 children [17].

In the midst of the increasing use of APs in children, AP polypharmacy is a particular area of concern. In some cases, using two or more medications to treat a mental illness may be more effective than monotherapy, especially if the mechanisms of action are complementary [18,19]. However, the concomitant use of two or more pharmacologically similar APs lacks scientific rationale and evidence. One may argue that using two similar agents may result in additive efficacy or rapid therapeutic response, but this argument is not supported by any compelling evidence or theoretical explanation [20,21]. Instead, AP polypharmacy increases the risk of drug overdosing and adverse side effects, such as hyperlipidemia or type 2 diabetes [20–23].

Several risk factors of AP polypharmacy have been discussed elsewhere. Non-elderly patients (age < 65) [24,25], patients in an inpatient setting [26,27], particularly those with a longer stay [26,28], and schizophrenia [29–31] are reported as being associated with AP polypharmacy. The impact of patient sex on AP polypharmacy is inconclusive [24,27,32]. However, a majority of these studies primarily focus on adult populations, and AP polypharmacy trends in children are underexplored.

The purpose of this study was to assess the U.S. national trends in AP polypharmacy among children and young adults in office-based or hospital outpatient department settings. More specifically, we carried out three specific objectives: (1) evaluate the yearly trends in AP polypharmacy use amongst 6- to 24-year-old patients in the U.S.; (2) identify frequently used AP agents and the primary mental diagnoses in AP polypharmacy; and (3) assess the strength of association between AP polypharmacy and the characteristics of patients and providers.

2. Methods

2.1. Data Source

The cross-sectional dataset for the study was obtained from the National Ambulatory Medical Care Survey (NAMCS) and the National Hospital Ambulatory Medical Care Survey (NHAMCS) database. The NAMCS and NHAMCS are nationally representative surveys that collect samples on patient visits to office-based or hospital outpatient department-based providers who are primarily engaged in direct patient care. More specifically, the sampling process utilizes a three-stage probability design. The first stage of probability sampling is based on geographic segments, and the second stage involves the probability sampling of physician practices. Thirdly, within the sampled physician practices, random samples of patient visits are collected. Each NAMCS/NHAMCS record has a single sample weight that is calculated based on this three-stage probability design. The NAMCS/NHAMCS data contains patient demographics, physician specialty, other clinicians seen during the visits, diagnoses based on the International Classification of Diseases, Ninth Revision, Clinical Modification (ICD-9-CM), and up to eight prescribed drugs during the visit. Our study sample consisted of AP visits (refer to the succeeding text for details on defining AP visits) of patients who were 6 to 24 years of age between 2007 and 2011. We intended to estimate the national trends in non-emergent visits associated with AP prescriptions, and therefore, we excluded data from the hospital emergency department from the study. The rationale is that treatment strategies can be different between an emergency department setting and an office-based or hospital outpatient department setting. For example, pharmacotherapy in an emergency department setting is likely to be focused on treating a particular incident or episode in the short-term, rather than for the chronic management of mental illness with regular follow-up visits. Sample weights were applied in all analyses using Stata Version 13 (StataCorp, College Station, TX, USA, 2013). The data use for the study was approved by the Ferris State University Institutional Review Board, which oversees the ethical conduct of research at this institution.

2.2. National Trends in AP Polypharmacy

As the first objective of the study, we estimated the national AP visit rates and the national AP polypharmacy visit rates in each year between 2007 and 2011. Since the unit of observation of the dataset is the physician-patient encounter, the number of patients cannot be estimated. A patient visit was defined as an AP visit if one or more of the following medications were prescribed: (1) as typical APs, haloperidol, loxapine, thiothixene, trifluoperazine, chlorpromazine, fluphenazine, perphenazine, prochlorperazine, and thioridazine; and (2) as atypical APs, risperidone, olanzapine, quetiapine, ziprasidone, aripiprazole, paliperidone, asenapine, iloperidone, and clozapine. An AP polypharmacy visit was defined as an AP visit with two or more AP prescriptions. Drug prescriptions were identified using the Multum classification system (Cerner Corporation, Lexicon, Denver, CO, USA). The Multum classification utilizes a three-level nested category system in which drugs are coded in terms of their generic components and therapeutic classes.

2.3. Diagnoses and Frequently Used APs in AP Polypharmacy

As the second objective of the study, we identified mental disorder diagnoses (ICD-9-CM code 290–319) and frequently used AP agents associated with AP polypharmacy. If two or more mental disorder diagnoses were present, we identified a primary mental disorder diagnosis based on a previously developed hierarchy [1]. More specifically, the primary mental disorder diagnosis was assigned in the following order: (1) schizophrenia and other psychoses (295, 297–298); (2) pervasive developmental disorder or mental retardation (299, 317–319); (3) bipolar disorder (290.6, 296.1, 296.4–296.8, 301.13); (4) disruptive behavior disorder (312.0–312.4, 312.81, 312.82, 312.89, 312.9, 313.81); (5) attention-deficit/hyperactivity disorder (ADHD) (314); (6) depression/mood disorder, not otherwise specified (293.83, 296.2, 296.3, 296.9, 298.0, 300.4, 311); (7) anxiety disorder (293.84, 300.0, 300.2, 300.3, 309.3, 309.21, 309.81, 313.0, 313.2, 313.89); (8) adjustment disorder (308.0–308.2, 308.4, 308.9, 309.0–309.4, 309.82, 309.83, 309.89, 309.9); (9) communication and learning disorder (307.0, 307.9, 315.0–315.2, 315.31, 315.32, 315.39, 315.9); and (10) other mental disorders (290–319, not listed above). The assignment of primary mental disorder was mutually exclusive. We adopted this method because the ordering of the diagnostic group generally corresponds to the strength of clinical evidence for AP treatment in pediatrics [1,11].

2.4. Patient and Provider Characteristics Associated with AP Polypharmacy

We assessed the association between patient and provider characteristics and AP polypharmacy. As patient characteristics, age, sex, race, geographic region (Northeast, Midwest, South, and West), Metropolitan Statistical Area (MSA), primary payer source, median household income based on patient zip code, and % of adults with a Bachelor's degree or higher based on patient zip code were included in the model. As provider characteristics, we identified variables on health care providers (e.g., psychiatrist, mental health provider) and the type of health care services provided during the visit (e.g., psychotherapy, other mental health counseling). A mental health provider refers to psychologists, counselors, social workers, or therapists who provide mental health counseling.

Differences in patient and provider characteristics between monotherapy and polypharmacy visits were tested for statistical significance. We used chi-squared tests for categorical variables and *t*-tests for continuous variables. Also, univariate and multivariate logistic regression models were developed to estimate the strength of association between polypharmacy and patient and provider characteristics.

In the NAMCS/NHAMCS, between 2007 and 2011, approximately 18% of all patient visits did not have race information. For the observations missing race information, we used imputed values that were provided by the NAMCS/NHAMCS. The imputation methods used by the NAMCSNHAMCS are described in the Public Use Data File Documentation [33]. For variables of median household income based on patient zip code and % of adults with a Bachelor's degree or higher based on patient zip code, approximately 15% of all patient visits had missing data. Since the NAMCS/NHAMCS does not provide the patient zip code or imputation values for these variables, we created a missing data indicator for the variables and treated them as a separate category. Then, we conducted a sensitivity analysis by excluding missing values from the estimation to check whether the findings were robust.

3. Results

3.1. National Rates of AP Polypharmacy

Between 2007 and 2011, approximately 1.92 per 100 visits included one or more AP prescriptions (95% Confidence interval (95% CI) 1.65–2.25 per 100 visits, weighted count 16,131,721). Of these visits,

5% were visits related to AP polypharmacy (95% CI 3.77–7.78 weighted count 877,071). Year-by-year estimation is shown in Figure 1. Over the 5-year observation period, trends in AP visits and AP polypharmacy did not increase significantly. Although not significant, the AP visit rate appeared higher in 2009, as it was 2.53 per 100 visits (95% CI 1.93–3.31 per 100 visits), while it was between 1.71 and 1.90 per 100 visits in other years (i.e., 1.71; 95% CI 1.24–2.35 per 100 visits in 2008, 1.90; 95% CI 1.41–2.55 per 100 visits in 2011). As for AP polypharmacy, year-to-year variation ranged from 3% (95% CI 1.84–4.47 in 2010) to 7% (95% CI 3.12–14.76 in 2009).

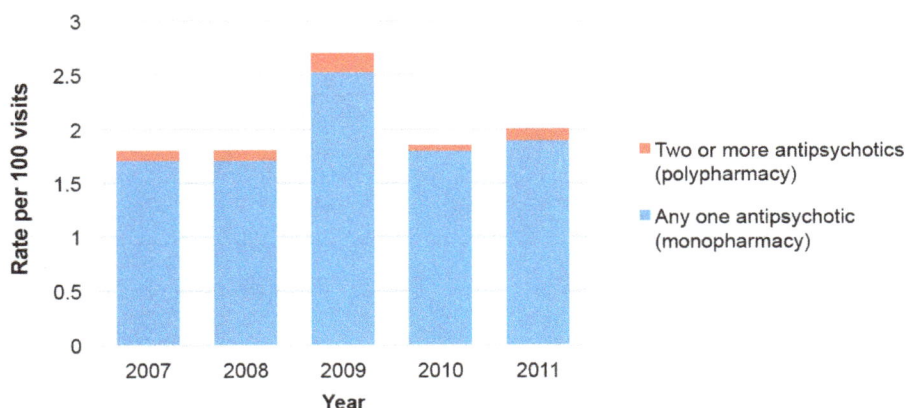

Figure 1. National antipsychotic (AP) visit rates and the proportion of AP polypharmacy between 2007 and 2011.

3.2. Common Mental Disorder Diagnoses and Drugs Used in AP Polypharmacy

Bipolar disorder and schizophrenia were the most common primary mental diagnoses in AP polypharmacy (24% and 22%, respectively) (Figure 2). Approximately 12% were patients diagnosed with ADHD, and 15% did not have any recorded mental disorder diagnosis.

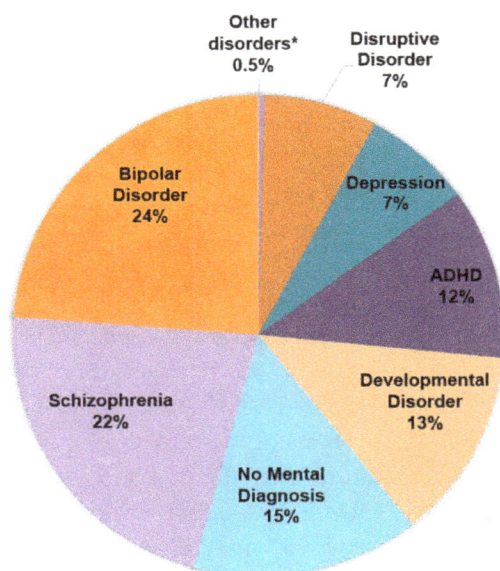

Figure 2. Primary mental disorder diagnoses in AP polypharmacy. Percentages may not total 100% due to rounding. * Anxiety disorder, adjustment disorder, communication and learning disorder, and other mental disorders.

In AP polypharmacy visits, the most common combination was to use two or more second-generation APs (80.63%, 95% CI 60.20–91.97). The combination of first- and second-generation APs accounted for 19.37% (95% CI 8.03–39.80) (Table 1). Among the drugs used in AP polypharmacy, quetiapine was the most frequently used agent (53.25%; 95% CI 37.45–68.41), followed by aripiprazole (48.46%; 95% CI 33.58–63.62) (Table 2).

Table 1. Frequently used antipsychotic classes in AP polypharmacy. *

Drug Class Used in AP Polypharmacy	%	95% Confidence Interval
Second generation only	80.63	60.20–91.97
First and second generations	19.37	8.03–39.80

* The number of observations for the "first generation only" category was very small (unweighted count = 5), and it was estimated to be less than 0.001% of AP polypharmacy visits.

Table 2. Frequently used antipsychotics in AP polypharmacy.

Drugs Used in AP Polypharmacy	%	95% Confidence Interval
First generation antipsychotics		
Haloperidol	12.19	3.08–37.77
Chlorpromazine	6.98	2.24–19.72
Prochlorperzine	0.11	0.02–0.83
Fluphenazine	0.09	0.01–0.65
Second generation antipsychotics		
Quetiapine	53.25	37.45–68.41
Aripiprazole	48.46	33.58–63.62
Olanzapine	26.1	13.60–44.21
Risperidone	26.41	15.18–41.89
Ziprasidone	23.17	9.99–45.04
Clozapine	8.09	2.77–21.40
Paliperidone	7.56	1.13–36.89

3.3. Factors Associated with AP Polypharmacy

Patient and provider characteristics were compared between AP monotherapy and AP polypharmacy visits (Table 3). Among those, the variables of patient age, whether mental health provider was seen (yes/no), and the number of non-AP prescribed were statistically significant. More specifically, a higher proportion of AP polypharmacy visits was made by young adult patients (age 19–24), and a smaller proportion was made by elementary school-aged children (age 6–12), compared to AP monotherapy visits ($p = 0.004$). Also, a higher proportion of AP polypharmacy visits involved a mental health provider during the visit than AP monotherapy visits. (20.57% versus 8.06%, $p = 002$). The average number of non-AP prescriptions was 2.45 in AP polypharmacy visits, while it was 2.02 in AP monotherapy visits ($p = 0.03$).

In the multivariate logistic regression model, the variables of age, race, number of non-AP prescriptions, schizophrenia, and ADHD were significantly associated with AP polypharmacy (Table 4). Young adults were more likely to have AP polypharmacy visits than elementary school-aged children (adjusted odds ratio (AOR) 3.43; 95% CI 1.07–11.02). Adolescents were not significantly different from elementary school-aged children in terms of the rate of AP polypharmacy (AOR 1.65; 95% CI 0.56–4.89). With respect to race, compared to white patients, black patients were significantly less likely to have AP polypharmacy (AOR 0.21; 95% CI 0.07–0.57). Also, compared to AP visits without any concomitant non-AP prescriptions, AP visits with one non-AP prescription were more likely to have AP polypharmacy (AOR 5.57; 95% CI 1.65–18.86). AP visits with two or more non-AP prescriptions showed a similar association with AP polypharmacy (two non-AP AOR 8.08; 95% CI 2.01-32.48, three or more non-AP AOR 6.67; 95% CI 2.07–21.53). As for primary mental disorder diagnosis, compared to AP visits with a bipolar disorder diagnosis, AP visits with a schizophrenia or an ADHD diagnosis were more likely to have AP polypharmacy (AOR 4.23; 95% CI 1.61–11.16, AOR 2.65; 95% CI 1.07–6.60, respectively). The variables of sex, geographic region, MSA, payer source, psychotherapy, other mental health counseling, health care provider, household income, and education level were not significantly associated with AP polypharmacy.

Table 3. National estimated visit rates of AP monotherapy and AP polypharmacy stratified by patient and provider characteristics between 2007 and 2011.

Characteristics	Monotherapy		Polypharmacy		p-Value *
	Weighted Count (in Thousands)	Weighted %	Weighted Count (in Thousands)	Weighted %	
Age					0.004
6–12 (Elementary school age)	4251	27.87	135	15.44	
13–18 Years (Adolescent)	5980	39.2	227	25.91	
19–24 (Young adult)	5023	32.93	514	58.66	
Sex					0.084
Female	5803	38.04	218	24.84	
Male	9452	61.96	659	75.16	
Race					0.365
White	12,255	80.34	760	86.62	
Black	2357	15.45	81	9.18	
Other/Unspecified	642	4.21	37	4.2	
Geographic region					0.685
Northeast	3485	22.85	273	31.1	
Midwest	3004	19.69	168	19.13	
South	5863	38.44	311	35.5	
West	2902	19.03	125	14.27	
MSA or non-MSA area					0.291
MSA	13,378	87.7	807	92.04	
non-MSA	1877	12.3	70	7.96	
Payer					0.152
Private	5666	37.45	276	31.53	
Medicaid	6576	43.46	316	36.03	
Other	2888	19.09	285	32.45	
Psychiatrist					0.317
Yes	8261	54.16	552	62.93	
No	6693	45.84	325	37.07	
Psychotherapy					0.077
Yes	4706	30.85	396	45.2	
No	10,549	69.15	481	54.8	
Other mental health counseling					0.872
Yes	3504	22.97	210	23.99	
No	11,751	77.03	667	76.01	
Mental health provider					0.002
Yes	1230	8.06	180	20.57	
No	14,025	91.94	697	79.43	
Number of non-AP (mean, SD)	2.02	0.08	2.45	0.20	0.03
Median household Income based on patient zip code					0.381
Quartile 1	3302	21.65	225	25.60	
Quartile 2	3294	21.59	78	8.93	
Quartile 3	3100	20.32	184	21.01	
Quartile 4	4271	28.01	331	37.77	
Missing data	1287	8.44	59	6.69	
% of Adults with a Bachelor's degree or higher based on patient zip code					0.911
Quartile 1	2973	19.49	154	17.52	
Quartile 2	3490	22.88	165	18.81	
Quartile 3	3103	20.34	217	24.73	
Quartile 4	4401	38.85	283	32.24	
Missing data	1287	8.44	59	6.69	

* Chi-squared tests were used for all variables, except the number of non-AP prescriptions (t-test). MSA: Metropolitan Statistical Area.

As a sensitivity analysis, we excluded observations missing either median household income based on patient zip code or % of adults with a Bachelor's degree or higher based on patient zip code from the estimation. As a result, the association between AP polypharmacy and these variables remained as not significant ($p > 0.05$) in the chi-squared tests and logistic regressions (Appendix A).

Table 4. Univariate and multivariate logistic regressions examining factors associated with AP polypharmacy.

Characteristics	Unadjusted Odds Ratio	95% Confidence Interval	Adjusted Odds Ratio *	95% Confidence Interval
Age				
6–12 (Elementary school age)	1	Reference	1	Reference
13–18 (Adolescent)	0.54	0.28–1.05	1.65	0.56–4.89
19–24 (Young adult)	2.89	1.67–5.01	3.43	1.07–11.02
Sex				
Male	1	Reference	1	Reference
Female	0.54	0.26–1.10	0.51	0.22–1.17
Race				
White	1	Reference	1	Reference
Black	0.55	0.27–1.15	0.21	0.07–0.57
Other/Unspecified	1	0.26–3.82	0.87	0.16–4.79
Payer				
Private	1	Reference	1	Reference
Medicaid	0.82	0.41–1.62	1.27	0.54–3.01
Other	2.06	0.98–4.32	2.27	1.00–5.18
Psychotherapy	1.85	0.93–3.69	1.57	0.69–3.59
Other mental health counseling	1.06	0.53–2.11	0.98	0.45–2.13
Mental health provider	2.95	1.45–6.00	2.24	0.86–5.65
Psychiatrist	1.44	0.71–2.93	1.75	0.78–3.94
Number of non-AP				
None	1	Reference	1	Reference
One	0.91	0.49–1.69	5.57	1.65–18.86
Two	1.42	0.57–3.56	8.08	2.01–32.48
Three or More	1.25	0.63–2.46	6.67	2.07–21.53
Primary mental disorder diagnosis				
Bipolar disorder	1	Reference	1	Reference
Schizophrenia	3.39	1.76–6.53	4.23	1.61–11.16
Developmental disorder	1.39	0.54–3.54	1.17	0.42–3.31
Disruptive disorder	0.65	0.24	1.02	0.32–3.24
Depression	0.38	0.16–0.89	0.3	0.12–0.76
Anxiety disorder	0.68	0.30–1.51	0.61	0.20–1.82
Learning disorder	1.48	0.35–6.27	0.92	0.16–5.38
ADHD	1.64	0.85–3.20	2.65	1.07–6.60
Other mental disorder	1.33	0.51–3.48	1.26	0.42–3.72
No mental disorder diagnosis	0.78	0.24–2.57	2.2	0.75–6.48

* The multivariate logistic regression model adjusted for geographic region, MSA, median household income, and % of adults with a Bachelor's degree or higher based on patient zip codes, in addition to the variables above.

4. Discussion

The purpose of the study was: (1) to estimate the national trends in AP polypharmacy among 6- to 24-year-old patients in the U.S.; (2) to identify frequently used AP agents and diagnoses related to AP polypharmacy; and (3) to assess the strength of association between AP polypharmacy and patient/provider characteristics.

Although not significant, the rate of AP visits and the proportion of AP polypharmacy appeared increased in 2009 and decreased in 2010. Several factors may have affected this trend. For example, in 2009, two second-generation AP agents, iloperidone and asenapine, were newly approved by the U.S. Food and Drug Administration (FDA), and aripiprazole was additionally approved for the treatment of autistic spectrum disorder. New approvals of APs and drug indications could have temporarily increased the rate of AP prescription and polypharmacy in 2009. In addition, new findings of clinical trials and observational studies associated with APs, changes in practice guidelines, pharmaceutical marketing, and public education about the effectiveness and risks of APs would potentially have increased or decreased the rate of AP prescription to a certain extent.

Bipolar disorder and schizophrenia were the two most prevalent primary mental diagnoses among AP polypharmacy visits (24% and 22%, respectively). Approximately 12% of AP polypharmacy visits had ADHD. However, unlike bipolar disorder or schizophrenia, none of the APs are approved for the treatment of ADHD by the FDA. While the off-label use of APs in ADHD patients has been reported in a number of studies, our study further extends the concern to AP polypharmacy. It is concerning that a risk of unnecessary harm from AP misuse is imposed on ADHD patients, not only from the off-label use perspective but also from the polypharmacy perspective.

Approximately 15% of AP polypharmacy visits did not have any mental disorder diagnosis. It should be noted that the NAMCS/NHAMCS collects only up to three diagnosis codes, and therefore, if a patient has three or more physical disorder diagnoses, it is possible that a mental disorder diagnosis is not captured in the dataset due to limited space in the survey. However, in our study sample, of the AP polypharmacy visits without any mental disorder diagnosis, 83% had two or fewer diagnoses. This means that approximately 12% of AP polypharmacy visits did not have any mental disorder diagnosis, and limited space in the survey was not the reason for it.

The most common combination of AP polypharmacy was to use two or more second-generation APs (80.63%). This trend can be explained by that second-generation APs have no or reduced extrapyramidal symptoms compared to the first-generation APs. When second-generation APs were introduced, they were marketed as relatively safer agents than the pre-existing first-generation APs [5,6]. However, great caution is needed before using second-generation APs, since they have serious side effects, including hyperlipidemia and type 2 diabetes [20–23]. Furthermore, the concomitant use of two or more second-generation antipsychotics may only increase the risk of those adverse events.

Among AP visits, polypharmacy visits were significantly associated with young adults than elementary school-aged children, and black patients than white patients. Also, patients who had one or more non-AP prescriptions in addition to their AP prescription were significantly more likely to be classified as AP polypharmacy. Interestingly, when adjusted for other covariates, primary payer source, household income, and education-related factors were not significantly associated with AP polypharmacy. In previous studies, the initiation of AP treatment in young patients was significantly associated with socioeconomic factors, such as having Medicaid as the primary payer source [3,4,23]. These findings suggest that, when it comes to AP polypharmacy, individuals' comorbidities and the complexity of the physical/mental conditions play a more important role than previously reported risk factors.

Some limitations should be noted. First, the unweighted count of AP polypharmacy in each year was small ($n < 30$), and therefore, the yearly estimation of AP polypharmacy can be potentially unreliable. In order to address the small sample size problem, we combined five-years' worth of data (2007–2011) and used it to carry out the objectives of the study. Nonetheless, caution is needed when interpreting the results of the study, particularly for the yearly estimation (Figure 1). Second, the NAMCS/NHAMCS collects the cross-sectional sample of office-based or hospital outpatient department visits and it does not establish the sequence of events. For example, our analysis cannot infer that the concurrent prescription of non-AP drugs caused the AP polypharmacy. Instead, we only suggest that the number of non-AP prescriptions is positively associated with the likelihood of AP polypharmacy. In addition, due to the cross-sectional nature of the study dataset, our study cannot exclude the short-term, temporary use of two or more APs from the definition of AP polypharmacy. This could overestimate the true rate of AP polypharmacy because it is common to have a short overlap period when a patient switches APs. Third, our study sample only includes non-emergent office-based or hospital outpatient department visit data, and it does not include emergency room or inpatient visit data. This would result in the underestimation of AP polypharmacy rates. It is because AP polypharmacy occurs most frequently in schizophrenia or bipolar disorder patients, and patients with these conditions are more frequently hospitalized. Therefore, it should be noted that the findings of the study should not be applied to an emergency room or inpatient visits. Fourth, we conducted a multivariate logistic regression model to adjust for a number of potential confounders, but it is limited to variables that are observable and available in the dataset. While our model includes variables that were identified in prior studies, we cannot rule out the possibility of having a confounding bias.

In conclusion, between 2007 and 2011, approximately 2% of office-based or hospital outpatient department visits made by 6- to 24-year-old patients included one or more AP prescriptions. Of these visits, 5% were AP polypharmacy visits. The most common combination of AP polypharmacy was to use two or more second-generation APs concomitantly. Also, bipolar disorder and schizophrenia were the two most frequent primary mental diagnoses among AP polypharmacy visits. The factors associated with AP polypharmacy were: older age (young adults), black, having one or more non-AP prescriptions, and having schizophrenia or ADHD.

Acknowledgments: No funding was provided for this study. We would like to thank reviewers for providing detailed and insightful comments.

Author Contributions: All authors contributed to the design of the study and the analysis of the results. Meghan Burgess and Minji Sohn wrote the manuscript. Mohamed Bazzi provided revisions and comments.

Appendix A

Table A1. Sensitivity analysis of national estimated visit rates of AP monotherapy and AP polypharmacy stratified by patient and provider characteristics between 2007 and 2011.

Characteristics	Monotherapy		Polypharmacy		p-Value *
	Weighted Count (in Thousands)	Weighted %	Weighted Count (in Thousands)	Weighted %	
Age					0.004
6–12 (Elementary school age)	4251	27.87	135	15.44	
13–18 Years (Adolescent)	5980	39.2	227	25.91	
19–24 (Young adult)	5023	32.93	514	58.66	
Sex					0.084
Female	5803	38.04	218	24.84	
Male	9452	61.96	659	75.16	
Race					0.365
White	12,255	80.34	760	86.62	
Black	2357	15.45	81	9.18	
Other/Unspecified	642	4.21	37	4.2	
Geographic region					0.685
Northeast	3485	22.85	273	31.1	
Midwest	3004	19.69	168	19.13	
South	5863	38.44	311	35.5	
West	2902	19.03	125	14.27	
MSA or non-MSA area					0.291
MSA	13,378	87.7	807	92.04	
non-MSA	1877	12.3	70	7.96	
Payer					0.152
Private	5666	37.45	276	31.53	
Medicaid	6576	43.46	316	36.03	
Other	2888	19.09	285	32.45	
Psychiatrist					0.317
Yes	8261	54.16	552	62.93	
No	6693	45.84	325	37.07	
Psychotherapy					0.077
Yes	4706	30.85	396	45.2	
No	10,549	69.15	481	54.8	
Other mental health counseling					0.872
Yes	3504	22.97	210	23.99	
No	11,751	77.03	667	76.01	
Mental health provider					0.002
Yes	1230	8.06	180	20.57	
No	14,025	91.94	697	79.43	
Number of non-AP (mean, SD)	2.02	0.08	2.45	0.20	0.03

Table A1. *Cont.*

Characteristics	Monotherapy		Polypharmacy		p-Value *
	Weighted Count (in Thousands)	Weighted %	Weighted Count (in Thousands)	Weighted %	
Median household Income based on patient zip code					0.341
Quartile 1	3302	23.64	225	27.44	
Quartile 2	3294	23.58	78	9.57	
Quartile 3	3100	22.20	184	22.51	
Quartile 4	4271	30.58	331	40.48	
% Adults with Bachelor's degree or higher based on patient zip code					0.894
Quartile 1	2973	21.29	154	18.78	
Quartile 2	3490	24.99	165	20.16	
Quartile 3	3103	22.22	217	26.51	
Quartile 4	4401	31.51	283	34.55	

* Chi-squared tests were used for all variables, except the number of non-AP prescriptions (t-test).

Table A2. Sensitivity analysis of univariate and multivariate logistic regressions examining factors associated with AP polypharmacy.

Characteristics	Unadjusted Odds Ratio	95% Confidence Interval	Adjusted Odds Ratio *	95% Confidence Interval
Age				
6–12 (Elementary school age)	1	Reference	1	Reference
13–18 (Adolescent)	0.54	0.28–1.05	1.50	0.50–4.50
19–24 (Young adult)	2.89	1.67–5.01	3.57	1.08–11.78
Sex				
Male	1	Reference	1	Reference
Female	0.54	0.26–1.10	0.53	0.22–1.27
Race				
White	1	Reference	1	Reference
Black	0.55	0.27–1.15	0.23	0.09–0.60
Other/Unspecified	1	0.26–3.82	1.07	0.23–5.11
Payer				
Private	1	Reference	1	Reference
Medicaid	0.82	0.41–1.62	1.45	0.62–3.37
Other	2.06	0.98–4.32	2.11	0.91–4.90
Psychotherapy	1.85	0.93–3.69	1.71	0.74–3.94
Other mental health counseling	1.06	0.53–2.11	1.02	0.47–2.25
Mental health provider	2.95	1.45–6.00	2.16	0.83–5.62
Psychiatrist	1.44	0.71–2.93	1.40	0.66–2.96
Number of non-AP				
None	1	Reference	1	Reference
One	0.91	0.49–1.69	5.28	1.53–18.20
Two	1.42	0.57–3.56	7.28	1.78–29.66
Three or More	1.25	0.63–2.46	6.30	1.94–20.47
Primary mental disorder diagnosis				
Bipolar disorder	1	Reference	1	Reference
Schizophrenia	3.39	1.76–6.53	4.53	1.69–12.13
Developmental disorder	1.39	0.54–3.54	1.21	0.43–3.40
Disruptive disorder	0.65	0.24	1.51	0.33–4.04
Depression	0.38	0.16–0.89	0.33	0.13–0.83
Anxiety disorder	0.68	0.30–1.51	0.67	0.22–2.07
Learning disorder	1.48	0.35–6.27	0.99	0.18–5.61
ADHD	1.64	0.85–3.20	2.83	1.13–7.11
Other mental disorder	1.33	0.51–3.48	1.11	0.35–3.51
No mental disorder diagnosis	0.78	0.24–2.57	2.16	0.70–6.66

* The multivariate logistic regression model adjusted for geographic region, MSA, median household income and % of adults with a Bachelor's degree or higher based on patient zip codes, in addition to variables above.

References

1.   Olfson, M.; Crystal, S.; Huang, C.; Gerhard, T. Trends in antipsychotic drug use by very young, privately insured children. *J. Am. Acad. Child Adolesc. Psychiatry* **2010**, *49*, 13–23. [CrossRef] [PubMed]

2.   Harrison, J.N.; Cluxton-Keller, F.; Gross, D. Antipsychotic medication prescribing trends in children and adolescents. *J. Pediatr. Health Care* **2012**, *26*, 139–145. [CrossRef] [PubMed]

3.   Burcu, M.; Safer, D.J.; Zito, J.M. Antipsychotic prescribing for behavioral disorders in US youth: Physician specialty, insurance coverage, and complex regimens. *Pharmacoepidemiol. Drug Saf.* **2016**, *25*, 26–34. [CrossRef] [PubMed]

4.   Sohn, M.; Moga, D.C.; Blumenschein, K.; Talbert, J. National trends in off-label use of atypical antipsychotics in children and adolescents in the United States. *Medicine (Baltimore)* **2016**, *95*, e3784. [CrossRef] [PubMed]

5.   Feltus, M.S.; Gardner, D.M. Second generation antipsychotics for schizophrenia. *Can. J. Clin. Pharmacol.* **1999**, *6*, 187–195. [PubMed]

6.   Correll, C.U.; Leucht, S.; Kane, J.M. Lower Risk for Tardive Dyskinesia Associated with Second-Generation Antipsychotics: A Systematic Review of 1-Year Studies. *Am. J. Psychiatry* **2004**, *161*, 414–425. [CrossRef] [PubMed]

7.   Zito, J.M.; Safer, D.J.; dosReis, S.; Magder, L.S.; Gardner, J.F.; Zarin, D.A. Psychotherapeutic medication patterns for youths with attention-deficit/hyperactivity disorder. *Arch. Pediatr. Adolesc. Med.* **1999**, *153*, 1257–1263. [CrossRef] [PubMed]

8.   Vitiello, B.; Correll, C.; van Zwieten-boot, B.; Zuddas, A.; Parellada, M.; Arango, C. Antipsychotics in children and adolescents: Increasing use, evidence for efficacy and safety concerns. *Eur. Neuropsychopharmacol.* **2009**, *19*, 629–635. [CrossRef] [PubMed]

9.   Olfson, M.; Blanco, C.; Liu, S.M.; Wang, S.; Correll, C.U. National trends in the office-based treatment of children, adolescents, and adults with antipsychotics. *Arch. Gen. Psychiatry* **2012**, *69*, 1247–1256. [CrossRef] [PubMed]

10. Burcu, M.; Zito, J.M.; Ibe, A.; Safer, D.J. Atypical Antipsychotic Use among Medicaid-Insured Children and Adolescents: Duration, Safety, and Monitoring Implications. *J. Child Adolesc. Psychopharmacol.* **2014**, *24*, 112–119. [CrossRef] [PubMed]

11. Cooper, W.O.; Hickson, G.B.; Fuchs, C.; Arbogast, P.G.; Ray, W.A. New Users of Antipsychotic Medications Among Children Enrolled in TennCare. *Arch. Pediatr. Adolesc. Med.* **2004**, *158*, 753. [CrossRef] [PubMed]

12. Kamble, P.; Chen, H.; Sherer, J.T.; Aparasu, R.R. Use of antipsychotics among elderly nursing home residents with dementia in the US: An analysis of National Survey Data. *Drugs Aging* **2009**, *26*, 483–492. [CrossRef] [PubMed]

13. Alexander, G.C.; Gallagher, S.A.; Mascola, A.; Moloney, R.M.; Stafford, R.S. Increasing off-label use of antipsychotic medications in the United States, 1995–2008. *Pharmacoepidemiol. Drug Saf.* **2011**, *20*, 177–184. [CrossRef] [PubMed]

14. Schröder, C.; Dörks, M.; Kollhorst, B.; Blenk, T.; Dittmann, R.W.; Garbe, E.; Riedel, O. Outpatient antipsychotic drug use in children and adolescents in Germany between 2004 and 2011. *Eur. Child Adolesc. Psychiatry* **2017**, *26*, 413–420. [CrossRef] [PubMed]

15. Cooper, W.O.; Arbogast, P.G.; Ding, H.; Hickson, G.B.; Fuchs, D.C.; Ray, W.A. Trends in Prescribing of Antipsychotic Medications for US Children. *Ambul. Pediatr.* **2006**, *6*, 79–83. [CrossRef] [PubMed]

16. Pathak, P.; West, D.; Martin, B.C.; Helm, M.E.; Henderson, C. Evidence-based use of second-generation antipsychotics in a state Medicaid pediatric population, 2001–2005. *Psychiatr. Serv.* **2010**, *61*, 123–129. [CrossRef] [PubMed]

17. Seida, J.C.; Schouten, J.R.; Boylan, K.; Newton, A.S.; Mousavi, S.S.; Beaith, A.; Vandermeer, B.; Dryden, D.M.; Carrey, N. Antipsychotics for children and young adults: A comparative effectiveness review. *Pediatrics* **2012**, *129*, e771–e784. [CrossRef] [PubMed]

18. Casey, D.E.; Daniel, D.G.; Wassef, A.A.; Tracy, K.A.; Wozniak, P.; Sommerville, K.W. Effect of divalproex combined with olanzapine or risperidone in patients with an acute exacerbation of schizophrenia. *Neuropsychopharmacology* **2003**, *28*, 182–192. [CrossRef] [PubMed]

19. Tohen, M.; Vieta, E.; Calabrese, J.; Ketter, T.A.; Sachs, G.; Bowden, C.; Mitchell, P.B.; Centorrino, F.; Risser, R.; Baker, R.W.; et al. Efficacy of olanzapine and olanzapine-fluoxetine combination in the treatment of bipolar I depression. *Arch. Gen. Psychiatry* **2003**, *60*, 1079–1088. [CrossRef] [PubMed]

20. Stahl, S.M. Focus on antipsychotic polypharmacy: Evidence-based prescribing or prescribing-based evidence? *Int. J. Neuropsychopharmacol.* **2004**, *7*, 113–116. [CrossRef] [PubMed]

21. Barnes, T.R.E.; Paton, C. Antipsychotic Polypharmacy in Schizophrenia. *CNS Drugs* **2011**, *25*, 383–399. [CrossRef] [PubMed]

22. Bobo, W.V.; Cooper, W.O.; Stein, C.M.; Olfson, M.; Graham, D.; Daugherty, J.; Fuchs, D.C.; Ray, W.A. Antipsychotics and the risk of type 2 diabetes mellitus in children and youth. *JAMA Psychiatry* **2013**, *70*, 1067–1075. [CrossRef] [PubMed]

23. Sohn, M.; Talbert, J.; Blumenschein, K.; Moga, D.C. Atypical antipsychotic initiation and the risk of type II diabetes in children and adolescents. *Pharmacoepidemiol. Drug Saf.* **2015**, *24*, 583–591. [CrossRef] [PubMed]

24. Aparasu, R.R.; Jano, E.; Bhatara, V. Concomitant antipsychotic prescribing in US outpatient settings. *Res. Soc. Adm. Pharm.* **2009**, *5*, 234–241. [CrossRef] [PubMed]

25. Kogut, S.J.; Yam, F.; Dufresne, R. Prescribing of Antipsychotic Medication in a Medicaid Population: Use of Polytherapy and Off-Label Dosages. *J. Manag. Care Pharmacy* **2005**, *11*, 17–24. [CrossRef] [PubMed]

26. Gilmer, T.P.; Dolder, C.R.; Folsom, D.P.; Mastin, W.; Jeste, D.V. Antipsychotic polypharmacy trends among Medicaid beneficiaries with schizophrenia in San Diego County, 1999–2004. *Psychiatr. Serv.* **2007**, *58*, 1007–1010. [CrossRef] [PubMed]

27. Kreyenbuhl, J.A.; Valenstein, M.; McCarthy, J.F.; Ganoczy, D.; Blow, F.C. Long-term antipsychotic polypharmacy in the VA health system: Patient characteristics and treatment patterns. *Psychiatr. Serv.* **2007**, *58*, 489–495. [CrossRef] [PubMed]

28. Ghio, L.; Natta, W.; Gotelli, S.; Ferrannini, L. Antipsychotic utilisation and polypharmacy in Italian residential facilities: A survey. *Epidemiol. Psychiatr. Sci.* **2011**, *20*, 171–179. [CrossRef] [PubMed]

29. Millier, A.; Sarlon, E.; Azorin, J.-M.; Boyer, L.; Aballea, S.; Auquier, P.; Toumi, M. Relapse according to antipsychotic treatment in schizophrenic patients: A propensity-adjusted analysis. *BMC Psychiatry* **2011**, *11*, 24. [CrossRef] [PubMed]

30. Procyshyn, R.M.; Honer, W.G.; Wu, T.K.Y.; Ko, R.W.Y.; McIsaac, S.A.; Young, A.H.; Johnson, J.L.; Barr, A.M. Persistent antipsychotic polypharmacy and excessive dosing in the community psychiatric treatment setting: A review of medication profiles in 435 Canadian outpatients. *J. Clin. Psychiatry* **2010**, *71*, 566–573. [CrossRef] [PubMed]

31. Correll, C.U.; Frederickson, A.M.; Kane, J.M.; Manu, P. Does antipsychotic polypharmacy increase the risk for metabolic syndrome? *Schizophr. Res.* **2007**, *89*, 91–100. [CrossRef] [PubMed]

32. Molina, J.D.; Lerma-Carrillo, I.; Leonor, M.; Pascual, F.; Blasco-Fontecilla, H.; González-Parra, S.; López-Muñoz, F.; Alamo, C. Combined treatment with amisulpride in patients with schizophrenia discharged from a short-term hospitalization unit: A 1-year retrospective study. *Clin. Neuropharmacol.* **2009**, *32*, 10–15. [CrossRef] [PubMed]

33. Center for Disease Control and Prevention. Ambulatory Health Care Data. Available online: http://www.cdc.gov/nchs/ahcd.htm (accessed on 8 May 2017).

6

A Comparison of Parametric and Non-Parametric Methods Applied to a Likert Scale

Constantin Mircioiu [1] and Jeffrey Atkinson [2,*]

[1] Pharmacy Faculty, University of Medicine and Pharmacy "Carol Davila" Bucharest, Dionisie Lupu 37, Bucharest 020021, Romania; constantin.mircioiu@yahoo.com
[2] Pharmacolor Consultants Nancy, 12 rue de Versigny, Villers 54600, France
* Correspondence: jeffrey.atkinson@univ-lorraine.fr

Academic Editor: Nick Shaw

Abstract: A trenchant and passionate dispute over the use of parametric versus non-parametric methods for the analysis of Likert scale ordinal data has raged for the past eight decades. The answer is not a simple "yes" or "no" but is related to hypotheses, objectives, risks, and paradigms. In this paper, we took a pragmatic approach. We applied both types of methods to the analysis of actual Likert data on responses from different professional subgroups of European pharmacists regarding competencies for practice. Results obtained show that with "large" (>15) numbers of responses and similar (but clearly not normal) distributions from different subgroups, parametric and non-parametric analyses give in almost all cases the same significant or non-significant results for inter-subgroup comparisons. Parametric methods were more discriminant in the cases of non-similar conclusions. Considering that the largest differences in opinions occurred in the upper part of the 4-point Likert scale (ranks 3 "very important" and 4 "essential"), a "score analysis" based on this part of the data was undertaken. This transformation of the ordinal Likert data into binary scores produced a graphical representation that was visually easier to understand as differences were accentuated. In conclusion, in this case of Likert ordinal data with high response rates, restraining the analysis to non-parametric methods leads to a loss of information. The addition of parametric methods, graphical analysis, analysis of subsets, and transformation of data leads to more in-depth analyses.

Keywords: ranking; Likert; parametric; non-parametric; scores

1. Introduction

Statistical methods have the following as prime functions: (1) the design of hypotheses and of experimental procedures and the collection of data; (2) the synthetic presentation of data for easy, clear, and meaningful understanding; and (3) the analysis of quantitative data to provide valid conclusions on the phenomena observed. For these three main functions, two types of methods are usually applied: parametric and non-parametric. Parametric methods are based on a normal or Gaussian distribution, characterized by the mean and the standard deviation. The distribution of results is symmetric around the mean, with 95% of the results within two standard deviations of the mean. Nonparametric statistics are not based on such parameterized probability distributions or indeed on any assumptions about the probability distribution of the data. Parametric statistics are used with continuous, interval data that shows equality of intervals or differences. Non-parametric methods are applied to ordinal data, such as Likert scale data [1] involving the determination of "larger" or "smaller," i.e., the ranking of data [2].

Discussion on whether parametric statistics can be used in a valid, robust fashion for the presentation and analysis of non-parametric data has been going on for decades [3–6]. Theoretical simulations using computer-generated data have suggested that the effects of the non-normality of distributions, unequal variances, unequal sample size, etc. on the robustness of parametric methods are not determinant [7], except in cases of very unusual distributions with a low number of data.

Regarding ordinal Likert data, the theoretical discussion of "parametric versus non-parametric" analysis continues [8,9]. In this paper, we will investigate this from a practical angle using real Likert data obtained in a recent study on pharmacy practitioners' ranking of competencies required for pharmacy practice [10]. The differences and similarities amongst the different subgroups of pharmacists are discussed in detail in the latter paper. In this paper, we ask a specific question on statistical methodology: does the significance of the differences within and amongst subgroups of practitioners in the rankings of the importance of competencies for practice diverge with the type of analysis (parametric or non-parametric) used? We will use the data for community pharmacists and their comparison with those for industrial pharmacists as an example.

The history behind the choice of dataset for this article is as follows. The PHAR-QA project had as primary endpoint the estimation of the core competencies for pharmacy graduate students that are by and large accepted by all subgroups whatever the statistical method used; this is presented in the results section. The secondary end-point consisted in the differences between professional subgroups and we found clear differences between groups whatever the statistical method used. As is suggested by the significance of the interaction term, these differences amongst subgroups are largely centered on particular competencies (see results). This paper follows those already published on this PHAR-QA survey, and its primary purpose is to compare the use and conclusions of parametric and non-parametric analyses.

2. Experimental Section

The data analyzed were from an on-line survey involving 4 subgroups of respondents:

1. community pharmacists (CP, $n = 183$),
2. hospital pharmacists (HP, $n = 188$),
3. industrial pharmacists (IP, $n = 93$), and
4. pharmacists in other occupations (regulatory affairs, consultancy, wholesale, ..., OP, $n = 72$).

Respondents were asked to rank 50 competencies for practice on a 4-point Likert scale:

1 = Not important = Can be ignored.
2 = Quite important =Valuable but not obligatory.
3 = Very important = Obligatory (with exceptions depending upon field of pharmacy practice).
4 = Essential = Obligatory.

There was a "cannot rank" check box as well as a possibility of choosing not to rank at all (blank). The questionnaire response rate was calculated as the distribution between "cannot rank + choose not to rank" versus "rank (1 + 2 + 3 + 4)."

Analysis was carried out on the numbers of values for each of the 4 ranks for each of the 50 competencies. Data were also transformed into binary scores = obligatory/total% = (numbers of values for Ranks 3 and 4)/total number of values for ranks, as a percentage [11]. Such transformation leads to a loss of information but a gain in granularity and in understanding.

Results are presented in three sections starting with reflections on the distribution of the data. This is followed by a section of parametric and non-parametric presentation of the data and a final section on parametric and non-parametric analyses of the data. Data were analyzed using GraphPad software [12] and in-house Excel spreadsheets.

3. Results and Discussion

3.1. Distribution of the Data

The questionnaire response rate between "cannot rank + choose not to rank" versus "rank" was globally 14.5:85.5 ($n = 536$ respondents); there were no significant differences in response rate amongst the four subgroups (chi-square, $p > 0.05$). This aspect was not pursued further given that the vast majority of respondents (86%) were able to understand and reply to the 50 questions on competencies. It can be inferred that differences in distributions of ranking values were not based on misunderstanding of questions.

There were no differences amongst subgroups in the response rate for individual competencies (= number of responses/50) (chi-square, $p > 0.05$). Missing values were not replaced.

The distributions of the ranking data are shown in Figure 1.

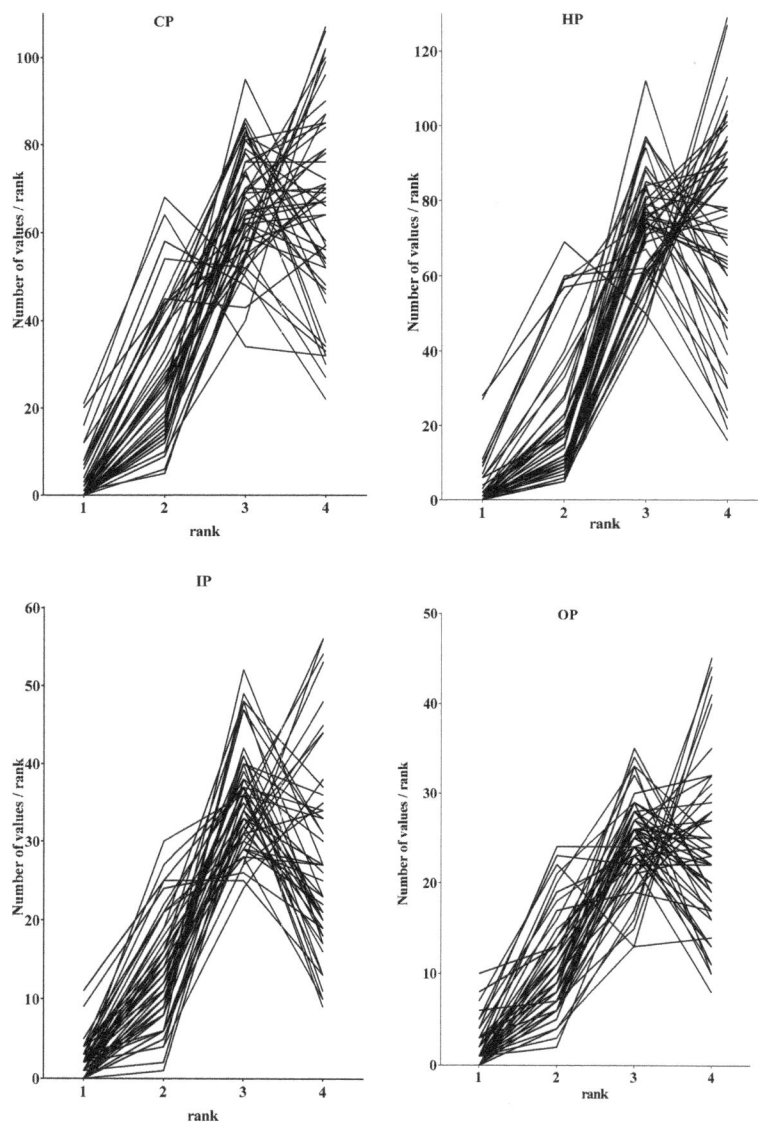

Figure 1. Distributions of ranking data (number of values/rank) for each of the 50 ranked competencies (lines). The four subgroups are as follows: community pharmacists (CP, $n = 183$ respondents, top left); hospital pharmacists (HP, $n = 188$, top right); industrial pharmacists (IP, $n = 93$, bottom right); pharmacists in other occupations such as regulatory affairs, consultancy, and wholesale (OP, $n = 72$, bottom left).

Visual inspection of the four graphs reveals that there were no outliers. Distributions visually suggested a non-Gaussian distribution, i.e., neither continuous nor bell-shaped. Given the small numbers of bins involved ($n = 4$ ranks), tests of normality of distribution such as the Kolmogorov–Smirnov test were not performed.

Distributions were, however, very similar in all four subgroups. They were of two types: inverted "j" or "linear/exponential"; both types of distribution were skewed to the left, i.e., to higher ranking values (on the right of each graph). In order to estimate the numbers of each type of distribution in individual subgroups of pharmacists, the "inverted j" was defined as having a negative value for "number of values for Rank 4–number of values for Rank 3", and the "linear/exponential" was defined as having a positive value for Rank 4–Rank 3.

The "inverted j" distribution was defined as having a negative value for "number of values for Rank 4–number of values for Rank 3", and the "linear/exponential" distribution was defined as having a positive value for "number of values for Rank 4–number of values for Rank 3."

Table 1 shows the numbers of "inverted j" and "linear/exponential" distributions. Chi-square analysis showed a difference between IP and the other three subgroups ($p < 0.05$). This is also seen in the visual inspection of the graphical representation in Figure 1. Distributions of negative and positive values were normal in all four subgroups; means of values "Rank 4–Rank 3" were not different from zero ($p > 0.05$).

Figure 2 contains the values for the differences in "number of values for Rank 4–number of values for Rank 3" for 50 competencies in the four subgroups. There were two clusters of negative values for competencies 13–30 and 38–50, indicating distributions of the "inverted j" form and two clusters of positive values for competencies 1–13 and 31–37, indicating "linear/exponential" distributions of ranking data. Thus, although sample distributions of ranks within competencies are not normal, they are similar in form from one competency to another, and one subgroup of pharmacists to another.

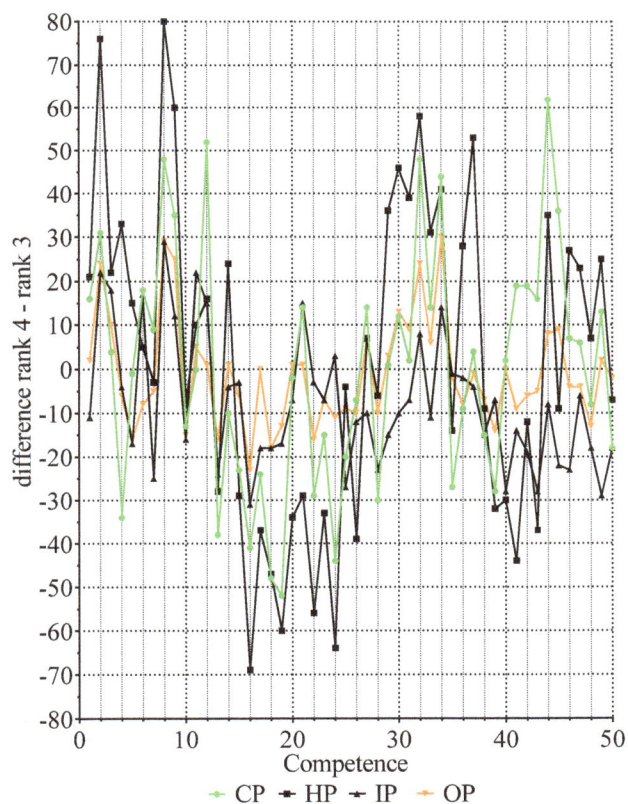

Figure 2. Values for the difference Rank 4–Rank 3 for all four subgroups. The four subgroups are as follows: community pharmacists (CP, $n = 183$ respondents, green circles); hospital pharmacists (HP, $n = 188$, red squares); industrial pharmacists (IP, $n = 93$, blue triangles); pharmacists in other occupations such as regulatory affairs, consultancy, and wholesale (OP, $n = 72$, orange inverted triangles).

Table 1. Numbers of negative and positive values for "number of values for Rank 4–number of values for Rank 3", range, means, standard deviations, and Kolmogorov–Smirnov test for normality, in the four subgroups of pharmacists.

Subgroup	CP	HP	IP	OP
Numbers of inverted j distributions	24	25	39	28
Numbers of linear/exponential distributions	26	25	11	22
Mean of values Rank 4–Rank 3	0.2	1.6	−7.7	−1.1
Standard deviation	27	37	15	12
Kolmogorov–Smirnov (KS) normality test				
KS distance	0.085	0.11	0.12	0.12
Passed normality test (alpha = 0.05)?	Yes	Yes	Yes	Yes

The situation here is one of similar distributions with different numbers of values (ranging from 72 for OP to 188 for HP). Boneau [7], using simulated data, found that, if numbers were large enough (>15), such a situation should not be problematic in terms of parametric analysis. Below, we shall determine whether this statement applies to the actual data.

3.2. Presentation and Analysis of Within-Subgroup Data

The question asked here is as follows: Within a given subgroup (CP will be used as an example), are there significant differences amongst the 50 competencies?

Graphic presentations of the medians, means, and scores of data for the ranking of the 50 competencies by CP, HP, IP, and OP are given in Figure 3.

For CP, whichever form of graphical presentation is used, the major features were the same, namely, that competencies 2, 8, 9, 12, 27, 32, 34, 42, 44, and 45 were ranked higher, and competencies 20 and 39 lower, than the others. The graphs for means and scores visually suggest that there may be significant differences amongst the other 38 competencies as more discriminant information is gathered by the use of parametric statistics (means) and data transformation (scores).

Although somewhat skewed to the right, the distributions of the means and scores were not significantly different from normal (Shapiro–Wilk and Kolmogorov–Smirnov test, $p < 0.05$). The number of bins was too small to test the distribution of medians (Figure 4).

To test for significant differences amongst rankings for comparisons between competencies across subgroups, we used (1) parametric 1-way ANOVA followed by the Bonferroni multiple comparisons test and (2) non-parametric Kruskal–Wallis analysis followed by the Dunn multiple comparisons test. Both analyses showed that there was a significant effect of "competency" (Table 2); both analyses gave the same very low p-values.

There were 8095 data points analyzed with 1055 missing values (11.5% of total (= 50 × 183 = 9150)). Missing values were not replaced.

Table 2. Parametric (top) and non-parametric (bottom) analyses of the significance of the effect of competency using the ranking data for CP ($n = 183$).

	Parametric				
1-Way ANOVA	**Sum of Squares**	**Degrees of Freedom**	**Mean Square**	**F (49, 8045)**	**p-Value**
Treatment (competencies)	611.2	49	12.47	22.99	$p < 0.0001$
Residual	4365	8045	0.5426		
Total	4976	8094			
Non-Parametric					
Kruskal–Wallis Test					
p-value (for competencies)					<0.0001
Kruskal–Wallis statistic					720.8

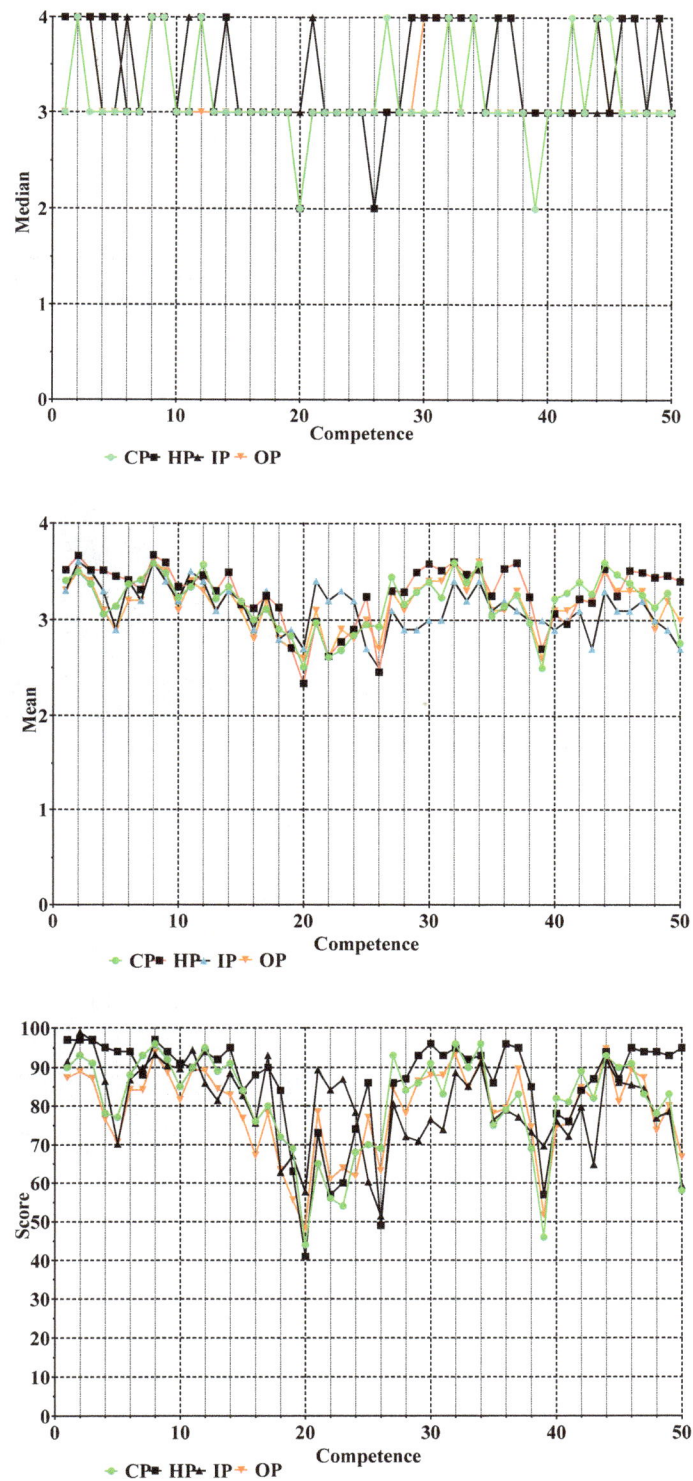

Figure 3. Graphic presentation of the data for the ranking of the 50 competencies. The four subgroups are as follows: community pharmacists (CP, n = 183 respondents, green circles), hospital pharmacists (HP, n = 188, red squares), industrial pharmacists (IP, n = 93, blue triangles), and pharmacists in other occupations such as regulatory affairs, consultancy, and wholesale (OP, n = 72, orange inverted triangles).

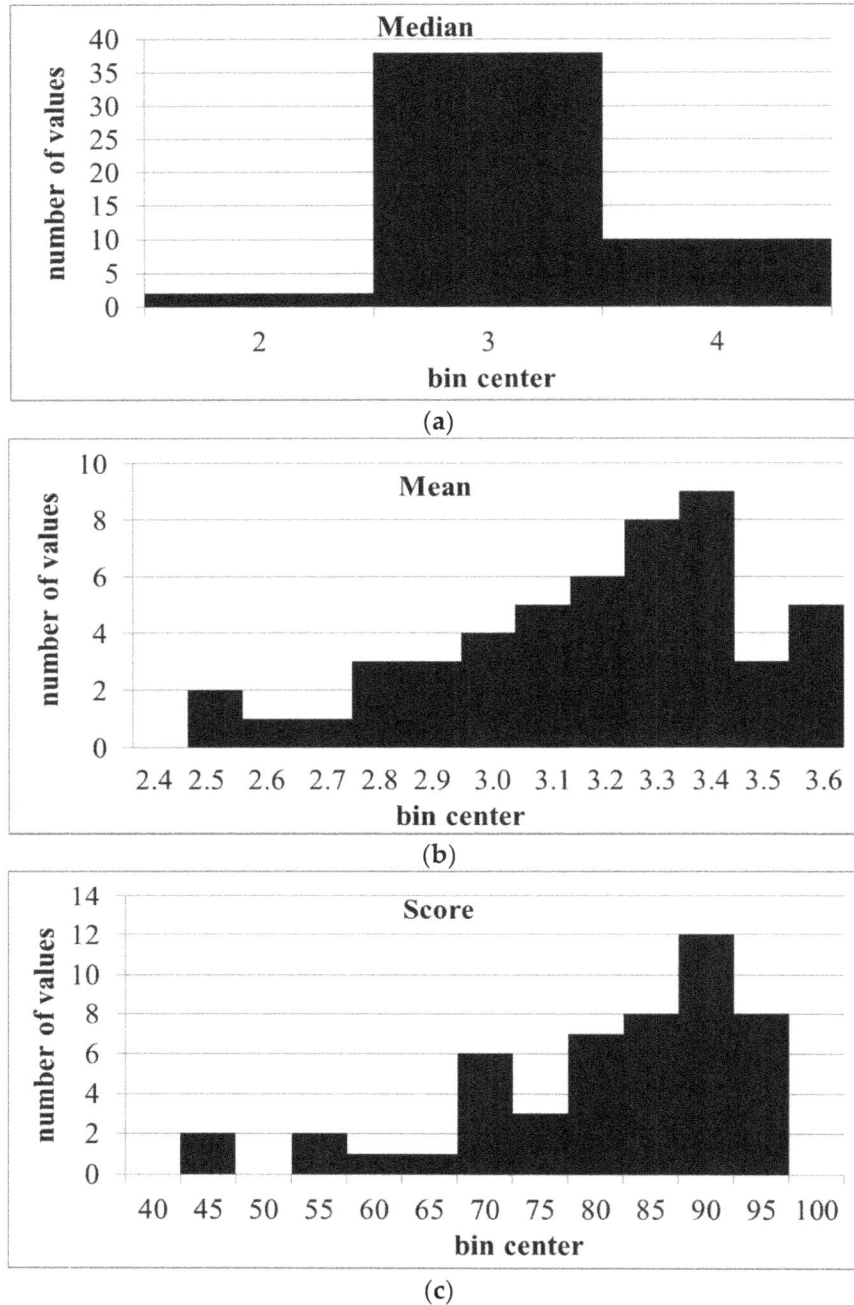

Figure 4. Distributions of medians, means, and scores of ranks for competencies given by CP (same data as in Figure 3). (**a**): medians; (**b**): means; (**c**): scores.

The total number of possible multiple comparisons amongst the 50 competencies was 1225. There was agreement between the parametric and non-parametric tests in the case of a conclusion of "not significant" (756 cases) (Table 3). The Bonferroni test revealed a significant difference in $469/1225 = 38\%$ of the comparisons. There was disagreement between the parametric Bonferroni test and the non-parametric Dunn test in 76 (6%) of these cases, the Bonferroni producing a significant result but not the Dunn test (Table 3).

Table 3. Comparison of the significance of the differences amongst rankings for competencies within subgroups obtained by the parametric Bonferroni and the non-parametric Dunn tests (data for CP).

		Dunn	Dunn	
		Significant	Not significant	Total
Bonferroni	Significant	393	76	469
Bonferroni	Not significant	0	756	756
	Total	393	832	1225

The similarity of difference of competency-ranking (Table 3) by parametric and non-parametric methods can be formally assessed by the kappa test [13].

In this case, P_o = (proportion of observed agreement) = 0.94 and P_r = (proportion of random agreement) = 0.54.

$$\kappa = \frac{p_o - p_r}{1 - p_r} = 0.86$$

As we obtained a value 0.86, this can be considered as very good agreement.

In summary, both tests revealed significant and non-significant differences. In the majority of cases, the tests indicated the same result. The parametric Bonferroni test detected more significant differences than the non-parametric Dunn test, showing that the parametric test was more discriminate.

3.3. Presentation and Analysis of Amongst-Subgroup Data

The question asked was as follows: Are there significant differences between subgroups for one or several of the 50 competencies?

Figure 3 (above) shows the ranking data for the four subgroups in the form of medians (upper), means (middle), and scores (lower). Differences amongst subgroups are difficult to see in the case of medians. Means reveal granularity in results for the different subgroups. This shows, for example, that results for competencies 21–23 and 28–30 as ranked by IP (triangles) appear different from those of the other subgroups such as CP (circles). Such differences are accentuated in the graph of scores.

Individual ranking data for each competency in each subgroup were analyzed using a parametric two-way ANOVA with Sidak's multiple comparisons test, and the non-parametric Friedman test with Dunn's multiple comparisons test analyses (Table 4), in order to determine differences amongst subgroups.

The parametric two-way ANOVA revealed a significant effect of competency, subgroup, and the interaction "subgroup–competency" (Table 4). The percentage variation for competency was much greater than that for subgroup, suggesting that global differences amongst competencies were much greater than those amongst subgroups. Sidak's multiple comparisons test (Table 4) showed a significant difference between CP and IP or OP. Although the interaction "subgroup–competency" is highly significant, this type of analysis does not permit any conclusion as to which specific competencies are significantly different between two given subgroups (this will be dealt with later using the parametric multiple t-test and the non-parametric chi-square test). It could be argued that the interaction effect (F-value = 3.6) could be a spurious consequence of the relatively large primary competency effect (F-value = 38). We consider that the interaction effect is not spurious. The interaction effect is real since there are special clusters of competencies that are ranked differently in different professional subgroups (see Figure 3, e.g., CP versus IP for competencies 21–23).

Table 4. Parametric (upper) and non-parametric (lower) analyses of ranking data for four subgroups of pharmacists. (**a**) Parametric two-way ANOVA and Sidak's multiple comparisons test for differences amongst subgroups (number of missing values: 14,328). (**b**) Non-parametric Friedman analysis with Dunn's multiple comparisons test for differences amongst subgroups.

(a)

ANOVA Table	Sum of Squares	% of Total Variation	Degrees of Freedom	Mean Square	F	p
Interaction: competency–subgroup	289	2.1	147	2.0	F (147, 22,872) = 3.6	p < 0.0001
Competency	1032	7.3	49	21	F (49, 22,872) = 38	p < 0.0001
Subgroup	17	0.12	3	5.7	F (3, 22,872) = 10	p < 0.0001
Residual	12,517		22,872	0.55		

Sidak's Multiple Comparisons Test, Comparisons with CP Only Are Given	Difference of Means	95% Confidence Limits of Difference	p-Value Summary
CP versus HP	0.0087	−0.019 to 0.036	Not significant
CP versus IP	0.0630	0.029 to 0.098	p < 0.0001
CP versus OP	0.0520	0.014 to 0.090	p < 0.01

(b)

Friedman Statistic						10.05
p-value						0.0182
Number of subgroups						4

Dunn's Multiple Comparisons Test, Comparisons with CP Only Are Given	Rank Sum 1	Rank Sum 2	Sum Difference	N1	N2	p
CP versus HP	139.0	139.0	0.0	50	50	p > 0.05
CP versus IP	139.0	106.0	33.00	50	50	p > 0.05
CP versus OP	139.0	116.0	23.00	50	50	p > 0.05

The large number of missing values in this two-way ANOVA (38% of total) emphasizes the unbalanced nature of the analysis with numbers per subgroup ranging from 188 (HP) to 72 (OP). This can often occur in real-life surveys.

Non-parametric Friedman analysis (Table 4) also revealed a significant overall effect of subgroup, but Dunn's multiple comparisons test failed to reveal any significant effect of any specific combination of subgroup. It was thus less discriminant than Sidak's parametric multiple comparisons test. Furthermore, the Friedman test does not allow for the evaluation of the significance of interactions and so again provides less information than the two-way ANOVA.

Differences in specific competencies between two given subgroups were analyzed using the parametric multiple t-test and the non-parametric chi-square test. Amongst the multitude of potential combinations, data are shown (Table 5) for the comparisons between CP and IP for the six competencies revealed in Figure 3 above.

Table 5. Comparison of the chi-square test with the parametric t-test for the differences in competencies between CP and IP. For both tests, all values are $p < 0.05$.

Competency	t-Test	Chi-Square
21	3.49	17.2
22	4.99	22.9
23	5.18	27.9
28	2.93	10.4
29	3.63	13.7
30	3.47	12.1

In this example, it can be seen that the use of a parametric or a non-parametric test leads to the same conclusion regarding statistical significance (Table 5). As can be observed in Figure 5, the correlation between the t-test and chi-square test is good and approximately linear.

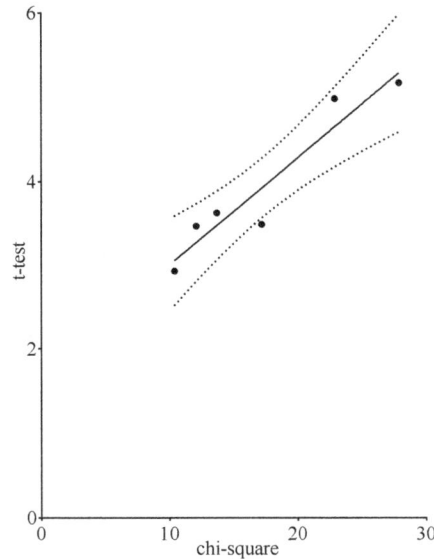

Figure 5. Correlation between the chi-square test and t-test for the competencies given in Table 5 in the comparison CP versus IP. (t-test = ((0.13 × chi-square) + 1.73), r^2 = 0.91).

4. Conclusions

Likert data from an actual survey are neither continuous nor Gaussian in distribution, and numbers per subgroup vary widely. In spite of this, parametric analyses are "robust" [14] as judged from the observation that parametric and non-parametric analyses lead to similar conclusions regarding statistical significance. The explanation for this may lie in the fact that numbers are large and distributions are similar.

Graphical representation in the form of scores provided an easier visual appreciation of differences. The calculation of scores, however, leads to a loss of information as a 4-point Likert scale is transformed into a binary scale. We suggest that this could be "compensated" by determining the difference between scores on the basis of a non-parametric chi-square test on the original ranking data.

Applying parametric analysis of real survey data leads practically in all cases to the same conclusions as those drawn from applying non-parametric analyses. Thus, the advantages of parametric analysis [15], which as seen above is more discriminant, can be exploited in a robust fashion. Several authors have criticized this position and argued on theoretical grounds that parametric analysis of ordinal data such as Likert rankings is inappropriate [4]. Others, after extensive analysis, have reached different conclusions. Thus, Glass et al. [16] concluded that "the flight to non-parametrics was unnecessary principally because researchers asked 'are normal theory ANOVA assumptions met?' instead of 'how important are the inevitable violations of normal theory ANOVA assumptions?'" In this paper, we have attempted to follow the same pragmatic approach. Likewise, Norman [9], after dissecting the argument that parametric analysis cannot be used for ordinal Likert scales, reached the conclusion that "parametric statistics are robust with respect to violations of these assumptions parametric methods can be utilized without concern for 'getting the wrong answer.'" Finally, Carifio and Perla [17], after considering the arguments, counter-arguments and empirical evidence found "many persistent claims and myths about 'Likert scales' to be factually incorrect and untrue."

In the light of the above, we suggest that, in the case presented here, the use of scores for graphical representation plus chi-square for analysis of Likert data, which (1) facilitates the visual appreciation of the data and (2) avoids the futile "parametric" versus "non-parametric" debate, assured the best mosaic of statistical tests combined with phenomenological analysis.

In our example, sample sizes are large (=/>72) and the question can be asked as to how sample size could affect our conclusions. It is certain that, according to the laws of large numbers, experimental frequencies tend in probability to theoretical probability, but the rapidity of such convergence was not our aim. The problem of sample size was discussed by Boneau [7], who suggested that "samples of sizes of 15 are generally sufficient to undo most of the damage inflicted by violation of assumptions. Only in extreme cases involving distributions differing in skew [authors' note: as was the case in our example] would it seem that slightly larger sizes are prescribed say, 30, for extreme violations." It should be noted, however, as discussed by Norman [9], that, "Nowhere is there any evidence that non-parametric tests are more appropriate than parametric tests when sample sizes get smaller." Curtis et al. argued—on theoretical grounds—that (more or less equal) numbers per group is also an important factor for ensuring robustness of statistical analysis [18]. Again, in our pragmatic approach, sample sizes varying from 72 to 188 did not appear to affect the issue.

Another possible issue concerns homogeneity of variance given that the IP data show some differences in distribution to those of the other three subgroups. This does not seem to be a problem given the similarities between the parametric and non-parametric analyses of CP versus IP. This is in agreement with the work of Boneau [7], on simulated data, who concluded "that for a large number of different situations confronting the researcher, the use of the ordinary t test and its associated table will result in probability statements which are accurate to a high degree, even though the assumptions of homogeneity of variance and normality of the underlying distributions are untenable. This large number of situations has the following general characteristics: (a) the two sample sizes are equal or nearly so (authors' note: this was not the case in our example); (b) the assumed underlying population distributions are of the same shape or nearly so."

Acknowledgments: With the support of the Lifelong Learning programme of the European Union: 527194-LLP-1-2012-1-BE-ERASMUS-EMCR. This project has been funded with support from the European Commission. This publication reflects the views only of the author; the Commission cannot be held responsible for any use that may be made of the information contained therein.

Author Contributions: J.A. and C.M. conceived the project; J.A. made the initial calculations and analyses; these were then checked by C.M., who suggested further analyses; J.A. wrote the manuscript that was corrected by C.M.; J.A. and C.M. participated equally in the revision of the manuscript.

References

1. Likert, R. A technique for the measurement of attitudes. *Arch. Psychol.* **1932**, *22*, 5–55.
2. Stevens, S.S. On the theory of scales of measurement. *Science* **1946**, *103*, 677–680. [CrossRef] [PubMed]
3. Feinstein, A.R. *Clinical Biostatistics. Chapter 16: On Exorcising the Ghost of Gauss and the Curse of Kelvin*; Mosby: Saint Louis, MO, USA, 1977.
4. Kuzon, W.M.; Urbanchek, M.G.; McCabe, S. The seven deadly sins of statistical analysis. *Ann. Plast. Surg.* **1996**, *37*, 265–272. [CrossRef] [PubMed]
5. Knapp, T.R. Treating ordinal scales as interval scales: An attempt to resolve the controversy. *Nurs. Res.* **1990**, *39*, 121–123. [CrossRef] [PubMed]
6. Gardner, P.L. Scales and statistics. *Rev. Educ. Res.* **1975**, *45*, 43–57. [CrossRef]
7. Boneau, C.A. The effects of violations of assumptions underlying the *t*-test. *Psychol. Bull.* **1960**, *57*, 49–64. [CrossRef] [PubMed]
8. Jamieson, S. Likert scales; how to (ab)use them. *Med. Educ.* **2004**, *38*, 1212–1218. [CrossRef] [PubMed]
9. Norman, G. Likert scales, levels of measurement and the "laws" of statistics. *Adv. Health Sci. Educ.* **2010**, *15*, 625–632. [CrossRef] [PubMed]
10. Atkinson, J.; De Paepe, K.; Sánchez Pozo, A.; Rekkas, D.; Volmer, D.; Hirvonen, J.; Bozic, B.; Skowron, A.; Mircioiu, C.; Marcincal, A.; et al. The PHAR-QA Project: Competence Framework for Pharmacy Practice—First Steps. The Results of the European Network Delphi Round 1. *Pharmacy* **2015**, *3*, 307–329. [CrossRef]
11. Marz, R.; Dekker, F.W.; van Schravendijk, C.; O'Flynn, S.; Ross, M.T. Tuning research competencies for Bologna three cycles in medicine: Report of a MEDINE2 European consensus survey. *Perspect. Med. Educ.* **2013**, *2*, 181–195. [CrossRef] [PubMed]

12. GraphPad Prism 7 for Biostatistics, Curve Fitting and Scientific Graphing. 2017. Available online: https://www.graphpad.com/ (accessed on 10 January 2017).
13. Landis, J.R.; Koch, G.G. The measurement of observer agreement for categorical data. *Biometrics* **1977**, *33*, 159–174. [CrossRef] [PubMed]
14. Box, G.E.P. Non-normality and tests on variances. *Biometrika* **1953**, *40*, 318–335. [CrossRef]
15. Gaito, J. Non-parametric methods in psychological research. *Psychol. Rep.* **1959**, *5*, 115–125. [CrossRef]
16. Glass, G.V.; Peckham, P.D.; Sanders, J.R. Consequences of Failure to Meet Assumptions Underlying the Fixed Effects Analyses of Variance and Covariance. *Rev. Educ. Res.* **1972**, *42*, 237–288. [CrossRef]
17. Carifio, J.C.; Perla, R.J. Ten Common Misunderstandings, Misconceptions, Persistent Myths and Urban Legends about Likert Scales and Likert Response Formats and their Antidotes. *J. Soc. Sci.* **2007**, *3*, 106–116. [CrossRef]
18. Curtis, M.J.; Bond, R.A.; Spina, D.; Ahluwalia, A.; Alexander, S.P.A.; Giembycz, M.A.; Gilchrist, A.; Hoyer, D.; Insel, P.A.; Izzo, A.A.; et al. Experimental design and analysis and their reporting: New guidance for publication in BJP. *Br. J. Pharmacol.* **2015**, *172*, 3461–3471. [CrossRef] [PubMed]

7

Adherence to Oral Anticancer Medications: Evolving Interprofessional Roles and Pharmacist Workforce Considerations

Gennaro A. Paolella [1], Andrew D. Boyd [2], Scott M. Wirth [3], Sandra Cuellar [3], Neeta K. Venepalli [4] and Stephanie Y. Crawford [5,*]

[1] Naval Medical Center San Diego, United States Navy, San Diego, CA 92101, USA; gpaolella@comcast.net

[2] Department of Biomedical and Health Information Sciences, University of Illinois at Chicago, Chicago, IL 60612, USA; boyda@uic.edu

[3] Department of Pharmacy Practice, Ambulatory Pharmacy Services, University of Illinois at Chicago, Chicago, IL 60612, USA; swirth1@uic.edu(S.M.W.); scuell1@uic.edu (S.C.)

[4] Department of Medicine, Hematology/Oncology, University of Illinois at Chicago, Chicago, IL 60612, USA; nkv@uic.edu

[5] Department of Pharmacy Systems, Outcomes and Policy, University of Illinois at Chicago, Chicago, IL 60612, USA

* Correspondence: crawford@uic.edu

Abstract: Interprofessional care is exhibited in outpatient oncology practices where practitioners from a myriad of specialties (e.g., oncology, nursing, pharmacy, health informatics and others) work collectively with patients to enhance therapeutic outcomes and minimize adverse effects. Historically, most ambulatory-based anticancer medication therapies have been administrated in infusion clinics or physician offices. Oral anticancer medications (OAMs) have become increasingly prevalent and preferred by patients for use in residential or other non-clinic settings. Self-administration of OAMs represents a significant shift in the management of cancer care and role responsibilities for patients and clinicians. While patients have a greater sense of empowerment and convenience when taking OAMs, adherence is a greater challenge than with intravenous therapies. This paper proposes use of a qualitative systems evaluation, based on theoretical frameworks for interdisciplinary team collaboration and systems science, to examine the social interactionism involved with the use of intravenous anticancer treatments and OAMs (as treatment technologies) by describing patient, organizational, and social systems considerations in communication, care, control, and context (i.e., Kaplan's 4Cs). This conceptualization can help the healthcare system prepare for substantial workforce changes in cancer management, including increased utilization of oncology pharmacists.

Keywords: communication; team effectiveness; medication adherence; oncology workforce; oncology pharmacist; applied theory; systems science

1. Introduction

Pharmacologic anticancer therapies are increasingly shifting from clinic-based infusions to orally-administered medications by patients and/or their informal caregivers, thereby changing patient and health professional roles, responsibilities, and priorities [1,2]. Awareness of the evolving interprofessional roles, as well as social and technological interplay, can facilitate improved adherence with prescribed anticancer therapeutic regimens. This paper describes a conceptualization of the social interactionism dynamics involved in cancer care management with emphasis on the changing workforce requirements for pharmacists.

An estimated 15.5 million Americans are living with cancer, and 1.69 million Americans were expected to be diagnosed with some form of cancer in 2017 [3,4]. The historical mainstay of pharmacologic treatment has been ambulatory, infusion-based chemotherapy. While oral formulations (e.g., tablets and capsules) of anticancer drugs have been on the market for decades, Food and Drug Administration (FDA) approval of capecitabine in April 1998 marked the start of a new wave of major advancements in oral anticancer therapies in the U.S., including a flurry of approvals of targeted oral anticancer medications (OAMs) that continues to this day. Tyrosine kinase inhibitors, histone deacetylase inhibitors, vascular endothelial growth factor (VEGF) inhibitors, and mammalian target of rapamycin (mTOR) inhibitors [5–7] are just a few examples of novel OAMs. One-third of anticancer therapies on the U.S. market are available in oral formulations [8,9], and OAMs represent 25–30% of anticancer drugs in pipeline development [7]. When clinically appropriate and equally efficacious [10,11], patients prefer OAMs over intravenous (IV) therapy because OAMs provide patients with a greater sense of control over their care, convenience, improved quality of life, decreased lost time traveling to clinical appointments, reduced need for invasive procedures, and fewer distractions from work and social activities [1,12–15]. Safe handling of all anticancer medications, including OAMs, is important for patients and their caregivers, in addition to healthcare professionals [16–20].

Medication adherence is the degree to which patient behavior and action corresponds with the agreed upon therapeutic regimen from the healthcare practitioner with respect to timing, dosage, and frequency [21,22]. Consequences of nonadherence are well documented in chronic diseases and lead to increased healthcare utilization, e.g., unnecessary doctor visits, emergency room visits, and hospitalizations [23–25], resulting in additional costs of $100 to $300 billion annually within the U.S. [26]. Medication adherence is an indicator of therapeutic response in cancer care management [27]. For instance, one study found that patients with chronic myeloid leukemia with >90% adherence to imatinib demonstrated increased probability of a six-year 3-log reduction of disease compared to patients with adherence levels ≤90% (94.5% vs. 28.4%, $p < 0.001$) [28]. Consequences of non-adherent behavior also include development of resistance, increased burden for patients and caregivers, disease progression, and death [10].

While patients with cancer display higher motivation towards medication adherence, challenges remain [23,24,27,29,30]. Adherence estimates for patients taking OAMs range from less than 20% to 100%, but are typically between 50% and 90% [7,30–33]. OAM adherence levels are lower than IV anticancer therapies [14]. Reasons for nonadherence to OAMs include complex treatment regimens, intolerable side effects, inconvenient clinic visits, unfilled prescription refills, inadequate supervision, problematic patient–clinician communications, socioeconomic factors, and high medication costs [1,7,12,27,34,35]. Additionally, an estimated 10% of patients on newly-prescribed OAMs never pick up the prescription to start treatment, which could lead to dire consequences [36,37].

2. The Oncology Workforce

The swift rate of OAM development, FDA approval, and prescribing over the past 15 years has changed ambulatory-care service modes. Healthcare professionals should anticipate operational system changes and needed strategies and procedures (e.g., communications, task flow, relationship building and team coordination) to effectuate improved adherence, planned therapeutic outcomes, and high-value care [17,38–42]. Increased oncology services and care provided by nurses, nurse practitioners and physician assistants have been highlighted [41,43]. Sessions and colleagues noted increased utilization of highly knowledgeable, specially-trained oncology pharmacists can help optimize cancer care and help address projected workforce needs in cancer management [44]. Those authors noted the extensive knowledge that oncology clinical pharmacists bring to the healthcare team, such as expertise in pharmacotherapy, toxicities, monitoring, and pharmacoeconomics. Through contributions to multidisciplinary teams, clinical oncology pharmacists should be prepared for the changing healthcare landscape and new practice models to facilitate improved outcomes for patients with cancer [45].

The scope of practice document from the Hematology/Oncology Pharmacy Association noted the integral role of hematology/oncology pharmacists in cancer care teams in a variety of roles [46,47]. Common services and care provided by oncology pharmacists include developing therapeutic plans, collaboration with oncologists in medication selection/adjustment, adverse drug reaction prevention and monitoring, laboratory test ordering and monitoring, drug compounding, dispensing, supply management, patient counseling, patient/family and provider education, addressing drug insurance requests, research, and assisting in the development of evidence-based guidelines [48–52].

Currently, most pharmacists have limited formal education and training in hematology and oncology. In the U.S., student pharmacists typically receive a block of lectures on oncology medications in the required core course on therapeutics or a standalone required course, and typically only about 30% are exposed to oncology practice through four-to-six week Advanced Pharmacy Practice Experience clerkship electives [53]. The pathway to becoming an oncology pharmacist often includes on-the-job training. Knowledge and skills can be obtained through specialized postgraduate pharmacy residency training or other structured traineeship, and a competency-based approach has been called for in efforts to expand the workforce in cancer care [54].

The highest level of credentialing for pharmacists in cancer care is recognition as a Board of Pharmacy Specialties (BPS) board certified oncology pharmacist (BCOP), a designation that requires extensive postgraduate training in oncology pharmacy and passing of the Oncology Pharmacy Specialty Certification Examination (and periodic recertification requirements) [55]. A total of 2265 pharmacists were designated as BCOP in 2016 [56], which represented less than one percent of the approximately 305,510 pharmacists in the U.S. [57]. Some states recognize pharmacists as providers that are able to prescribe or administer drugs under a scope of practice or collaborative practice agreement. With relatively few pharmacists recognized as oncology specialists and the huge demand for oncology pharmacist services, workforce solutions are needed to achieve high-value patient care. Subsequent sections of this article describe collaborative models (with the patient, within the profession, and via interdisciplinary collaborations) that are needed for optimal patient care management.

3. Patients as Cancer-Care Providers

A cautious approach to cancer therapy management is warranted. Patients taking OAMs (in their home or other non-institutional or non-clinic settings) are consuming drugs with a high potential for toxicity [58]. OAMs can cause intolerable side effects and/or possible adverse effects that necessitate ongoing monitoring and assessment [1,59]. OAMs require special handling and can involve complicated dosage regimens. For example, some patients receive OAMs where two medications are to be taken on given days, but only one medication on other days, or with on–off cycling in dosage regimens (mono or combination therapy). Accurate dosing may necessitate numerous pill combinations. Some OAMs must be taken with food, while others should not be taken within several hours of eating. Patients with cancer are often prescribed additional medications to treat multiple comorbidities such as hypertension, hyperlipidemia, depression, and pain, or shorter-term drug regimens to manage side effects of anticancer medications such as chemotherapy-induced nausea and vomiting. The totality of dose, schedule, and administration of medications becomes extremely complicated, even in a healthcare proficient patient. Cancer patients with low health literacy may experience greater written and spoken communication difficulties, be at higher risk for self-medication errors, and benefit from counseling and education on OAM use from healthcare professionals who are sensitive to their communication needs [60,61].

Preventable errors with the potential for patient injury with home-based cancer medication management have been observed at rates similar to or higher than what occurs in hospitals [62,63]. Patients with chronic diseases are required to be "effective self-managers of their illness" [64] and co-creators in care management [65]. Patients must be well-managed by clinicians for early detection of adverse effects that merit counseling and/or dosage or medication adjustments or other untoward conditions that raise the likelihood of non-adherence and poor patient outcomes [66]. Patient education and behavioral interventions can be vital in efforts to achieve treatment goals with OAM regimens, and interdisciplinary care efforts should be well planned and evaluated to promote medication adherence, which should improve cancer survival. A conceptualized model of the interactive patient and healthcare professional roles across the course of treatment can foster improved patient-centered care [40]. Oncology pharmacists are essential for expedition of initial therapy start, subsequent therapeutic management decisions, foreseeable prevention of adverse effects, and ongoing provision of high quality, patient centered and evidence based care [44,47,67,68]. Integration of oncology pharmacists into the cancer care team and healthcare model is vital for effective delivery of care for patients [69]. Demonstrated examples include oncology pharmacists' impact with respect to patient care services, supportive care services, and interventions on inappropriate polypharmacy and potentially inappropriate medication use [20,70–73].

4. Cancer Care Management Using a Theoretical Lens

D'Amour and colleagues reviewed published conceptual frameworks for interdisciplinary team collaboration, identifying four major commonalities—"sharing" (shared responsibilities, decision-making, data, interdisciplinary perspectives), "partnering" (based on effective communication and trust), "interdependency", and "empowerment" of team members regardless of title or function [74]. While these considerations underpin the essence of interprofessional collaboration, a proactive practical model is needed to ensure smooth care processes and increase adherence for patients taking OAMs to maximize therapeutic effectiveness and minimize safety concerns and delayed drug therapy from nonadherence [12,66]. Adaptive systems theory for dealing with uncertainties in the system [75] and systems-based practice (knowing how an individual action affects functioning and outcomes in other aspects of the system) in a complex healthcare environment or clinical microsystem subsumes core elements of "interdependency" and "interrelationships"—such as interdisciplinary sharing and partnering, as well as individual empowerment [76].

Systems science provides qualitative methods for evaluating healthcare delivery that can be applied in the pharmacological care of oncology patients. "Systems science" refers to the interactive, dynamic, and multilevel (individual, community, and societal) interrelated pathways that should be considered in a macro view of problem solving [77]. Theoretical knowledge from systems science can be contextualized by considering the social systems of people and how they interact with others and with their environments, i.e., "situated cognition" [78]. While the need for IV site access with attendant care by healthcare professionals is obviated with patient self-administration of OAMs [58], the need for coordinated care persists. By comparatively assessing oral and IV treatment modalities using a qualitative systems evaluation, researchers and members of the oncology care team can redesign systems for optimal patient care. A qualitative systems evaluation considers the social dimension, which includes individual factors (including cultural issues) and both institutional/organizational and trans-organizational levels (i.e., beyond the cancer clinic or oncology pharmacy in our application) in the workflow and process flow [79]. Social interactionism weaves the interplay between organizational systems, social interactions, and technology [78,80].

In applying social interactionism, "Kaplan's 4Cs" (as originally developed by Bonnie Kaplan) denote sociotechnical relationships within a healthcare setting and changes in the ways departments linked by computer systems communicate, the impact on management and organizational control, and care delivery prompted by a technology within the organizational context. In short, Kaplan's 4Cs assess communication, care, control, and context [81]. "Communication" refers to how systems implementation of the technology alters information flows within a system, including patient-provider communications. Communication is a critical aspect of healthcare and technology as new care delivery techniques interrupt existing communication pathways. The "care" segment conveys how the technology impacts service delivery and health outcomes. Conclusions as to how patients are affected are limited to the care segment. "Control" describes how a technology affects the workflow of users and management. Control is the sense that the provider or patient can make choices or actions that influence the health outcomes. "Context" pertains to the circumstance in which a technology is adopted (i.e., systems implementation in the specific organizational practice setting and how decisions are made with the knowledge of the individuals). Context is the overall situation of the patient, care plan, delivery of care, and healthcare team. Context allows patients to receive personalized treatment instead of just following a flowchart. Application of Kaplan's 4Cs to dynamic social systems processes and evolving technologies can help provide an evidence-based model in evaluations of systems and outcomes [82]. For example, the social interactionist framework of Kaplan's 4Cs was used in a small European study to evaluate patient survey responses and general practitioner interviews about usability of a smartphone app to improve adherence for patients with diabetes [83,84].

This paper considers IV anticancer therapies and OAM treatment modalities as 'technologies', different from but analogous to the health informatics technology originally described in the context of social interactionism. Applying Kaplan's 4Cs to an entire treatment modality (i.e., OAMs and IV anticancer therapies) substantially expands the scope of this evaluation tool. Use of Kaplan's 4Cs represents a practical application of social interactionism, i.e., small theoretical programmatic application for quality improvement [85]. The enhanced roles that patients and caregivers assume with prescribed OAMs, as well as patient experiences, warrant consideration of the different aspects encompassed by the 4Cs. Table 1 summarizes the comparisons described below.

Table 1. Social Interactionism Comparisons for Intravenous (IV) and Oral Anticancer Therapies.

	Patients	Oncologists and Other Healthcare Professionals
Communication		
IV Therapies	Interactive, face-to-face communication of relevant information	Opportunity to educate and counsel patients directly during therapy; interdisciplinary teamwork Information for cancer care management potentially limited within system
Oral Therapies	Receive extensive amounts of information (e.g., administration, side effects) from oncology team in order to independently deliver, monitor, and safely handle oral anticancer medications. Increased communication with outside providers and practitioners who might not be cancer care specialists	Opportunity to educate and counsel patients at their respective health and digital literacy levels with the intention of better self-management Non-verbal communication of patients unobservable during drug administration with the medication administered at home. Visual ques such as body fatigue, stress, and overall gestalt require patient to initiate conversation.
Care		
IV Therapies	Role in care delivery centered around keeping clinic appointments and reporting events that occur between episodes of care. Outcomes tied to performance of interdisciplinary healthcare team, cancer response to IV therapies, and patient transportation to clinic	Direct observation of intermittent, IV drug administration, checking of patient parameters (e.g., weight, laboratory values), and direct team monitoring and support services
Oral Therapies	Expanded roles for patients and/or informal caregivers (e.g., self-administration of medication, monitoring, contacting healthcare professionals if problems) Increased care provision outside cancer center or oncology practice, e.g., specialty pharmacy	Service delivery diffused across providers within and outside oncology healthcare teams Pharmacists might lack access to patient data needed to check important clinical parameters.
Control		
IV Therapies	Limited control over care delivery	Controlled environment for service and drug delivery More standardized protocols and procedures, safety checks
Oral Therapies	Patients empowered over drug administration, side effect and symptom management	More limited knowledge of medication adherence by patients Potentially reduced opportunities for patient monitoring

Table 1. *Cont.*

	Patients	Oncologists and Other Healthcare Professionals
Context		
IV Therapies	Care coordination in hospital or clinic Fewer patient responsibilities in direct therapy	Financial and operational mainstay of infusion-based oncologist practice
Oral Therapies	Potentially higher out-of-pocket costs for patients Need to partner with oncologists or pharmacists for timely drug procurement	Less social interactionism among healthcare practitioners Pharmacy benefit management controls

5. Communication

Effective communication in oncology care provision is defined as the open expression of opinions, concerns, and questions in the form of dialog among patients and the healthcare team; nonverbal cues also demonstrate levels of message understanding, comfort, and emotion [86]. Patients receiving infusion therapy relay concerns as appropriate, often via a real-time interactive question-and-answer format with their practitioners, as well as a visual assessment of body language. Concerns are typically evaluated through interdisciplinary teamwork by oncology nurses or pharmacists and shared with the appropriate health professional(s) within the same facility or center. Thus, patients with cancer receiving IV therapy have extended contact with healthcare professionals within the same setting on an ongoing basis. This allows patients to communicate face-to-face, receive advice directly from providers during infusion times, and build relationships with providers. In one study, time spent discussing health-related quality of life between oncologists and patients correlated with the number of previous appointments [87]. Regardless of setting, patient-centered interpersonal communication in oncology care is essential in delivering a high quality patient experience [88–90]. Clinicians should solicit and provide feedback to ascertain if messages are received as intended. Topics addressed between clinicians and patients (and possibly their family or other caregivers) typically include cancer treatment plan, need for treatment adherence, anticipated side effects, monitoring and reporting adverse events.

In contrast to IV therapy, OAM management offers opportunities and new challenges to build patient-health care provider communications and support systems. For example, patients taking OAMs require extensive educational interventions and counseling focused on drug administration instructions, side effects and symptom management, possible dosage adjustments per advice of the oncologist, storage and safe handling, drug interactions, and interdisciplinary supportive care [16,19,20]. This extensive educational intervention and counseling may be provided by oncology pharmacists, however that is not always the case. In some instances, oncologists or their staff initiate patient-centered education about OAMs [12] that may require additional work resources. Some literature suggests the complexity of communicating the necessary breadth and depth of information about OAMs to patients requires additional time and effort from mid-level providers, often requiring role expansion without organizational compensation for such services [1,12]. Even within the inpatient setting, medical information shared between providers during the handover process has been found to be inadequate (i.e., restricted and incomplete) [91]. Barring effective communication with patients and/or pharmacists, prescribers may be unaware of actual usage dates for OAM regimens. Improved communication and interprofessional collaboration in sharing knowledge about start-up and follow-up dates of OAM regimens (dispensing and actual patient behavior) are needed for effective monitoring of therapeutic effects and safety concerns [12]. Oncologists, nurses, and pharmacists need to be in sync with this information, as with IV therapy, to optimize OAM therapy. In addition, updated clinic or office procedures may be needed to establish quality initiatives in documenting patient start dates and discontinuation dates for OAMs [92]. Electronic tools, such as mobile apps, may help pharmacists and other healthcare professionals in providing patient education and assessing adherence, while assisting patients in medication management [15,93,94]. Published interventions include interactive telephone interventions spearheaded by nurses, medication management appointments combined with side effect monitoring by pharmacists, patient-centered applications to increase OAM adherence, and creation of an entire clinic solely dedicated to OAMs [34,93,95,96]. Despite the potential of such initiatives to enhance patient care, systematic constructs (i.e., communication flow, care delivery, social dynamics, and work environment) that coexist with an intervention may alter or even compromise effectiveness. Applying systems science-based theoretical frameworks can address and lead to solutions that overcome such barriers as patient-centered factors would be considered along with institutional processes and social interaction systems beyond the organization. Fundamentally, the interpersonal communication models between the infused therapies and OAMs have undergone a significant change. The communication with the pharmacist will be the most current information and the last interaction unless the patient initiates additional communication with the care team. If the patient is anxious, has questions or is hesitant, then the oncology pharmacist (or possibly other pharmacist such as those employed in specialty pharmacies) will be the last healthcare practitioner to engage and/or communicate concerns with the larger healthcare team. Specifically, the pharmacist is positioned to identify medication issues before, during, and after initiation of OAM therapy. Issues such as medication adherence, medication changes, and medication tolerability in a cancer patient are dynamic variables that require the careful attention and subsequent communication to the healthcare team.

6. Care

Patients prescribed OAMs need to realize the critical role they play in self-care. Tasks historically satisfied by oncologists, nurses, or oncology pharmacists (in physician offices or associated clinics) are relegated to patients and/or caregivers who are distanced from treating clinicians during drug administration. This represents a material shift in the management of cancer care from a provider-driven intermittent infusion model to a chronic disease model [97]. Studies are needed to assess the effects this transition has on cancer patient outcomes and care delivery. At present, trends observed in other chronic diseases help guide therapy management.

Outpatient oncology centers provide patient care services and more safety checks in a structured environment for drug administration, monitoring, and supportive services. Patients receiving IV therapy have generous opportunity to take advantage of these services given the increased frequency and routine time required for infusion appointments. The frequency of care allows clinicians to have multiple patient evaluations for comparison purposes as well as a familiarity with all staff and clinicians of a center. While all essential care is documented, the interaction frequency can lead to more opportunities to better understand the social context of the patient (e.g., their caregivers and social support, transportation issues).

Although patients taking OAMs might receive oncology care in the same facility where the medicines are dispensed, the oral medication self-administration reduces opportunities for direct observation and care provision. Consequently, the roles of patients and/or informal caregivers in drug administration and monitoring is expanded. This could lead to similar diminished treatment outcomes from nonadherence as observed within other chronic diseases [7]. To prepare themselves better for (self-)administration of OAMs, patients and caregivers might seek care from health professionals outside of the practitioners actively involved in their direct treatment in oncologist offices and cancer clinics. For example, patients might direct questions to an extended network of practitioners providing base support in other ways (e.g., spiritual advisors, social workers, friends and family) or seek social support from a wider community network such as patient advocates, friends, or medical information staff in the pharmaceutical industry [40,98,99]. Patients who receive care external to an oncology center may be more likely to report adverse events to their primary care physicians or community pharmacists [100]. Many professionals outside of an oncology practice may have limited or no experience with OAMs [101]. Regardless of experience level, coordinating multidisciplinary cancer care becomes inherently more difficult as the number of providers increases [1].

Patients taking any form of chemotherapy or OAMs are at heightened risk of experiencing side effects or life-threatening adverse effects and should be educated about symptoms and the need to report promptly to their oncologist, oncology nurse, or pharmacist. It is imperative that patients know how to appropriately react, when to seek medical attention, and, if necessary, seek emergency care. This is especially true for patients taking OAMs as they are self-managing drug therapy largely away from oncology care providers. Drug toxicities have greater potential to go untreated until future clinic appointments. Oncology pharmacists are in a unique position to identify OAM medication side effects (or more serious adverse effects) because of repeated access to the patient. Interactions with pharmacists may occur either at the point of OAM dispensing or at the clinical site.

7. Control

Intravenous therapies are administered in environments where members of the healthcare team have almost complete control over the therapy administered. Attending clinic appointments as scheduled is largely under patient control if access to services is possible. Healthcare systems typically implement rigorous workflow measures to ensure patient safety and mitigate medication errors [98]. Organizations can ensure that health professionals comply with institutional policies based on insurance reimbursement requirements, care guidelines, and other organizational policies. Medication reconciliations and provider notes can be easily accessed in the patient record for oncologists to make care decisions, and organizations can more readily assess quality assurance. Such organizational control becomes shared with patients and caregivers when an OAM is prescribed.

As a result of the complexity of OAM therapies, accreditation standards for specialty pharmacies have been developed by organizations such as the Accreditation Commission for Health Care (ACHC), Center for Pharmacy Practice Accreditation (CPPA), and URAC [102–104]. In general, these accreditation standards improve medication management and improve quality of care provided by pharmacists [105].

Care regimens for patients taking OAMs require better relations and coordination among diverse healthcare practitioners. The oncology pharmacy workforce should be well trained (e.g., certification as BCOP and/or enhanced professional development and continuing education for other pharmacists engaged in oncology care) to enhance this coordination by providing consistent management across all areas of medication provision and monitoring. This would allow for the same level of care when medications are dispensed from outside pharmacies (i.e., specialty pharmacies not located within the same institution), but medication management is coordinated by clinic-based oncology pharmacists. A less fragmented, more seamless transition of care across all levels of OAM management (education, dispensing, professional communication, follow-up) may eliminate confusion for patients, minimize the potential for errors, and increase confidence in their ability to appropriately self-administer their OAMs. Pharmacists have the opportunity to improve this process through enhanced communication with outside providers or pharmacies, the patient, and the primary care team.

Greater control over drug administration with OAMs can instill feelings of empowerment among patients [13]. Essentially, patients must become effective self-managers for their disease. Providers might have limited knowledge of patient medication adherence aside from word of mouth and review of refill histories.

8. Context

Interdisciplinary interactions among oncologists, nurses, pharmacists and others within medical centers and/or oncology-clinics are generally well facilitated for patients receiving IV medications. All individuals making decisions regarding the infused medications have enough information to provide adequate context about the patient and the status of the cancer to decide the next step. Health system infrastructures for care coordination provides less context for patients taking OAMs. Patients might need to obtain OAMs through a specialty pharmacy or other pharmacy setting. Different pharmacy outlets have varying services available pertaining to adherence monitoring, medication therapy management, prior authorization experience, and patient assistance programs [12]. Dispensing of OAMs in data-poor environments (e.g., without the ability to access patient medical history, care plan) and in settings where pharmacists are not specifically trained in managing complex OAM therapies represents a challenge to successful patient outcomes, given that providers must be able to provide adequate patient counseling and education in the absence of essential context and patient information.

Additionally, reimbursement for OAMs is managed through different payment schemes than IV therapies. In non-institutional settings, IV anticancer drugs are usually billed through major insurances as part of the medical benefit plan using a fee-for-service system. A highly substantial percentage of revenue in private oncology practices stems from infused therapy administration and monitoring [1]. Conversely, covered OAMs are billable through the prescription drug benefit, usually administered by third-party pharmacy benefits managers (PBMs) [12,106]. Patients taking OAMs have historically incurred increased out-of-pocket cost sharing expenses for deductibles, copayments, and coverage gaps [107]. High costs of OAMs can be prohibitive as typical prescription costs for monthly courses of therapy are $1500 for traditional oral chemotherapy and from $3000 to over $11,000 per month for targeted OAMs [1,108–111]. As of December 2017, 43 states and the District of Columbia enacted "parity laws" placing caps on out-of-pocket costs for OAMs or requiring health plans to provide more equitable cost-sharing provisions to ensure comparable coverage for both IV and OAM treatments [112,113]. State parity laws, however, have not consistently demonstrated patient protection from high out-of-pocket costs for OAMs [114]. Federal U.S. parity legislation, i.e., H.R. 1409, Cancer Drug Parity Act of 2017 [115], has been proposed to mandate that group and individual health plans offer patient cost sharing options that are at least equivalent for OAMs as for IV therapies under the medical benefit. Economic evaluations are inconsistent with respect to cost-effectiveness of targeted OAMs versus targeted IV therapies of comparable efficacy [12,107,110,114].

PBMs commonly institute administrative requirements (e.g., prior authorization) from the pharmacist or oncologist prior to initiating and continuing OAM coverage. Patients taking OAMs have increased responsibility in partnering with their pharmacists and oncologists to manage timely drug procurement as treatment delays might occur in the payment authorization processes. The procedures needed for timely drug procurement and refills may be confusing to patients without adequate education by healthcare practitioners. The change in contextual awareness needs to be explicitly included in the oncology pharmacist's plan and collaboration with the oncology team. Non-specialist pharmacists in other ambulatory settings may need additional oncology training and education (in OAM regimens, continuity of care as team members, and handling/disposal of OAM drugs) in order better coordinate specialized clinical care with reimbursement and procurement strategies [116,117].

9. Conclusions

Optimal care for patients with cancer involves team science, including consideration of complex social and organizational phenomena in the interdependent, multilevel healthcare systems [118]. Prescribing oral anticancer therapies presents larger implications on care delivery than merely altering the route in which a drug is administered. Healthcare systems will become increasingly incentivized to provide adherence-boosting initiatives and monitoring for patients taking OAMs as value-based reimbursement models take precedence over fee-for-service models [119,120]. Utilization of new technologies in complex healthcare systems is dependent upon good interprofessional team performance and adaptable shared mental models to address potential performance failures [99,121]. The Kaplan 4C evaluation highlights mutual relationships across treatment modalities, people, tasks, and organizational and social structures. The Kaplan 4Cs can be used as a practical application for planning care continuity and appreciating the evolving requirements on both the patients and the healthcare system and creating new paradigms for pharmacists. In collaboration with medical oncologists and other team members, oncology pharmacists should participate in efforts to optimally manage cancer medications and to minimize or prevent medication-related adverse events.

Changes in oncology care will have implications for new directions in the use of workforce and in workforce training. Oncology pharmacists have the ability to play a central role in the management of OAMs due to their extensive knowledge in medication administration, monitoring, and reimbursement. Their impact will be determined by their ability to be proactive in providing patient education, coordinating care among healthcare providers and dispensers, and their communication and follow-up with the patients who are in control of administering OAMs. To help meet patient demand, the oncology pharmacist workforce needs to help educate non-specialist pharmacists and other healthcare professionals. Oncology pharmacists should collaborate and share information with others involved in providing oncology care to patients, such as pharmacists practicing in specialty clinics. In conclusion, oncology pharmacists have an increased role in interdisciplinary patient care, patient care management, educational intervention and counseling for patients, and information provision to other healthcare professionals.

Acknowledgments: The development of this manuscript was funded by the McKesson Foundation. The authors alone are responsible for the content and writing of the article.

Author Contributions: Gennaro A. Paolella, Andrew D. Boyd, and Stephanie Y. Crawford conceived and designed the paper. All authors, i.e., Gennaro A. Paolella, Andrew D. Boyd, Scott M. Wirth, Sandra Cuellar, Neeta K. Venepalli, and Stephanie Y. Crawford, wrote and reviewed the final paper.

References

1. Weingart, S.N.; Brown, E.; Bach, P.B.; Eng, K.; Johnson, S.A.; Kuzel, T.M.; Langbaum, T.S.; Leedy, R.D.; Muller, R.J.; Newcomer, L.N.; et al. NCCN Task Force Report: Oral chemotherapy. *J. Natl. Compr. Cancer Netw.* **2008**, *6* (Suppl. 3), S1–S14.

2. Krzyzanowska, M.K.; Powis, M. Extending the quality and safety agenda from parenteral to oral chemotherapy. *J. Oncol. Pract.* **2015**, *11*, 198–201. [CrossRef] [PubMed]

3. American Cancer Society. Cancer Facts & Figures. Available online: https://www.cancer.org/content/dam/cancer-org/research/cancer-facts-and-statistics/annual-cancer-facts-and-figures/2017/cancer-facts-and-figures-2017.pdf (accessed on 28 February 2018).

4. Siegel, R.L.; Miller, K.D.; Jemal, A. Cancer Statistics. 2017. *Cancer J. Clin.* **2017**, *67*, 7–30. [CrossRef] [PubMed]

5. Aisner, J. Overview of the changing paradigm in cancer treatment: Oral chemotherapy. *Am. J. Health Syst. Pharm.* **2007**, *64*, S4–S7. [CrossRef] [PubMed]

6. Masui, K.; Gini, B.; Wykosky, J.; Zanca, C.; Mischel, P.S.; Furnari, F.B.; Cavenee, W.K. A tale of two approaches: Complementary mechanisms of cytotoxic and targeted therapy resistance may inform next-generation cancer treatments. *Carcinogenesis* **2013**, *34*, 725–738. [CrossRef] [PubMed]

7. Geynisman, D.M.; Wickersham, K.E. Adherence to targeted oral anticancer medications. *Discov. Med.* **2013**, *15*, 231–241. [PubMed]

8. Hershman, D.L. Sticking to it: Improving outcomes by increasing adherence. *J. Clin. Oncol.* **2016**, *34*, 2440–2442. [CrossRef] [PubMed]

9. IMS Institute for Healthcare Informatics. *Global Oncology Trend Report: A Review of 2015 and Outlook to 2020*; IMS Institute for Healthcare Informatics: Parsippany, NY, USA, 2016.

10. Hall, A.E.; Paul, C.; Bryant, J.; Lynagh, M.C.; Rowlings, P.; Enjeti, A.; Small, H. To adhere or not to adhere: Rates and reasons of medication adherence in hematological cancer patients. *Crit. Rev. Oncol.* **2016**, *97*, 247–262. [CrossRef] [PubMed]

11. Liu, G.; Franssen, E.; Fitch, M.I.; Warner, E. Patient preferences for oral versus intravenous palliative chemotherapy. *J. Clin. Oncol.* **1997**, *15*, 110–115. [CrossRef] [PubMed]

12. Betcher, J.; Dow, E.; Khera, N. Oral Chemotherapy in Patients with Hematological Malignancies-Care Process, Pharmacoeconomic and Policy Implications. *Curr. Hematol. Malig. Rep.* **2016**, *11*, 288–294. [CrossRef] [PubMed]

13. Wood, L. A review on adherence management in patients on oral cancer therapies. *Eur. J. Oncol. Nurs.* **2012**, *16*, 432–438. [CrossRef] [PubMed]

14. Seal, B.S.; Anderson, S.; Shermock, K.M. Factors Associated with Adherence Rates for Oral and Intravenous Anticancer Therapy in Commercially Insured Patients with Metastatic Colon Cancer. *J. Manag. Care Spec. Pharm.* **2016**, *22*, 227–235. [CrossRef] [PubMed]

15. Burhenn, P.S.; Smudde, J. Using tools and technology to promote education and adherence to oral agents for cancer. *Clin. J. Oncol. Nurs.* **2015**, *19*, 53–59. [CrossRef] [PubMed]

16. Cass, Y.; Connor, T.H.; Tabachnik, A. Safe handling of oral antineoplastic medications: Focus on targeted therapeutics in the home setting. *J. Oncol. Pharm. Pract.* **2017**, *23*, 350–378. [CrossRef] [PubMed]

17. Goodin, S.; Griffith, N.; Chen, B.; Chuk, K.; Daouphars, M.; Doreau, C.; Patel, R.A.; Schwartz, R.; Tames, M.J.; Terkola, R.; et al. Safe handling of oral chemotherapeutic agents in clinical practice: Recommendations from an international pharmacy panel. *J. Oncol. Pract.* **2011**, *7*, 7–12. [CrossRef] [PubMed]

18. Griffin, E. Safety considerations and safe handling of oral chemotherapy agents. *Clin. J. Oncol. Nurs.* **2003**, *7*, 25–29. [CrossRef] [PubMed]

19. Hartigan, K. Patient education: The cornerstone of successful oral chemotherapy treatment. *Clin. J. Oncol. Nurs.* **2003**, *7*, 21–24. [CrossRef] [PubMed]

20. Valgus, J.; Jarr, S.; Schwartz, R.; Rice, M.; Bernard, S.A. Pharmacist-led, interdisciplinary model for delivery of supportive care in the ambulatory cancer clinic setting. *J. Oncol. Pract.* **2010**, *6*, e1–e4. [CrossRef] [PubMed]

21. World Health Organization. *Adherence to Long Term Therapies: Evidence for Action*; World Health Organization: Geneva, Switzerland, 2003.

22. Cramer, J.A.; Roy, A.; Burrell, A.; Fairchild, C.J.; Fuldeore, M.J.; Ollendorf, D.A.; Wong, P.K. Medication compliance and persistence: Terminology and definitions. *Value Health* **2008**, *11*, 44–47. [CrossRef] [PubMed]

23. Hohneker, J.; Shah-Mehta, S.; Brandt, P.S. Perspectives on adherence and persistence with oral medications for cancer treatment. *J. Oncol. Pract.* **2011**, *7*, 65–67. [CrossRef] [PubMed]

24. Partridge, A.H.; Avorn, J.; Wang, P.S.; Winer, E.P. Adherence to therapy with oral antineoplastic agents. *J. Natl. Cancer Inst.* **2002**, *94*, 652–661. [CrossRef] [PubMed]

25. Gebbia, V.; Bellavia, G.; Ferrau, F.; Valerio, M.R. Adherence, compliance and persistence to oral antineoplastic therapy: A review focused on chemotherapeutic and biologic agents. *Expert Opin. Drug Saf.* **2012**, *11* (Suppl. 1), S49–S59. [CrossRef] [PubMed]

26. Iuga, A.O.; McGuire, M.J. Adherence and health care costs. *Risk Manag. Healthc. Policy* **2014**, *7*, 35–44. [CrossRef] [PubMed]

27. Ruddy, K.; Mayer, E.; Partridge, A. Patient adherence and persistence with oral anticancer treatment. *Cancer J. Clin.* **2009**, *59*, 56–66. [CrossRef] [PubMed]

28. Marin, D.; Bazeos, A.; Mahon, F.X.; Eliasson, L.; Milojkovic, D.; Bua, M.; Apperley, J.F.; Szydlo, R.; Desai, R.; Kozlowski, K.; et al. Adherence is the critical factor for achieving molecular responses in patients with chronic myeloid leukemia who achieve complete cytogenetic responses on imatinib. *J. Clin. Oncol.* **2010**, *28*, 2381–2388. [CrossRef] [PubMed]

29. Barthelemy, P.; Asmane-De la Porte, I.; Meyer, N.; Duclos, B.; Serra, S.; Dourthe, L.M.; Ame, S.; Litique, V.; Giron, C.; Goldbarg, V.; et al. Adherence and patients' attitudes to oral anticancer drugs: A prospective series of 201 patients focusing on targeted therapies. *Oncology* **2015**, *88*, 1–8. [CrossRef] [PubMed]

30. Greer, J.A.; Amoyal, N.; Nisotel, L.; Fishbein, J.N.; MacDonald, J.; Stagl, J.; Lennes, I.; Temel, J.S.; Safren, S.A.; Pirl, W.F. A systematic review of adherence to oral antineoplastic therapies. *Oncologist* **2016**, *21*, 354–376. [CrossRef] [PubMed]

31. Bassan, F.; Peter, F.; Houbre, B.; Brennstuhl, M.J.; Costantini, M.; Speyer, E.; Tarquinio, C. Adherence to oral antineoplastic agents by cancer patients: Definition and literature review. *Eur. J. Cancer Care* **2014**, *23*, 22–35. [CrossRef] [PubMed]

32. Puts, M.T.; Tu, H.A.; Tourangeau, A.; Howell, D.; Fitch, M.; Springall, E.; Alibhai, S.M. Factors influencing adherence to cancer treatment in older adults with cancer: A systematic review. *Ann. Oncol.* **2014**, *25*, 564–577. [CrossRef] [PubMed]

33. Verbrugghe, M.; Verhaeghe, S.; Lauwaert, K.; Beeckman, D.; Van Hecke, A. Determinants and associated factors influencing medication adherence and persistence to oral anticancer drugs: A systematic review. *Cancer Treat. Rev.* **2013**, *39*, 610–621. [CrossRef] [PubMed]

34. Spoelstra, S.L.; Given, B.A.; Given, C.W.; Grant, M.; Sikorskii, A.; You, M.; Decker, V. An intervention to improve adherence and management of symptoms for patients prescribed oral chemotherapy agents: An exploratory study. *Cancer Nurs.* **2013**, *36*, 18–28. [CrossRef] [PubMed]

35. Nilsson, J.L.; Andersson, K.; Bergkvist, A.; Bjorkman, I.; Brismar, A.; Moen, J. Refill adherence to repeat prescriptions of cancer drugs to ambulatory patients. *Eur. J. Cancer Care* **2006**, *15*, 235–237. [CrossRef] [PubMed]

36. Accordino, M.K.; Hershman, D.L. Disparities and challenges in adherence to oral antineoplastic agents. *Am. Soc. Clin. Oncol.* **2013**, *33*, 271–276. [CrossRef] [PubMed]

37. Streeter, S.B.; Schwartzberg, L.; Husain, N.; Johnsrud, M. Patient and plan characteristics affecting abandonment of oral oncolytic prescriptions. *J. Oncol. Pract.* **2011**, *7*, 46s–51s. [CrossRef] [PubMed]

38. Gustafson, E. Analyzing trends in oral anticancer agents in an academic medical facility. *J. Hematol. Oncol. Pharm.* **2015**, *5*, 34–37.

39. Neuss, M.N.; Polovich, M.; McNiff, K.; Esper, P.; Gilmore, T.R.; LeFebvre, K.B.; Schulmeister, L.; Jacobson, J.O. 2013 updated American Society of Clinical Oncology/Oncology Nursing Society chemotherapy administration safety standards including standards for the safe administration and management of oral chemotherapy. *Oncol. Nurs. Forum* **2013**, *40*, 225–233. [CrossRef] [PubMed]

40. Ueno, N.T.; Ito, T.D.; Grigsby, R.K.; Black, M.V.; Apted, J. ABC conceptual model of effective multidisciplinary cancer care. *Nat. Rev. Clin. Oncol.* **2010**, *7*, 544–547. [CrossRef] [PubMed]

41. Erikson, C.; Salsberg, E.; Forte, G.; Bruinooge, S.; Goldstein, M. Future supply and demand for oncologists: Challenges to assuring access to oncology services. *J. Oncol. Pract.* **2007**, *3*, 79–86. [CrossRef] [PubMed]

42. American Society of Clinical Oncology. The State of Cancer Care in America, 2016: A Report by the American Society of Clinical Oncology. *J. Oncol. Pract.* **2016**, *12*, 339–383. [CrossRef]

43. Polansky, M.; Ross, A.C.; Coniglio, D. Physician Assistant Perspective on the ASCO Workforce Study Regarding the Use of Physician Assistants and Nurse Practitioners. *J. Oncol. Pract.* **2010**, *6*, 31–33. [CrossRef] [PubMed]

44. Sessions, J.K.; Valgus, J.; Barbour, S.Y.; Iacovelli, L. Role of oncology clinical pharmacists in light of the oncology workforce study. *J. Oncol. Pract.* **2010**, *6*, 270–272. [CrossRef] [PubMed]

45. Avery, M.; Williams, F. The importance of pharmacist providing patient education in oncology. *J. Pharm. Pract.* **2015**, *28*, 26–30. [CrossRef] [PubMed]

46. Hematology/Oncology Pharmacy Association. *Scope of Hematology/Oncology Pharmacy Practice*; Hematology/Oncology Pharmacy Association: Chicago, IL, USA, 2013.

47. Holle, L.M.; Boehnke Michaud, L. Oncology pharmacists in health care delivery: Vital members of the cancer care team. *J. Oncol. Pract.* **2014**, *10*, e142–e145. [CrossRef] [PubMed]

48. Hematology/Oncology Pharmacy Association. The Role of Hematology/Oncology Pharmacists. Available online: http://www.hoparx.org/images/hopa/advocacy/Issue-Briefs/HOPA-_About_Hem_Onc_Pharmacist_Issue_Brief.pdf (accessed on 5 December 2017).

49. Holle, L.M.; Harris, C.S.; Chan, A.; Fahrenbruch, R.J.; Labdi, B.A.; Mohs, J.E.; Norris, L.B.; Perkins, J.; Vela, C.M. Pharmacists' roles in oncology pharmacy services: Results of a global survey. *J. Oncol. Pharm. Pract.* **2017**, *23*, 185–194. [CrossRef] [PubMed]

50. Merten, J.A.; Shapiro, J.F.; Gulbis, A.M.; Rao, K.V.; Bubalo, J.; Lanum, S.; Engemann, A.M.; Shayani, S.; Williams, C.; Leather, H.; et al. Utilization of collaborative practice agreements between physicians and pharmacists as a mechanism to increase capacity to care for hematopoietic stem cell transplant recipients. *Biol. Blood Marrow Transplant.* **2013**, *19*, 509–518. [CrossRef] [PubMed]

51. Lewis, J. The oncology care pharmacist in health-system pharmacy. Available online: http://www.pharmacytimes.com/publications/health-system-edition/2017/january2017/the-oncology-care-pharmacist-in-healthsystem-pharmacy (accessed on 15 January 2017).

52. Ma, C.S.J. Role of pharmacists in optimizing the use of anticancer drugs in the clinical setting. *Integr. Pharm. Res. Prat.* **2014**, *3*, 11–24. [CrossRef]

53. Kwon, J.; Ledvina, D.; Newton, M.; Green, M.R.; Ignoffo, R. Oncology pharmacy education and training in the United States schools of pharmacy. *Curr. Pharm. Teach. Learn.* **2015**, *7*, 451–457. [CrossRef]

54. Smith, A.P.; Lichtveld, M.Y.; Miner, K.R.; Tyus, S.L.; Gase, L.N. A competency-based approach to expanding the cancer care workforce: Proof of concept. *Medsurg Nurs.* **2009**, *18*, 38–49. [CrossRef] [PubMed]

55. Board of Pharmacy Specialties. Oncology Pharmacy. Available online: https://www.bpsweb.org/bps-specialties/oncology-pharmacy/ (accessed on 5 December 2017).

56. Board of Pharmacy Specialties. BPS 2016 Annual Report, Board Certified Pharmacists. Available online: http://board-of-pharmacy-specialties.dcatalog.com/v/2016-Annual-Report/#page=0 (accessed on 19 January 2018).

57. United States Department of Labor—Bureau of Labor Statistics. Occupational Employment AD Wages, Pharmacists. Available online: https://www.bls.gov/oes/current/oes291051.htm (accessed on 5 December 2017).

58. Birner, A. Safe administration of oral chemotherapy. *Clin. J. Oncol. Nurs.* **2003**, *7*, 158–162. [CrossRef] [PubMed]

59. Schneider, S.M.; Hess, K.; Gosselin, T. Interventions to promote adherence with oral agents. *Semin. Oncol. Nurs.* **2011**, *27*, 133–141. [CrossRef] [PubMed]

60. Busch, E.L.; Martin, C.; DeWalt, D.A.; Sandler, R.S. Functional health literacy, chemotherapy decisions, and outcomes among a colorectal cancer cohort. *Cancer Control* **2015**, *22*, 95–101. [CrossRef] [PubMed]

61. Davis, T.C.; Williams, M.V.; Marin, E.; Parker, R.M.; Glass, J. Health literacy and cancer communication. *Cancer J. Clin.* **2002**, *52*, 134–149. [CrossRef]

62. Walsh, K.E.; Roblin, D.W.; Weingart, S.N.; Houlahan, K.E.; Degar, B.; Billett, A.; Keuker, C.; Biggins, C.; Li, J.; Wasilewski, K.; et al. Medication errors in the home: A multisite study of children with cancer. *Pediatrics* **2013**, *131*, e1405–e1414. [CrossRef] [PubMed]

63. Schwappach, D.L.; Wernli, M. Medication errors in chemotherapy: Incidence, types and involvement of patients in prevention. A review of the literature. *Eur. J. Cancer Care* **2010**, *19*, 285–292. [CrossRef] [PubMed]

64. Wagner, E.H.; Austin, B.T.; Davis, C.; Hindmarsh, M.; Schaefer, J.; Bonomi, A. Improving chronic illness care: Translating evidence into action. *Health Aff.* **2001**, *20*, 64–78. [CrossRef] [PubMed]

65. McColl-Kennedy, J.R.; Vargo, S.L.; Dagger, T.S.; Sweeney, J.C.; van Kasteren, Y. Health care customer value cocreation practice styles. *J. Serv. Res.* **2012**, *15*, 370–389. [CrossRef]

66. McCue, D.A.; Lohr, L.K.; Pick, A.M. Improving adherence to oral cancer therapy in clinical practice. *Pharmacotherapy* **2014**, *34*, 481–494. [CrossRef] [PubMed]

67. Chan, M.Y.; Yu, A.K.; Lau, R.W.; Linh, E.; Chen, E.Y.; Birmingham, K. Clinical pharmacist integration into the oncology medical home. Abstract. *J. Clin. Oncol.* **2015**, *33*, e20703. [CrossRef]

68. Semchuk, W.M.; Sperlich, C. Prevention and treatment of venous thromboembolism in patients with cancer. *Can. Pharm. J.* **2012**, *145*, 24–29. [CrossRef] [PubMed]

69. Gatwood, J.; Gatwood, K.; Gabre, E.; Alexander, M. Impact of clinical pharmacists in outpatient oncology practices: A review. *Am. J. Health Syst. Pharm.* **2017**, *74*, 1549–1557. [CrossRef] [PubMed]

70. Alexander, M.D.; Rao, K.V.; Khan, T.S.; Deal, A.M.; Alexander, M.D.; Rao, K.V.; Khan, T.S.; Deal, A.M. ReCAP: Pharmacists' Impact in Hematopoietic Stem-Cell Transplantation: Economic and Humanistic Outcomes. *J. Oncol. Pract.* **2016**, *12*, 147–148. [CrossRef] [PubMed]

71. Bertsch, N.S.; Bindler, R.J.; Wilson, P.L.; Kim, A.P.; Ward, B. Medication Therapy Management for Patients Receiving Oral Chemotherapy Agents at a Community Oncology Center: A Pilot Study. *Hosp. Pharm.* **2016**, *51*, 721–729. [CrossRef] [PubMed]

72. Nightingale, G.; Hajjar, E.; Swartz, K.; Andrel-Sendecki, J.; Chapman, A. Evaluation of a pharmacist-led medication assessment used to identify prevalence of and associations with polypharmacy and potentially inappropriate medication use among ambulatory senior adults with cancer. *J. Clin. Oncol.* **2015**, *33*, 1453–1459. [CrossRef] [PubMed]

73. Prithviraj, G.K.; Koroukian, S.; Margevicius, S.; Berger, N.A.; Bagai, R.; Owusu, C. Patient Characteristics Associated with Polypharmacy and Inappropriate Prescribing of Medications among Older Adults with Cancer. *J. Geriatr. Oncol.* **2012**, *3*, 228–237. [CrossRef] [PubMed]

74. D'Amour, D.; Ferrada-Videla, M.; San Martin Rodriguez, L.; Beaulieu, M.-D. The conceptual basis for interprofessional collaboration: Core concepts and theoretical frameworks. *J. Interprof. Care* **2005**, *19*, 116–131. [CrossRef] [PubMed]

75. Sturmberg, J.P.; Martin, C.M.; Katerndahl, D.A. Systems and complexity thinking in the general practice literature: An integrative, historical narrative review. *Ann. Fam. Med.* **2014**, *12*, 66–74. [CrossRef] [PubMed]

76. Johnson, J.K.; Miller, S.H.; Horowitz, S.D. Systems-Based Practice: Improving the Safety and Quality of Patient Care by Recognizing and Improving the Systems in Which We Work. In *Advances in Patient Safety: New Directions and Alternative Approaches*; Henriksen, K., Battles, J.B., Keyes, M.A., Grady, M.L., Eds.; U.S. National Library of Medicine: Rockville, MD, USA, 2008.

77. Northridge, M.E.; Metcalf, S.S. Enhancing implementation science by applying best principles of systems science. *Health Res. Policy Syst.* **2016**, *14*, 74. [CrossRef] [PubMed]

78. Kaplan, B. Evaluating informatics applications—Some alternative approaches: Theory, social interactionism, and call for methodological pluralism. *Int. J. Med. Inform.* **2001**, *64*, 39–56. [CrossRef]

79. Kaplan, B.; Brennan, P.F.; Dowling, A.F.; Friedman, C.P.; Peel, V. Toward an informatics research agenda: Key people and organizational issues. *J. Am. Med. Inform. Assoc.* **2001**, *8*, 235–241. [CrossRef] [PubMed]

80. Berg, M. Implementing information systems in health care organizations: Myths and challenges. *Int. J. Med. Inform.* **2001**, *64*, 143–156. [CrossRef]

81. Kaplan, B. Addressing organizational issues into the evaluation of medical systems. *J. Am. Med. Inform. Assoc.* **1997**, *4*, 94–101. [CrossRef] [PubMed]

82. Kaplan, B.; Shaw, N.T. Future directions in evaluation research: People, organizational, and social issues. *Methods Inf. Med.* **2004**, *43*, 215–231. [PubMed]

83. Ross, P. What Patients Expect from Mobile Device? Available online: https://www.medetel.eu/download/2014/parallel_sessions/presentation/day2/Ross_What_Patients_Expect_from.pdf (accessed on 9 October 2017).

84. Sokolovska, J.; Gaisuta, R.; Puzaka, I.; Dekante, A.; Balode, B.; Zarina, L.; Grinsteine, M.; Vaivode, V.; Gailisa, U.; Geldnere, K.; et al. eMedic: Remote control of diabetes in patients on insulin treatment: eMedic pilot results from Latvia. In Proceedings of the International eHealth, Telemedicine and Health ICT Forum for Educational, Networking and Business, Geneva, Switzerland, 9–11 April 2014; pp. 77–78.

85. Davidoff, F.; Dixon-Woods, M.; Leviton, L.; Michie, S. Demystifying theory and its use in improvement. *BMJ Qual. Saf.* **2015**, *24*, 228–238. [CrossRef] [PubMed]

86. Pham, A.K.; Bauer, M.T.; Balan, S. Closing the patient-oncologist communication gap: A review of historic and current efforts. *J. Cancer Educ.* **2014**, *29*, 106–113. [CrossRef] [PubMed]

87. Rodriguez, K.L.; Bayliss, N.K.; Alexander, S.C.; Jeffreys, A.S.; Olsen, M.K.; Pollak, K.I.; Garrigues, S.K.; Tulsky, J.A.; Arnold, R.M. Effect of patient and patient-oncologist relationship characteristics on communication about health-related quality of life. *Psychooncology* **2011**, *20*, 935–942. [CrossRef] [PubMed]

88. Sinclair, S.; McClement, S.; Raffin-Bouchal, S.; Hack, T.F.; Hagen, N.A.; McConnell, S.; Chochinov, H.M. Compassion in Health Care: An Empirical Model. *J. Pain Symptom Manag.* **2016**, *51*, 193–203. [CrossRef] [PubMed]

89. Smyth, J.F. Communication within the context of multidisciplinary care. In *Communicating with Cancer Patients*; CRC Press: Boca Raton, FL, USA, 2014; pp. 36–42.

90. Balogh, E.P.; Ganz, P.A.; Murphy, S.B.; Nass, S.J.; Ferrell, B.R.; Stovall, E. Patient-centered cancer treatment planning: Improving the quality of oncology care. Summary of an Institute of Medicine workshop. *Oncologist* **2011**, *16*, 1800–1805. [CrossRef] [PubMed]

91. Braaf, S.; Rixon, S.; Williams, A.; Liew, D.; Manias, E. Medication communication during handover interactions in specialty practice settings. *J. Clin. Nurs.* **2015**, *24*, 2859–2870. [CrossRef] [PubMed]

92. McNamara, E.; Redoutey, L.; Mackler, E.; Severson, J.A.; Petersen, L.; Mahmood, T. Improving Oral Oncolytic Patient Self-Management. *J. Oncol. Pract.* **2016**, *12*, e864–e869. [CrossRef] [PubMed]

93. Hsu, G.I.-H.; Crawford, S.Y.; Paolella, G.; Cuellar, S.; Wirth, S.M.; Venepalli, N.K.; Wang, E.; Hughes, D.; Boyd, A.D. Design of customized mobile application for patient adherence to oral anticancer medications utilizing user-centered design. *J. Biocommun.* **2017**, *41*, 5–14. [CrossRef]

94. Passardi, A.; Rizzo, M.; Maines, F.; Tondini, C.; Zambelli, A.; Vespignani, R.; Andreis, D.; Massa, I.; Dianti, M.; Forti, S.; et al. Optimisation and validation of a remote monitoring system (Onco-TreC) for home-based management of oral anticancer therapies: An Italian multicentre feasibility study. *BMJ Open* **2017**, *7*, e014617. [CrossRef] [PubMed]

95. Holle, L.M.; Puri, S.; Clement, J.M. Physician-pharmacist collaboration for oral chemotherapy monitoring: Insights from an academic genitourinary oncology practice. *J. Oncol. Pharm. Pract.* **2016**, *22*, 511–516. [CrossRef] [PubMed]

96. Wong, S.F.; Bounthavong, M.; Nguyen, C.; Bechtoldt, K.; Hernandez, E. Implementation and preliminary outcomes of a comprehensive oral chemotherapy management clinic. *Am. J. Health Syst. Pharm.* **2014**, *71*, 960–965. [CrossRef] [PubMed]

97. Bedell, C.H. A changing paradigm for cancer treatment: The advent of new oral chemotherapy agents. *Clin. J. Oncol. Nurs.* **2003**, *7*, 5–9. [CrossRef] [PubMed]

98. Goldspiel, B.; Hoffman, J.M.; Griffith, N.L.; Goodin, S.; DeChristoforo, R.; Montello, C.M.; Chase, J.L.; Bartel, S.; Patel, J.T. ASHP guidelines on preventing medication errors with chemotherapy and biotherapy. *Am. J. Health Syst. Pharm.* **2015**, *72*, e6–e35. [CrossRef] [PubMed]

99. Page, J.S.; Lederman, L.; Kelly, J.; James, T.A. Teams and teamwork in cancer care delivery: Shared mental models to improve planning for discharge and coordination of follow-up care. *J. Oncol. Pract.* **2016**, *12*, 1053–1058. [CrossRef] [PubMed]

100. Gandhi, S.; Day, L.; Paramsothy, T.; Giotis, A.; Ford, M.; Boudreau, A.; Pasetka, M. Oral Anticancer Medication Adherence, Toxicity Reporting, and Counseling: A Study Comparing Health Care Providers and Patients. *J. Oncol. Pract.* **2015**, *11*, 498–504. [CrossRef] [PubMed]

101. Abbott, R.; Edwards, S.; Whelan, M.; Edwards, J.; Dranitsaris, G. Are community pharmacists equipped to ensure the safe use of oral anticancer therapy in the community setting? Results of a cross-country survey of community pharmacists in Canada. *J. Oncol. Pharm. Pract.* **2014**, *20*, 29–39. [CrossRef] [PubMed]

102. Accreditation Commission for Health Care. Pharmacy Accreditation. Available online: https://www.achc.org/pharmacy.html (accessed on 8 January 2018).

103. Center for Pharmacy Practice Accreditation. Specialty Pharmacy Practice Accreditation Program. Available online: https://www.pharmacypracticeaccredit.org/our-programs/specialty-pharmacy-practice-accreditation-program (accessed on 8 January 2018).

104. URAC. Specialty Pharmacy Accreditation. Available online: https://www.urac.org/accreditation-and-measurement/accreditation-programs/all-programs/specialty-pharmacy/ (accessed on 8 January 2018).

105. Stein, J.; Mann, J. Specialty pharmacy services for patients receiving oral medications for solid tumors. *Am. J. Health Syst. Pharm.* **2016**, *73*, 775–796. [CrossRef] [PubMed]

106. Howard, D.H.; Bach, P.B.; Berndt, E.R.; Conti, R.M. Pricing in the Market for Anticancer Drugs. *J. Econ. Perspect.* **2015**, *29*, 139–162. [CrossRef] [PubMed]

107. Benjamin, L.; Buthion, V.; Vidal-Trecan, G.; Briot, P. Impact of the healthcare payment system on patient access to oral anticancer drugs: An illustration from the French and United States contexts. *BMC Health Serv. Res.* **2014**, *14*, 274. [CrossRef] [PubMed]

108. Dusetzina, S.B. Drug pricing trends for orally administered anticancer medications reimbursed by commercial health plans, 2000–2014. *JAMA Oncol.* **2016**, *2*, 960–961. [CrossRef] [PubMed]

109. Raborn, M.L.; Pelletier, E.M.; Smith, D.B.; Reyes, C.M. Patient out-of-pocket payments for oral oncolytics: Results from a 2009 US claims data analysis. *J. Oncol. Pract.* **2012**, *8*, 9s–15s. [CrossRef] [PubMed]

110. Smieliauskas, F.; Chien, C.R.; Shen, C.; Geynisman, D.M.; Shih, Y.C. Cost-effectiveness analyses of targeted oral anti-cancer drugs: A systematic review. *Pharmacoeconomics* **2014**, *32*, 651–680. [CrossRef] [PubMed]

111. Tefferi, A.; Kantarjian, H.; Rajkumar, S.V.; Baker, L.H.; Abkowitz, J.L.; Adamson, J.W.; Advani, R.H.; Allison, J.; Antman, K.H.; Bast, R.C., Jr.; et al. In support of a patient-driven initiative and petition to lower the high price of cancer drugs. *Mayo Clin. Proc.* **2015**, *90*, 996–1000. [CrossRef] [PubMed]

112. Wang, B.; Joffe, S.; Kesselheim, A.S. Chemotherapy parity laws: A remedy for high drug costs? *JAMA Intern. Med.* **2014**, *174*, 1721–1722. [CrossRef] [PubMed]

113. Patients Equal Access Coalition. Oral Chemotherapy Access Legislative Map. Available online: http://peac.myeloma.org/oral-chemo-access-map/ (accessed on 5 December 2017).

114. Dusetzina, S.B.; Huskamp, H.A.; Winn, A.N.; Basch, E.; Keating, N.L. Out-of-Pocket and Health Care Spending Changes for Patients Using Orally Administered Anticancer Therapy After Adoption of State Parity Laws. *JAMA Oncol.* **2017**. [CrossRef] [PubMed]

115. H.R. 1409—Cancer Drug Parity Act of 2017. Available online: https://www.congress.gov/bill/115th-congress/house-bill/1409 (accessed on 15 January 2018).

116. Colquhoun, A. Is there a place for cancer therapy provided from community pharmacy? *Pharm. J.* **2011**, *286*, 144.

117. Khandelwal, N.; Duncan, I.; Ahmed, T.; Rubinstein, E.; Pegus, C. Oral chemotherapy program improves adherence and reduces medication wastage and hospital admissions. *J. Natl. Compr. Cancer Netw.* **2012**, *10*, 618–625. [CrossRef]

118. Salas, E. Team Science in Cancer Care: Questions, an Observation, and a Caution. *J. Oncol. Pract.* **2016**, *12*, 972–974. [CrossRef] [PubMed]

119. Centers for Medicare & Medicaid Services. Oncology Care Model. Available online: https://innovation.cms.gov/initiatives/oncology-care/ (accessed on 6 October 2017).

120. Cox, J.V.; Ward, J.C.; Hornberger, J.C.; Temel, J.S.; McAneny, B.L. Community oncology in an era of payment reform. *Am. Soc. Clin. Oncol.* **2014**, e447–e452. [CrossRef] [PubMed]

121. Rouse, W.B.; Cannon-Bowers, J.A. The role of mental models in team performance in complex systems. *IEEE Trans. Syst. Man Cybern.* **1992**, *22*, 1296–1308. [CrossRef]

8

Hospital Audit as a Useful Tool in the Process of Introducing Falsified Medicines Directive (FMD) into Hospital Pharmacy Settings

Urszula Religioni [1], Damian Swieczkowski [2,*] , Anna Gawrońska [3], Anna Kowalczuk [4], Mariola Drozd [5], Mikołaj Zerhau [6], Dariusz Smoliński [7], Stanisław Radomiński [8], Natalia Cwalina [2], David Brindley [9,10,11,12,13], Miłosz J. Jaguszewski [2] and Piotr Merks [14]

[1] Department of Public Health, Medical University of Warsaw, Banacha 1a, 02-097 Warsaw, Poland; urszula.religioni@gmail.com

[2] First Department of Cardiology, Medical University in Gdansk, Dębinki 7, 80-952 Gdańsk, Poland; ncwalina@gumed.edu.pl (N.C.), mjaguszewski@gumed.edu.pl (M.J.J.)

[3] Institute of Logistics and Warehousing, Ewarysta Estkowskiego 6, 61-755 Poznań, Poland; anna.gawronska@ilim.poznan.pl

[4] National Medicines Institute, Chełmska 30/34, 00-725 Warsaw, Poland; a.kowalczuk@nil.gov.pl

[5] Department of Applied Pharmacy, Medical University of Lublin, Chodźki 1, 20-093 Lublin, Poland; marioladrozd@umlub.pl

[6] Hospital Pharmacy, Mazowiecki Szpitala Specjalistyczny w Ostrołęce, Al. Jana Pawła II 120 A, 07-410 Ostrołęka, Poland; mikizerh@gmail.com

[7] Community Pharmacy, Poland; smolinski.d.a@gmail.com

[8] Quizit Sp. z. o. o., Unit Dose, Sprinterów 2/6, 94-022 Łódź, Poland; s.radominski@quizit.eu

[9] Department of Paediatrics, University of Oxford, Level 2, Children's Hospital, John Radcliffe, Headington, Oxford OX3 9DU, UK; david.brindley@paediatrics.ox.ac.u

[10] The Oxford—UCL Centre for the Advancement of Sustainable Medical Innovation (CASMI), The University of Oxford, Tavistock Square, London WC1H 9JP, UK

[11] Centre for Behavioural Medicine, UCL School of Pharmacy, University College London, BMA House, Tavistock Square, London WC1H 9JP, UK

[12] Harvard Stem Cell Institute, Cambridge, MA 02138, USA

[13] USCF-Stanford Centre of Excellence in Regulatory Science and Innovation (CERSI), San Francisco, CA 94158, USA

[14] Department of Pharmaceutical Technology, Faculty of Pharmacy Collegium Medicum in Bydgoszcz, Nicolaus Copernicus University in Torun, 85-089 Bydgoszcz, Poland; piotrmerks@gmail.com

* Correspondence: d.swieczkowski@gumed.edu.pl

Abstract: Background: Recently, the European Union has introduced the Falsified Medicines Directive (FMD). Additionally, in early 2016, a Delegated Act (DA) related to the FMD was published. The main objective of this study was to evaluate the usefulness of external audits in the context of implementing new regulations provided by the FMD in the secondary care environment. Methods: The external, in-person workflow audits were performed by an authentication company in three Polish hospital pharmacies. Each audit consisted of a combination of supervision (non-participant observation), secondary data analysis, and expert interviews with the use of an independently designed authorial Diagnostic Questionnaire. The questionnaire included information about hospital drug distribution procedures, data concerning drug usage, IT systems, medication order systems, the processes of medication dispensing, and the preparation and administration of hazardous drugs. Data analysis included a thorough examination of hospital documentation in regard to drug management. All data were subjected to qualitative analysis, with the aim of generating meaningful information through inductive inference. Results: Only one dispensing location in the Polish hospitals studied has the potential to be a primary authentication area. In the audited hospitals, an Automated Drug Dispensing System and unit dose were not identified during the study. Hospital wards contained an enclosed place within the department dedicated to drug storage under the direct supervision of senior nursing staff. An electronic order system was not available. In the largest center, unused medications are re-dispensed to different hospital departments, or may be sold to various institutions. Additionally, in one hospital pharmacy, pharmacists prepared parenteral nutrition and chemotherapeutic drugs for patients admitted to the hospital. Conclusions: External audits might prove beneficial in the course of introducing new regulations into everyday settings. However, such action should be provided before the final implementation of authentication services. To sum up, FMD can impact several hospital departments.

Keywords: hospital pharmacy; pharmacist; pharmaceutical law; point of authentication; patient safety; Falsified Medicines Directive

---

1. Introduction

According to the World Health Organization (WHO), approximately 10% of medicinal products available within legal distribution are falsified. The financial value of this market reaches over 45 billion Euros, when considered in a global perspective. This problem remains underrecognized, particularly in highly-developed countries, where experts estimate that ca. 50% of drugs purchased via the Internet are falsified [1–4]. For the time being, the most frequently falsified medicines are those for weight loss and erectile dysfunction, as well as steroid hormones [5–7]. Recently, authorities have identified an increased number of falsified medicines in other therapeutic groups, such as contraceptives, psychotropic drugs, or cardiovascular agents [8–10].

The falsification of medicinal products remains an international issue, and thus it is necessary for the global authorities that are responsible for the creation of regulation frameworks, e.g., the Food and Drug Administration (FDA) or the European Medicines Agency (EMA), to implement actions against this. Recently, the European Union introduced the Falsified Medicines Directive (FMD) [11]. Additionally, in early 2016, a Delegated Act (DA) related to the FMD was published. The DA included additional details and administrative procedures related to the new regulations. This information is particularly important for stakeholders involved in the pharmaceutical supply chain [12–14]. The most fundamental changes are based on authentication, i.e., the scanning of a unique identifier during the moment of drug dispensation. This step in authentication is associated with a new range of responsibilities for pharmacy staff [12]. The detailed regulations include a list of the drugs which must have a unique identifier, as well as a list of those which do not require authentication [12]. However, the differences between verification and authentication should be emphasized. Broadly speaking, drug verification could be performed at any time during drug distribution. Authentication leads to the withdrawal of unique identifiers from the system and should be done directly before the final dispensation [12]. All stakeholders involved in drug distribution both at the national and European level should create a depository of unique identifiers. This will require mutual understanding and effective cooperation [12]. These actions should be understood as an important step in ensuring the safety of European patients. Based on this regulation, hospital pharmacies in Europe have until February 2019 to launch authentication protocols and to complete successful harmonization with the new legislature [15,16]. One of the essential steps for the effective implementation of these regulations into routine practice subsets remains the introduction and continuous improvement of validated procedures, using Good Authentication Practice (GAP) [17].

So far, the implementation of FMD has been discussed in the context of the community pharmacy setting. However, as stated by Merks et al., the introduction of new regulations into hospital pharmacies might prove to be even more challenging [18]. For instance, it is necessary to find the most suitable place for decommissioning (withdrawal of a unique identifier from the system) and all new procedures must be harmonized with the existing framework used [18]. In Poland, hospital pharmacies are mainly responsible for drug distribution and as such, clinical activities are rare [19]. Hospitals pharmacists develop the list of drugs used in a particular hospital (under the direct supervision of physicians), order drugs from wholesalers, and supervise drug management on hospital wards [19]. From this perspective, hospital pharmacies are the center of creation for drug policies in hospitals [20]. Moreover, hospital pharmacists often prepare compounding formulations, e.g., pediatric dosages, chemotherapeutic agents, and intravenous medications including parenteral nutrition [19,20]. The head of the hospital pharmacy must be a fully qualified pharmacist with a specialization in hospital pharmacy and/or proper experience, as specified by Polish pharmaceutical law [21]. Depending on the hospital pharmacy location (for instance a regional or highly specialized medical center), the pharmacist's responsibilities might be different, e.g., not all hospitals prepare chemotherapeutic agents [18–20].

We evaluated the potential usefulness of external audits in regard to the implementation of the new regulations provided by the FMD into the routine hospital setting. Audits remain an important step in the process of understanding the impact of the FMD on the workflow within the hospital pharmacy setting.

2. Materials and Methods

In 2015, the research team conducted three independent audits in hospitals located in central Poland: two with <300 beds and one with >500 beds (convenience sampling). Each audit was followed by a second audit, which was performed by an external company experienced in authentication services. Each of the three hospitals has their own hospital pharmacy, which is not an obligatory prerequisite required by Polish pharmaceutical law. Audits focused on places in the hospital which may have a potential importance for the implementation of the FMD. In detail, a mixed-methods analysis, which included in-person workflow audits, was used. The collection of all relevant data was linked with chain distribution in the audited institutions. Each audit consisted of a combination of supervision (non-participant observation), secondary data analysis, and expert interviews with the use of an independently designed authorial Diagnostic Questionnaire. Data analysis included a thorough examination of hospital documentation in regard to drug management. This comprised of: hospital drug distribution procedures, data concerning drug usage, IT systems, medication order systems, the processes of medication dispensing, and the preparation and administration of hazardous drugs. The Diagnostic Questionnaire provided a general overview of the characteristics of each hospital pharmacy. All data was subjected to qualitative analysis, with the aim of generating meaningful information through inductive inference. This comprehensive analysis aided in obtaining specific and intersubjective features of the entire process. The supervision, secondary data analyses, and interviews allowed us to prepare reports that present optimal solutions for authentication in pharmacies. Finally, we provided recommendations for further steps in introducing FMD into the routine setting within the Polish healthcare system.

Ethics approval and consent to participate were not applicable.

3. Results

In the audited hospitals, no Automated Drug Dispensing Systems were identified within the pharmacy setting. It was documented that pharmacists did not dispense medications using a unit dose system. The hospital's drug supply was based on a standard chain distribution, with the majority of drugs purchased directly from their official producer or general wholesalers. The area of dispensing medicinal products in the hospitals was considered as a potential place of authentication. However, in the hospital with >500 beds, we identified possible additional methods of integration in using an authentication system, such as the use of mobile scanners. Hospital pharmacists often utilized shared packages, namely split packs, and for the most part, drugs were dispensed in bulk. Two of the audited hospital pharmacies did not provide compounded intravenous medications. One of the settings, however, did provide parenteral nutrition and chemotherapeutic preparations. Hospital wards were not directly supplied by the producers or wholesalers; the drug chain distribution was based on medicinal products available within the hospital pharmacies. On the hospital wards, we identified enclosed places that were dedicated to drug storage, and maintained under the direct supervision of senior nursing staff. An electronic ordering system was not used by any of the hospital wards, departments, or clinics. Ordering was based on traditional paper communication between wards and hospital pharmacies as authorized by the head of departments. In line with their internal protocols, hospital wards returned unused medications to the hospital pharmacy. The returned drugs could then be dispensed to other departments in the hospital, depending on current needs. However, drug suppliers required that medications were returned to the hospital pharmacy within seven days of dispensing, and that this prerequisite was fulfilled in an audited setting. All audited hospitals were part of a hospital network and coordinated broad-spectrum services within the group of institutions. The transition of medicinal products between various hospitals did not occur in any of the audited bodies. The hospitals did not use an external, outsourced administration. The results of our audits are summarized in Table 1.

Table 1. A summary of the results of audits.

Hospital	The Number of Hospitals Beds	Audits—Results
1 and 2	<300	Both hospitals had their own hospital pharmacy. We did not identify an Automated Drug Dispensing System nor the use of a unit dose. Hospital wards contained an enclosed place within the department dedicated to drug storage under the direct supervision of senior nursing staff. An electronic order system was not available. Hospital pharmacies did not provide compounded intravenous medications. Unused medications might be re-dispensed to different hospital departments. The hospitals are part of a hospital network; however, the individual hospital pharmacies did not provide drugs to different institutions.
3	>500	In this hospital there was only one hospital pharmacy. We did not identify an Automated Drug Dispensing System nor a unit dose distribution model. On the hospital wards, there was an enclosed place dedicated to drug storage under the direct supervision of senior nursing staff. An electronic order system was not available.

4. Discussion

To the best of our knowledge, this is the first report attempting to evaluate the usefulness of hospital audits during the process of FMD implementation within the hospital pharmacy, especially in countries where the pharmacist's position is limited to dispensing medications and where there is no history of well-established pharmaceutical care. We found that dispensaries are the most optimal places of authentication; however, we suggest that additional automated technology may be beneficial in larger hospital settings, e.g., those with more than 500 beds. We recommend that any unused medications be returned from the hospital wards to the pharmacy within 10 days from the moment of dispensation. Internal operation procedures need to be implemented. In this way, pharmacy staff can re-introduce the serialized unique identifier through the authentication system and decommission the unique identifier again when the package is dispensed. If more than 10 days have passed since the authentication was performed, the drug can still be returned to the hospital pharmacy, but can only be used in the physical institution that conducted the decommission operation. It should not be sold to other institutions or returned to the supplier. In our work, the audited hospitals did not use a more advanced distribution system e.g., unit dose. We should stress that this tendency is in accordance with previous studies in this field and noted as a national trend [22].

Moreover, we have provided some general recommendations on how to harmonize authentication with the standards currently used in hospital settings. All hospitals were considered as large. Due to this distinction, it is important to optimize internal procedures to ensure that products are not authenticated too early in the supply chain. Once medications are authenticated and a period of

10 days has elapsed, these products can no longer be returned to a manufacturer nor can they be transferred to another institution. In the context of dispensing drugs in bulk, we recommend selecting products from manufacturers that can produce aggregated codes, as this will reduce the time needed to authenticate products. Due to the fact that hospital pharmacies often use split packs, authentication must be conducted prior to opening a drug package, and the total content of the product needs to be kept at all times within the controlled environment of the hospital pharmacy. Of course, in this scenario, drugs cannot be transferred to any other area of the hospital, or be re-sold or transferred to another institution.

Ward stock can be maintained, as there is no need to change internal procedures within the hospital. If the hospital belongs to a trust/group of hospitals, and they legally all belong to the same institution, the authentication process can be performed in one of the hospital pharmacies. Drugs returned from hospital wards can be disposed of, if this is the normal policy of the hospital, or they can be reused, but only inside the same physical institution if the 10-day rule has passed. They cannot be re-sold or returned to the manufacturer.

Authentication of extemporaneously prepared medicines, intravenous and parenteral nutrition products, etc., should occur while assembling ingredients for the product before the final product is prepared by a qualified member of staff. A proper system to dispose of medicinal products needs to be put in place. The risk of reusing the packaging of products can be substantial depending on the setting. To summarize, authentication needs to be performed within the hospital pharmacy. Detailed records must be kept due to the possibility of product recall. Above mentioned recommendations are summarized in Table 2.

Table 2. A summary of recommendations.

	Recommendations
1	Dispensaries are the most optimal places of authentication; however, additional automated technology may be beneficial in larger hospital settings, e.g., those with more than 500 beds.
2	Any unused drugs are to be returned from the hospital wards to the pharmacy within 10 days from the moment of dispensation.
3	If more than 10 days have passed since the authentication has been performed, the drug can still be returned to the hospital pharmacy, but can only be used in the physical institution that conducted the decommission operation.
4	Authentication needs to be conducted before opening a drug package, and the total content of the product needs to be kept at all times within the controlled environment of the hospital pharmacy.
5	If the hospital belongs to a trust/group of hospitals, the authentication process can be done in one of the hospital pharmacies.
6	Authentication of extemporaneously prepared medicines, intravenous, and parenteral nutrition products, etc., should occur while assembling ingredients for the product before the final product is prepared by a qualified member of staff.
7	Authentication needs to be performed in the hospital pharmacy.
8	It is important to optimize internal procedures to ensure that products are not authenticated too early in the supply chain.

We believe that the implementation of FMD should be associated with amendments in the management of hospital pharmacies, as it will place new responsibilities on pharmacists and technicians employed within hospital pharmacies. Standard procedures should be introduced and harmonized with European laws, and further adjusted to the national practice [23]. Additionally, there is a strong need to adapt the protocols to the workflow available in a particular community or hospital pharmacy [24].

Here, we would like to stress the fact that GAP can be helpful in the successful implementation of a new framework for hospital pharmacies [17,25]. In line with GAP, our study suggested that the most desirable authentication should be provided by hospital pharmacists or technicians, at the final step of dispensing medications. Decommissioning procedures also need to occur. Moreover, whenever possible, manual authentication should be replaced by an automated process. By using scanners that read a 2D matrix, the risk of releasing a drug without authentication can be reduced, in accordance with lean management concepts. While legal regulations allow for the division of a drug package, the original container should not leave the dispensing point until its entire contents have been dispensed. Also, in instances when the hospital pharmacy contains a chemotherapeutic facility for compounding, the authentication of such products must be obtained before the drug is introduced in the clean room [17].

Our observations have several potential limitations. First, the process of drug authentication in the hospital setting remains in the early stages of development. A standard of best practices can only be achieved over time with the acquisition of experience and further conducted research. Secondly, our initial audits have been conducted only in three hospital pharmacies. Consequently, our findings cannot serve as an entirely accurate representation of all hospital pharmacies in Poland. However, we would like to emphasize that this is only a pilot study and again, further investigation is warranted. Moreover, we are still waiting for recommendations approved by national authorities, which will specify procedures in light of countrywide requirements [26].

5. Conclusions

FMD should be fully harmonized with national legal framework in accordance with the 2019 implementation deadline [18]. Currently, hospital pharmacies in Poland are not organized under the new regulations associated with the FMD [27]. The joint efforts of both pharmacists and hospital management staff are essential to the effective implementation of an innovative workflow in the hospital pharmacy setting. A pilot program of authentication should precede the final implementation. Preparations of standard operational procedures that are adjusted to national practice might prove very useful. External audits can be beneficial in this process and should be performed before introducing new tools into routine settings.

Acknowledgments: We thank Graham Smith and Mark De Simone from Aegate Ltd. for their contribution and support during the preparation of our paper. We express our sincere appreciation and thanks to the following organizations for providing their help and guidance at each stage of our research: the Royal Pharmaceutical Society (UK), the Polish National Pharmaceutical Chamber (Poland), and the Polish Pharmaceutical Society (Poland).

Author Contributions: Urszula Religioni designed the study and collected data. Damian Swieczkowski designed the study, prepared and revised the manuscript. Milosz Jaguszewski and Piotr Merks supervised the project. All authors contributed to the manuscript in a significant way. All authors of the manuscript have read and agreed to its content and are accountable for all aspects of the accuracy and integrity of the manuscript in accordance with ICMJE criteria.

References

1. World Health Organization—IMPACT. Counterfeit Medicines: An Update on Estimates. 2006. Available online: www.who.int/medicines/services/counterfeit/impact/TheNewEstimatesCounterfeit.pdf (accessed on 13 June 2017).
2. Griffiths, P.; Mounteney, J. Disruptive Potential of the Internet to Transform Illicit Drug Markets and Impact on Future Patterns of Drug Consumption. *Clin. Pharmacol. Ther.* **2017**, *101*, 176–178. [CrossRef] [PubMed]
3. Mackey, T.K.; Aung, P.; Liang, B.A. Illicit Internet availability of drugs subject to recall and patient safety consequences. *Int. J. Clin. Pharm.* **2015**, *37*, 1076–1085. [CrossRef] [PubMed]

4. Lee, K.S.; Yee, S.M.; Zaidi, S.T.R.; Patel, R.P.; Yang, Q.; Al-Worafi, Y.M. Long Chiau Ming Combating Sale of Counterfeit and Falsified Medicines Online: A Losing Battle. *Front. Pharmacol.* **2017**, *8*, 268. [CrossRef] [PubMed]

5. Kumar, B.; Baldi, A. The Challenge of Counterfeit Drugs: A Comprehensive Review on Prevalence, Detection and Preventive Measures. *Curr. Drug Saf.* **2016**, *11*, 112–120. [CrossRef] [PubMed]

6. Chiang, J.; Yafi, F.A.; Dorsey, P.J., Jr.; Hellstrom, W.J.G. The dangers of sexual enhancement supplements and counterfeit drugs to "treat" erectile dysfunction. *Transl. Androl. Urol.* **2017**, *6*, 12–19. [CrossRef] [PubMed]

7. Jackson, G.; Arver, S.; Banks, I.; Stecher, V.J. Counterfeit phosphodiesterase type 5 inhibitors pose significant safety risks. *Int. J. Clin. Pract.* **2010**, *64*, 497–504. [CrossRef] [PubMed]

8. Gibson, L. Drug regulatory study global treaty to tackle counterfeit drugs. *Br. Med. J.* **2004**, *328*, 486. [CrossRef] [PubMed]

9. Woosley, R.L.; Schwartz, P.J. Counterfeit drugs: A plot worthy of John le Carrè. *Int. J. Cardiol.* **2017**, *243*, 279–280. [CrossRef] [PubMed]

10. Fayzrakhmanov, N.F. Fighting trafficking of falsified and substandard medicinal products in Russia. *Int. J. Risk Saf. Med.* **2015**, *27*, S37–S40. [CrossRef] [PubMed]

11. Beninger, P. Opportunities for Collaboration at the Interface of Pharmacovigilance and Manufacturing. *Clin. Ther.* **2017**, *39*, 702–712. [CrossRef] [PubMed]

12. Commission Delegated Regulation (EU) 2016/161 of 2 October 2015 Supplementing Directive 2001/83/EC of the European Parliament and of the Council by Laying down Detailed Rules for the Safety Features Appearing on the Packaging of Medicinal Products for Human Use. 2015. Available online: http://ec.europa.eu/health/files/eudralex/vol-1/reg_2016_161/reg_2016_161_en.pdf (accessed on 8 September 2016).

13. Smith, G.; Smith, J.; Brindley, D. The Falsified Medicines Directive: How to secure your supply chain. *J. Generic Med.* **2014**, *11*, 169–172. [CrossRef] [PubMed]

14. Taaffe, T. European union has the falsified medicines directive. *BMJ* **2012**, *345*, e8356. [CrossRef] [PubMed]

15. EAHP Briefing. European Commission Publishes Falsified Medicines Directive Delegated Act. 2015. Available online: http://www.eahp.eu/news/EU-monitor/eahp-eu-monitor-25-august-2015 (accessed on 3 September 2017).

16. Borup, R.; Kaae, S.; Minssen, T.; Traulsen, J. Fighting falsified medicines with paperwork—A historic review of Danish legislation governing distribution of medicines. *J. Pharm. Policy Pract.* **2016**, *9*, 30. [CrossRef] [PubMed]

17. Naughton, B.D.; Smith, J.A.; Brindley, D.A. Establishing good authentication practice (GAP) in secondary care to protect against falsified medicines and improve patient safety. *Eur. J. Hosp. Pharm. Sci. Pract.* **2016**, *23*, 118–120. [CrossRef] [PubMed]

18. Merks, P.; Swieczkowski, D.; Byliniak, M.; Drozd, M.; Krupa, K.; Jaguszewski, M.; Brindley, D.A.; Naughton, B.D. The European Falsified Medicines Directive in Poland: Background, implementation and potential recommendations for pharmacists. *Eur. J. Hosp. Pharm. Sci. Pract.* **2016**. [CrossRef]

19. Farmacja Szpitalna—Niewykorzystany Potencjał. 2017. Available online: http://www.medexpress.pl/farmacja-szpitalna-niewykorzystany-potencjal-2/66062 (accessed on 22 October 2017).

20. Farmaceuta w Szpitalu. 2017. Available online: https://farmacja.pl/farmaceuta-w-szpitalu# (accessed on 22 October 2017).

21. Kierownik Apteki. 2017. Available online: http://e-prawnik.pl/artykuly/prawo-administracyjne/kierownik-apteki.html (accessed on 22 October 2017).

22. Religioni, U. *Rationalization Methods for Medicinal Products Management in Healthcare Facilities with Reference to Optimization of Medical Expenses*; Medical University of Warsaw: Warszawa, Poland, 2015.

23. Borup, R.; Traulsen, J. Falsified Medicines—Bridging the Gap between Business and Public Health. *Pharmacy* **2016**, *4*, 16. [CrossRef] [PubMed]

24. Naughton, B.; Roberts, L.; Dopson, S.; Chapman, S.; Brindley, D. Effectiveness of medicines authentication technology to detect counterfeit, recalled and expired medicines: A two-stage quantitative secondary care study. *BMJ Open* **2016**, *6*, e013837. [CrossRef] [PubMed]

25. Naughton, B.; Roberts, L.; Dopson, S.; Brindley, D.; Chapman, S. Medicine authentication technology as a counterfeit medicine-detection tool: A Delphi method study to establish expert opinion on manual medicine authentication technology in secondary care. *BMJ Open* **2017**, *7*, e013838. [CrossRef] [PubMed]

9

The Professional Culture of Community Pharmacy and the Provision of MTM Services

Meagen M. Rosenthal * (ID) and Erin R. Holmes

Department of Pharmacy Administration, School of Pharmacy, University of Mississippi, 223 Faser Hall, University, MS 38677-1848, USA; erholmes@olemiss.edu
* Correspondence: mmrosent@olemiss.edu

Abstract: The integration of advanced pharmacy services into community pharmacy practice is not complete. According to implementation research understanding professional culture, as a part of context, may provide insights for accelerating this process. There are three objectives in this study. The first objective of this study was to validate an adapted version of an organizational culture measure in a sample of United States' (US) community pharmacists. The second objective was to examine potential relationships between the cultural factors identified using the validated instrument and a number of socialization and education variables. The third objective was to examine any relationships between the scores on the identified cultural factors and the provision of MTM services. This study was a cross-sectional online survey for community pharmacists in the southeastern US. The survey contained questions on socialization/education, respondents' self-reported provision of medication therapy management (MTM) services, and the organizational culture profile (OCP). Analyses included descriptive statistics, a principle components analysis (PCA), independent samples *t*-test, and multivariate ordinal regression. A total of 303 surveys were completed. The PCA revealed a six-factor structure: social responsibility, innovation, people orientation, competitiveness, attention to detail, and reward orientation. Further analysis revealed significant relationships between social responsibility and years in practice, and people orientation and attention to detail and pharmacists' training and practice setting. Significant positive relationships were observed between social responsibility, innovation, and competitiveness and the increased provision of MTM services. The significant relationships identified between the OCP factors and community pharmacist respondents' provision of MTM services provides an important starting point for developing interventions to improve the uptake of practice change opportunities.

Keywords: professional culture; community pharmacy; advanced pharmacy services

1. Background

As quality measures permeate pharmacy practice, and pharmacists are afforded new legislated opportunities to provide clinical services, it is integral that all members of the pharmacy profession are ready, and able, to adapt to these changes [1]. Fortunately, evidence of pharmacists' clinical efficacy in helping to manage chronic conditions, such as diabetes, has been well documented [2]. In fact, there is even a growing body of evidence suggesting that pharmacists' independent prescribing is a safe and effective way to help patients with chronic conditions such as hypertension and hyperlipidemia to meet guideline targets [3–5]. Unfortunately, these practices have not spread to all members of the pharmacy profession, and by extension to patients.

For example, despite expressing interest in providing advanced pharmacy services such as medication therapy management (MTM) to patients, community pharmacists continue to struggle with a number of barriers including the lack of payment structures, support, and time [6].

Furthermore, pharmacists' lack of time to provide these services results in patients not seeking pharmacy services, and reinforces pharmacists' notion that patients do not want these services from pharmacists [7]. Some of these barriers are being addressed through national legislative efforts such as the "Pharmacy and Medically Underserved Areas Enhancement Act" (H.R.592), which, if passed, will allow pharmacists to seek reimbursement for the provision of clinical services [8]. While these fixes are incredibly important, alone they fail to address the complete context of community pharmacy practice.

Implementation research has found that merely providing healthcare professionals, like pharmacists, with clinical evidence in support of patient services is not enough to ensure its successful application by clinicians [9,10]. Research in this field suggests that the "context" in which the clinician finds themselves plays an integral role in the implementation process [10]. Context, in this case, includes aspects of the social, economic, political, legal, physical, and cultural environments into which a change is being proposed [10]. Therefore, access to reimbursement only addresses the legal, economic, and social aspects of pharmacists' context respectively. This study focuses on the potential impact of professional culture on the provision of medication therapy management (MTM) by community pharmacists.

Professional cultures are groups of people who share a pattern of values, beliefs, norms, and interpretations [11]. These values, beliefs, norms, and interpretations are developed through socialization and education processes [12]. The presence and importance of professional culture has been recognized by a number of authors [11,13,14]. Importantly, these authors also acknowledge that professional cultures exist within larger organizational cultures [11,15]. Preliminary work on professional culture has been conducted within healthcare settings examining the professional cultures of medicine, nursing, social work and pharmacy [16–20]. Some recent work has also established preliminary connections between various professional cultures' approaches to learning, the definitions of credibility and constructiveness, and how feedback was integrated into the various practices of these professions [14].

However, much of the previous work on professional culture in healthcare settings has been observational in nature, seeking to characterize the culture, rather than measuring and linking it with professional behaviors or actions. Recent work with pharmacists in Canada has uncovered a number of relationships between pharmacy's professional culture and the provision of clinical services by pharmacists [21]. In particular, respondents who saw greater value in the cultural factors innovation and competitiveness also provided an increased number of advanced pharmacy services such as medication reviews and immunizations [21]. Currently, there is limited research empirically examining the influence of professional culture of pharmacy on community pharmacists' behaviors in the United States (US). The purpose of this work is to begin to characterize the professional culture of community pharmacists, and to examine potential relationships between the factors of professional culture, socialization and education, and the provision of MTM services.

2. Objectives

There are three objectives in this study. The first objective of this study was to validate an adapted version of an organizational culture measure in a sample of US community pharmacists. The second objective was to examine potential relationships between the cultural factors identified using the validated instrument and a number of socialization and education variables. The third objective was to examine any relationships between the scores on the identified cultural factors and the provision of MTM services.

3. Materials and Methods

Study design: A cross-sectional online survey was used for the study. This study was approved as exempt under the University of Mississippi Institutional Review Board (protocol #15x-027).

Sample: The sample was comprised of community pharmacists from the southeastern US. The focus on community pharmacists was primarily based on potential differences between the professional cultures of community and hospital pharmacist given their distinct practice settings. The second reason for the focus on community pharmacy was based on the fact that most pharmacists in the US work in the community setting, meaning that any insights gained from this work would be applicable to a large proportion of the pharmacist population [22]. The target sample size for this study is 300, and is based on an examination of the literature, which states that this is the minimum threshold required to validate a survey instrument [23].

The sample was collected with the assistance of a health research and marketing firm called DMD Healthcare Research (http://deltamarketingdynamics.com). This company has access to a large, nationally representative, database of community pharmacist panelists. The advantage of approaching this company to complete data collection was a guarantee to achieve the sample size.

Procedure/data collection: Each of the 1457 randomly selected potential community pharmacist participants received an invitation email through DMD Healthcare Research which contained the survey link. The survey was administered in February of 2016, and data collection was completed within that month. A small monetary incentive was provided for each completed survey. The online survey was developed through Qualtrics Inc. online software system (Provo, UT, USA). This software houses all anonymous survey responses on its own secure server, which can be accessed through the license maintained by the University of Mississippi.

Survey: The online survey contained two sections. In the first section, the socialization and education variables and respondents' self-reported provision of MTM services were captured (see Supplement 1 for complete survey). The socialization and education variables were culled from the definition of professional culture and were chosen to capture community pharmacists' common experiences in becoming a pharmacist [12]. In particular, questions about how long the respondent had been in practice, his/her educational background, and current practice setting were asked. There were three of these questions. The questions for the provision of MTM services were generated through an examination of the definition of MTM offered by the American Pharmacists Association [24]. Questions in this survey focused on the number of immunizations, medication reviews, and disease management consultations provided in the previous month. These services were chosen because they correlate with measures used previously in the examination of Canadian pharmacists' professional culture and provision of advanced pharmacy services [21]. Three questions focused specifically on the number of each of the MTM services provided.

The second section of the survey contained the OCP. The OCP was originally designed to measure person-organization fit through an evaluation of overlapping cultural values [25]. In particular, the instrument was administered to employees to evaluate personal cultural values and then to managers of an organization to evaluate the organization's cultural values. The results of employees and managers were then compared to determine whether or not employee values matched with those of the organization [25]. This study was also replicated examining the fit between the culture of a hospital in Belgium and the culture of nursing staff working within the hospital [26]. Given the previous applications of this instrument evaluating individual, professional, and organizational cultures it was determined that an adapted version of the OCP could be applied to a preliminary evaluation of community pharmacists' professional culture in this study.

In this survey the instrument was adapted to begin with a statement prompting the respondent to consider, "To what extent pharmacy is recognized for its...", from "To what extent is your organization recognized for its..." [25]. Some examples of the 40 items of the OCP include adaptability, being innovative, being analytical, fairness, being results oriented, and being calm. All items were measured in a 5-point linear numeric scale from "not at all recognized" to "very much recognized". A previous validation of these items revealed seven cultural factors: innovation, supportiveness, social responsibility, competitiveness, stability, performance orientation, and reward orientation [25].

Unlike other culture measurement tools, reliability analyses of the previously identified cultural factors of the OCP have been undertaken [25]. The reliability scores for factors identified using the instrument have ranged between 0.77 and 0.88, depending upon the population under study [25].

Previous work using the OCP from Canada and identified five cultural factors: supportiveness, social responsibility, competitiveness, performance orientation, and reward orientation [21]. Reliability scores for these factors ranged from 0.92 for supportiveness, to 0.76 for performance orientation [21]. This survey was not pilot tested, however, as mentioned all survey questioned mirrored those administered in a previous survey conducted in Canada, and face validity tests were performed with experts in the field [21].

Analysis: All analyses were conducted using SPSS for Macintosh, version 22.0. An initial examination of the data from all MTM service variables revealed widely ranging mean and median scores (i.e., medication reviews mean = 19.09, median = 2.50; immunizations mean = 17.75, median = 10.00; disease management consultations mean = 3.04, median = 0). As such each of these items was recoded into categorical variables to more accurately reflect these wide ranges. Analyses of sample characteristics were completed using descriptive statistics.

The first objective to validate an adapted version of the OCP was analyzed using a principal component analysis (PCA), applying the guidelines outlined by Field (2009) [23]. A PCA was appropriate for this analysis because there is no way of knowing the number and kind of factors expected from this data. This analysis was followed by a reliability analysis, using Cronbach's Alpha, to determine the internal consistency of responses. Finally, the factors were scored by determining the mean using scale responses for each item.

The second objective to examine potential relationships between the cultural factors identified using the validated OCP and a number of socialization and education variables was measured using independent samples *t*-test for education and practice setting variables, and simple linear regression for years in practice [23]. The third objective to examine potential relationships between the cultural factors identified using the validated OCP and socialization and education variables was measured using multivariate ordinal regression, wherein the cultural factors were treated as the independent variables and pharmacists' responses to the MTM services questions were treated as dependent variables.

4. Results

A total of 303 US community pharmacists completed the survey, making the response rate 21%. Respondents had been in practice for an average of 23.4 years (SD = 12.1 years). Most respondents had completed a BSc in pharmacy (65%), and were working in a chain community pharmacy setting (65%). Compared to the wider community pharmacy population these respondents have been in practice longer, which accounts for the higher number of solely BSc Pharm trained respondents [27]. However, the breakdown of respondents working in chain versus independent pharmacies is consistent with the wider community pharmacy population [28,29]. The majority of respondents provided at least some advanced services to patients, with immunizations being the most frequently provided service (see Table 1 for complete details).

Objective 1. The PCA: The initial PCA was conducted on the 40 item OCP with orthogonal rotation (varimax). An examination of the factorability using the Kaiser-Meyer-Olkin (KMO) measure verified the sampling adequacy for the analysis, KMO = 0.91, and all items for individual values were > 0.86, which is well above the standard limit of 0.5. Bartlett's test of sphericity, which was x^2 (300) = 4049.12, $p < 0.0001$, indicated that correlations between items were sufficiently large for a PCA. A total of 15 items were eliminated because they did not have a primary factor loading of 0.4, and/or no cross-loading of 0.3 or above. The final PCA was conducted on 25 items using the previous approach. The KMO measure verified the sampling adequacy for the analysis, KMO = 0.90, and all items for individual values were > 0.78, which is still well above the standard limit of 0.5. Bartlett's test of sphericity, which was x^2 (300) = 3043.33, $p < 0.0001$, indicated that correlations between items were sufficiently large for the PCA. An eigenvalue analysis identified 6 components with a score over 1 and a combination of 63% total explained variance. After an examination of the scree plot, consideration of the large sample size, and the Kaiser's criterion, 6 factors were retained.

The items that clustered on each factor suggest that factor 1 represents *social responsibility*, factor 2 represents *innovation*, factor 3 represents *people orientation*, factor 4 represents *competitiveness*, factor 5 represents *attention to detail*, and factor 6 represents *reward orientation*. The internal consistency for each of the factors was relatively high ranging from a Cronbach's alpha of 0.73 for attention to detail to 0.82 for innovation.

Table 1. Respondent characteristics.

		Proportion (Frequency)
Highest level of education	BSc Pharm	65% (190)
	PharmD	35% (105)
	MSc Pharm	1% (4)
	Pharmacy residency	0.7% (2)
	Missing	0.3% (1)
Practice setting	Community pharmacy chain store	65% (195)
	Community pharmacy independent store	34% (104)
	Missing	1% (3)
Services	Immunizations	
	0	20% (61)
	1–20	59% (179)
	21<	20% (61)
	Missing	0.3% (1)
	Medication reviews	
	0	32% (96)
	1−10	49% (149)
	11−51<	17% (51)
	Missing	2% (6)
	Disease management consultations	
	0	58% (176)
	1−10	34% (104)
	11<	6% (18)
	Missing	1% (4)

Composite scores of each of the factors were created calculating the mean of the items comprising the factor, with higher scores indicting that respondents perceived greater value in the factor. The highest score was on shown on the factor attention to detail (M = 4.16, SD = 0.68), and the lowest score was on the factor innovation (M = 3.10, SD = 0.73). As outlined in Table 2 all of the factors were negatively skewed, however, both the skewness and kurtosis were well within the tolerable ranges for assuming a normal distribution [23].

Objective 2. Relationships between OCP factors and socialization/education variables: The examination of the relationship between the socialization/education variables and the six OCP factors revealed a number of significant relationships. To begin a simple linear regression found a significant relationship predicting respondents' valuing of the factor social responsibility based on pharmacists' years in practice (YiP) ($F(1, 286) = 9.64$, $p < 0.002$, with an R^2 of 0.033). That is, respondents predicted value in social responsibility is equal to 3.43 + 0.01 (YiP) points when it is measured in the OCP.

Next independent sample *t*-tests were conducted to examine the relationships between levels of pharmacists' education (BSc Pharm vs. PharmD), and practice setting (Chain vs. Independent), and the OCP factors. Pharmacists with BSc Pharmacy training perceived greater value in the factor people orientation (M = 3.56, SE = 0.055), than pharmacists with PharmD training (M = 3.36, SE = 0.07). However, pharmacists with PharmD training perceived greater value in the factor attention to detail (M = 4.27, SE = 0.07), than pharmacists with BSc Pharmacy training (M = 4.10, SE = 0.05). Pharmacists practicing in independent pharmacies perceived greater value in social responsibility (M = 3.88, SE = 0.05), than pharmacists working in chain pharmacy settings (M = 3.57, SE = 0.05). Additionally, pharmacists working in independent pharmacies also perceived greater value in people orientation (M = 3.65, SE = 0.08), than pharmacists working in chain pharmacy settings (M = 3.41, SE = 0.05). See Table 3 for complete results.

Objective 3. Relationships between OCP factors and MTM service provision: As first step to exploring objective three, ordinal regression models were run with each of the socialization/education variables to determine if confounding was possible. The only significant relationship noted here was that pharmacists from the chain community pharmacy setting were more likely to provide a greater number of immunizations per month, than pharmacists working in an independent community pharmacy setting (OR 7.24, 95% CI 4.02–13.03). However, all of the socialization/education variables were used in subsequent modeling.

Table 2. Descriptive statistics for the 6 OCP factors (*N* = 300).

	Factor Loadings	Mean (SD)	Skewness (SE)	Kurtosis (SE)	Cronbach's α
Social responsibility		3.67 (0.71)	−0.23 (0.14)	−0.19 (0.28)	00.81
Having a good reputation	0.74	4.11 (0.85)			
An emphasis on quality	0.71	4.09 (0.88)			
Being socially responsible	0.67	3.63 (0.92)			
Being calm	0.60	3.14 (1.1)			
Developing friends at work	0.60	3.42 (0.96)			
Innovation		3.10 (0.73)	0.25 (0.14)	−0.16 (0.28)	0.82
Being innovative	0.78	3.42 (0.96)			
Being reflective	0.73	3.20 (0.87)			
Being quick to take advantage of opportunities	0.71	3.28 (1.0)			
Adaptability	0.68	3.37 (0.95)			
Risk taking	0.61	2.71 (1.0)			
People orientation		3.49 (0.75)	−0.13 (0.14)	−0.28 (0.28)	0.77
Tolerance	0.74	3.40 (0.90)			
Informality	0.74	3.06 (1.0)			
Fairness	0.64	3.69 (0.98)			
Taking individual responsibility	0.54	3.78 (0.99)			
Competitiveness		3.67 (0.69)	−0.19 (0.14)	−0.21 (0.29)	0.76
Being results oriented	0.73	3.94 (0.91)			
Being aggressive	0.73	3.22 (1.0)			
Achievement orientation	0.63	3.65 (0.95)			
Being competitive	0.57	3.91 (0.92)			
Confronting conflict directly	0.44	3.61 (0.97)			
Attention to detail		4.16 (0.68)	−0.59 (0.14)	−0.35 (0.28)	0.73
Being rule oriented	0.81	4.24 (0.85)			
Paying attention to detail	0.71	4.39 (0.79)			
Being analytical	0.70	3.84 (0.88)			
Reward orientation		3.20 (0.85)	−0.06 (0.14)	−0.11 (0.28)	0.75
Security of employment	0.76	3.50 (0.97)			
High pay for good performance	0.75	3.08 (1.1)			
Offers of praise for good performance	0.64	3.01 (1.1)			

SD = Standard deviation, SE = Standard error; Scale: from 1 not at all recognized to 5 very much recognized.

Table 3. Independent sample *t*-tests between level of education and practice setting, and OCP factors.

	BSc Pharm N = 190	PharmD ˆ N = 105
Cultural factors	Mean (SE)	Mean (SE)
Social responsibility	3.76 (0.05)	3.53 (0.07)
Innovation	3.20 (0.05)	3.17 (0.07)
People orientation	3.56 (0.06) *	3.35 (0.07) *
Competitiveness	3.69 (0.05)	3.64 (0.07)
Attention to detail	4.10 (0.05) *	4.27 (0.07) *
Reward orientation	3.20 (0.06)	3.20 (0.09)
	Chain N = 195	*Independent N = 104*
Cultural factors	Mean (SE)	Mean (SE)
Social responsibility	3.57 (0.05) ***	3.88 (0.07) ***
Innovation	3.17 (0.05)	3.24 (0.08)
People orientation	3.41 (0.05) **	3.65 (0.08) **
Competitiveness	3.73 (0.05)	3.58 (0.07)
Attention to detail	4.17 (0.05)	4.14 (0.07)
Reward orientation	3.17 (0.06)	3.26 (0.09)

* *p* < 0.05, ** *p* < 0.01, *** *p* < 0.001; SE = Standard error; Scale: From 1 not at all recognized to 5 very much recognized;
ˆ Only those respondents with either a BSc Pharm or a PharmD were included in this analysis.

The adjusted ordinal regression models for the OCP factors and immunizations, medication reviews, and disease state consultations, identified a number of significant relationships (see Table 4). More specifically, those respondents who perceived value in the factors social responsibility, innovation, and competitiveness were more likely to provide immunizations than those respondents who perceived less value in these factors. Respondents who perceived value in the factor innovation were more likely to provide a higher number of medication reviews per month (OR 1.92, 95% CI 1.40–2.65). However, respondents who perceived value in the factor attention to detail were less likely to provide a higher number of medication reviews per month (OR 0.67, 95% CI 0.47–0.94). Finally, only innovation was significantly associated with disease state consultations. In particular, those respondents who perceived value in innovation were more likely to provide disease state consultations (OR 1.72, 95% CI 1.25–2.46).

Table 4. Results of multivariate ordinal regression of pharmacy services and OCP factors.

Service ^ (DV)	OCP Factor (IV)	Odds Ratio *	CI (95%)
Immunizations	Practice setting	7.24	4.02–13.03
	Social responsibility	1.46	1.03–2.06
	Innovation	1.58	1.14–2.21
	Competitiveness	1.75	1.22–2.52
Medication reviews	Innovation	1.92	1.40–2.65
	Attention to detail	0.67	0.47–0.94
Disease state consultations	Innovation	1.75	1.25–2.46

^ All services integrated into the models as previously developed categorical variables; * Only statistically significant odds ratios presented in this table; DV = dependent variable; IV = independent variable.

5. Discussion

This work provides some preliminary insights into the professional culture of community pharmacy in the US using the OCP, and how it may influence community pharmacists' provision of MTM services. The study identified six distinct cultural factors including: social responsibility, innovation, people orientation, competitiveness, attention to detail, and reward orientation. Respondents to the survey saw the greatest value in the factor attention to detail. When compared to previous Canadian data, the sample of US pharmacists also saw greater value in social responsibility and competitiveness, and also identified two new factors people orientation and attention to detail [21].

The regression models found that those respondents seeing greater value in the factors social responsibility, innovation, and competitiveness provided a higher number of immunizations. Furthermore, those respondents seeing greater value in innovation also provided more medication reviews and disease state consultations. When compared to Canadian data, a similarly positive relationship was noted for the factors competitiveness and innovation, and the provision of advanced pharmacy services [21]. Moreover, two other studies conducted in the US, one examining organizational factors influencing pharmacy practice change, and another examining influence on pharmacy service provision, found that entrepreneurial orientation and innovation were both positive influences on the provision of advanced pharmacy services [30].

Contrarily, respondents from this survey who saw greater value in attention to detail provided fewer medication reviews. This inverse relationship was unique to the US sample of community pharmacists. It is also worth noting that when compared to BScPharm trained respondents, PharmD trained respondents also saw greater value in this factor. A partial explanation for this emphasis within the PharmD trained population may be a function of the increased attention to the mitigation of medication errors that had taken place in the profession when transitioning to this training model [31]. It is also important to recognize that in and of itself attention to detail is not a negative cultural factor, as it likely contributes to pharmacists' ability to accurately fill patients' prescriptions. Rather it may be influenced by other contextual factors within the community pharmacy environment. For example, time constraints, as noted in other research, might result in pharmacists' dedicating the limited time they have to ensuring that patients' prescriptions are correct [7].

Taken together, all of these findings show an important overlap between social responsibility and competitiveness, which were also identified by the majority of survey respondents as being important, and the provision of immunizations to patients. A recent study found that from 2007 to 2013 the number of influenza vaccinations dispensed in community pharmacies increased from 3.2 to 20.9 million, showing that the respondents' perceptions of these factors, and self-reported provision of immunizations, are likely based on the actual care of patients [32].

However, the inverse relationship between attention to detail and the number of medication reviews provided, and that innovation was seen to be less important by most respondents, though connected with the higher provision of both medication reviews and disease state consultations, is potentially problematic. If the profession wishes to see the continued expansion of its scope of practice, and payment for these services, ensuring that the majority of pharmacists are actively providing these services is essential.

There are a number of ways in which innovation could be fostered in community pharmacists. To begin current community pharmacists and pharmacy students could be provided skills through coursework encouraging innovative thinking for problem resolution, reflective thinking, risk taking, and adaptability. In fact, this is training is already taking place through programs like Educating Pharmacists in Quality (EPIQ), which was developed and offered free of charge by the Pharmacy Quality Alliance [33]. As part of this program students learn how to "measure, improve, and report quality of care" [33]. However, perhaps a more explicit integration of the items comprising the factor innovation is possible?

It is also important to recognize that the reach of these programs is not complete. As such, this research should be extended and developed to apply the findings from this study to determine how to best help pharmacists transition their practices. This research, will go beyond simply mandating pharmacists to be more innovative. Rather it will be of key importance to account for the entire context in which pharmacists practice, as advocated for by implementation research [9,10]. A systematic review of implementation research studies in allied health professions identified 12 pharmacy-specific before-after and cohort studies, which primarily provided educational material to facilitate the integration of evidence into practice [34]. In addition to being of low methodological quality, these studies also make the underlying assumption that community pharmacists do not implement evidence because they lack appropriate education [34]. While this may be an important component of non-implementation, these studies have failed to account for structural barriers including poor workflow and staffing management that prevent pharmacists from taking adequate time to interact directly with patients in need of further intervention.

Two examples of studies furthering the objective of more fully accounting for the entire context of community pharmacy practice include: a qualitative study examining community pharmacists' perceptions of barriers and facilitators to targeted organizational structure adaptations to enhance the provision of medication adherence programming, and a cluster randomized trial to employ a facilitation intervention to improve the provision of medication management services in the community setting [35,36]. Moreover, the cluster randomized trial observed a decrease in the number of medication management services offered during the influenza vaccination season [36]. This means that future studies need to consider not only the time of year when interventions are implemented, but also consider how to deal with patients in need of medication reviews during this time period.

Study limitations: There are a few limitations to this study. First the use of the healthcare research firm to administer the survey may have consequences with respect to the generalizability of the survey results. However, given the correlations with previous Canadian findings it seems reasonable to suggest that this sample is not completely out of sync with the community pharmacy population in the US. Second, this work makes the assumption that at least part of the decision to provide MTM services rests with the pharmacist [21]. Without question, there are structural issues like high dispensing volumes, which were not accounted for in this study, that make it difficult for pharmacists to take on new practice opportunities, but this influence is not complete [6]. Third, MTM does not encompass all clinical services that community pharmacists may provide. As such, it is possible that possible relationships between the OCP and clinical services were missed. Fourth, while the sample of respondents from the southeastern US was randomly selected the characteristics of non-responders was not tracked. As such, the generalization of these findings to all community pharmacists should be approached with caution. Finally, the OCP provides just one perspective on the professional culture of community pharmacists in the US. To obtain a more complete vision of this professional culture additional work will need to be completed in this area.

6. Conclusions

The professional culture of pharmacy is an important part of the context of community pharmacy practice, of which a better understanding is required to ensure the successful integration of new practice opportunities into this setting. This validation of the OCP in a sample of community pharmacists from the US identified 6 cultural factors: social responsibility, innovation, people orientation, competitiveness, attention to detail, and reward orientation. A number of significant relationships were also observed between the factors and pharmacists' self-reported provision of MTM services like immunizations. This knowledge about the professional culture of community pharmacists provides further insight into the context of this environment, which when added to knowledge of structural barriers will improve pharmacists' ability to successfully implement new pharmacy services into their practices.

Acknowledgments: This project was funded by the American Association of Colleges of Pharmacy (AACP) New Investigator Award (206)—The content is the solely the responsibility of the authors and does necessarily represent the official views of the AACP.

Author Contributions: M.M.R. and E.H. conceived and designed the study; M.M.R. collected the data; M.M.R. and E.R.H. analyzed the data; M.M.R. and E.R.H. wrote the paper.

References

1.   Academy of Managed Care Pharmacy; American Pharmacists Association. Medicare star ratings: Stakeholder proceedings on community pharmacy and managed care partnerships in quality. *J. Am. Pharm. Assoc.* **2014**, *54*, 228–240.

2.   Santschi, V.; Chiolero, A.; Paradis, G.; Colosimo, A.L.; Burnaud, B. Pharmacist interventions to improve cardiovascular disease risk factors in diabetes: A systematic review and meta-analysis of randomized controlled trials. *Diabetes Care* **2012**, *12*, 2706–2717. [CrossRef] [PubMed]

3.   Houle, S.K.D.; Chuck, A.W.; McAlister, F.A.; Tsuyuki, R.T. Effect of a Pharmacist-Managed Hypertension Program on Health System Costs: An Evaluation of the Study of Cardiovascular Risk Intervention by Pharmacists—Hypertension (SCRIP-HTN). *Pharmacotherapy* **2012**, *32*, 527–537. [CrossRef] [PubMed]

4.   Tsuyuki, R.T.; Rosenthal, M.; Pearson, G. A randomized trial of a community-based approach to dyslipidemia management: Pharmacist prescribing to achieve cholesterol targets (RxACT study). *Can. Pharm. J.* **2016**, *149*, 283–292. [CrossRef] [PubMed]

5.   Latter, S.; Blenkinsopp, A.; Smith, A.; Chapmann, S.; Tinelli, M.; Gerard, K.; Little, P.; Celino, N.; Granby, T.; Nicholas, P.; et al. *Evaluation of Nurse and Pharmacist Independent Prescribing*; Department of Health Policy Research Programme: London, UK, 2010.

6.   Mossialos, E.; Courtin, E.; Naci, H.; Benrimoj, S.; Bouvy, M.; Farris, K.; Noyce, P.; Sketris, I. From "retailers" to health care proviers: Transforming the role of community pharmacists in chronic disease management. *Health Policy* **2015**, *119*, 628–639. [CrossRef] [PubMed]

7.   Schommer, J.; Gaither, C. A segmentation analysis for pharmacists' and patients views of pharmacists' role. *Res. Soc. Adm. Pharm.* **2014**, *10*, 508–528. [CrossRef] [PubMed]

8. Menigham, T. Provider Status Legislation Reintroduced: Your Voice Matters. Available online: http://www.pharmacistsprovidecare.com/CEOBlog/provider-status-legislation-reintroduced-your-voice-matters (accessed on 14 February 2017).

9. Brehaut, J.C.; Eva, K.W. Building theories of knowledge translation interventions: Use the entire menu of constructs. *Implement. Sci.* **2012**, *7*, 114. [CrossRef] [PubMed]

10. Peters, D.; Adam, T.; Alonge, O.; Agyepong, I.; Tran, N. Implementation resarch: What is it and how to do it? *Implement. Sci.* **2013**, *347*, f6753.

11. Bloor, G.; Dawson, P. Understanding professional culture in organizational context. *Organ. Stud.* **1994**, *15*, 275–295. [CrossRef]

12. Livigni, R. Occupational subcultures in the workplace. *Clin. Sociol. Rev.* **1994**, *12*, 290–291.

13. Vandenberghe, C. Organizational culture, person-culture fit, and turnover: A replication in the healthcare industry. *J. Organ. Behav.* **1999**, *20*, 175–184. [CrossRef]

14. Watling, C.; Drissen, E.; van der Vleuten, C.; Vanstone, M.; Lingard, L. Beyond individualism: Professional culture and its influence on feedback. *Med. Educ.* **2013**, *47*, 585–594. [CrossRef] [PubMed]

15. Hofstede, G. Indentifying organizational subcultures: An emperical approach. *J. Manag. Stud.* **1998**, *35*, 1–12. [CrossRef]

16. Boutin-Foster, C.; Foster, J.; Konopasek, L. Physician, know thyself: The professional culture of medicine as a framework for teaching cultural competence. *Acad. Med.* **2008**, *83*, 106–111. [CrossRef] [PubMed]

17. Roberts, C.S. Conflicting professional values in social work and medicine. *Health Soc. Work* **1989**, *14*, 211–218. [CrossRef] [PubMed]

18. Hopkins, A.; Solomon, J.; Abelson, J. Shifting boundaries in professional care. *J. R. Soc. Med.* **1996**, *89*, 364–371. [CrossRef] [PubMed]

19. Al Hamarneh, Y.; Rosenthal, M.; McElnay, J.; Tsuyuki, R. Pharmacists' perceptions of their professional role: Insights into hospital pharmacy culture. *Can. J. Hosp. Pharm.* **2011**, *64*, 31–35. [PubMed]

20. Rosenthal, M.; Breault, R.; Austin, Z.; Tsuyuki, R. Pharmacists' Self Perception of Their Professional Role: Insights into community pharmacy culture. *J. Am. Pharm. Assoc.* **2011**, *51*, 363–367. [CrossRef] [PubMed]

21. Rosenthal, M.; Tsao, N.W.; Tsuyuki, R.T.; Marra, C.A. Identifying relationships between the professional culture of pharmacy, pharmacists' personality traits, and the provision of advanced pharmacy services. *Res. Soc. Adm. Pharm.* **2016**, *12*, 56–67. [CrossRef] [PubMed]

22. Albanese, N.P.; Rouse, M.J. Scope of contemporary pharmacy practice: Roles, responsibilities, and functions of pharmacists and pharmacy technicians. *J. Am. Pharm. Assoc.* **2010**, *50*, e35–e69. [CrossRef] [PubMed]

23. Field, A. *Discovering Statistics Using SPSS Statistics*, 3rd ed.; Sage: Thousand Oaks, CA, USA, 2009.

24. American Pharmacists Association; National Association of Chain Drug Stores Foundation. Medication therapy management in pharmacy practice: Core elements of an MTM service model (version 2.0). *J. Am. Pharm. Assoc.* **2008**, *48*, 341–353.

25. Sarros, J.; Gray, J.; Densten, I.; Cooper, B. The organizational culture profile revisited and revised: An Australian perspective. *Aust. J. Manag.* **2005**, *30*, 159–182. [CrossRef]

26. Cable, D.M.; Judge, T.A. Interviewers' perceptions of person—Organization fit and organizational selection decisions. *J. Appl. Psychol.* **1997**, *82*, 546–561. [CrossRef] [PubMed]

27. DATAUSA: Pharmacists. Available online: https://datausa.io/profile/soc/291051/ (accessed on 20 March 2018).

28. Pharmacies in the United States. Available online: https://en.wikipedia.org/wiki/Pharmacies_in_the_United_States (accessed on 20 March 2018).

29. Qato, D.; Zenk, S.; Woilder, J.; Harrington, R.; Gaskin, D.; Alexander, C. The availability of pharmacies and pharmacy services in the United States: 2007–2015. *Value Health* **2017**, *19*, A268. [CrossRef]

30. Doucette, W.; Nevins, J.; Gaither, C.; Kreling, D.H.; Mott, D.A.; Pedersen, C.A.; Schommer, J.C. Organizational factors influencing pharmacy practice change. *Res. Soc. Adm. Pharm.* **2012**, *8*, 274–284. [CrossRef] [PubMed]

31. Folli, H.L.; Poole, R.L.; Benitz, W.E.; Russo, J.C. Medication error prevention by clinical pharmacists in two children's hospitals. *Pediatrics* **1987**, *79*, 718–722. [PubMed]

32. McConeghy, K.; Wing, C. A national examination of pharmacy-based immunization statutes and thier association with influenza vaccinations and preventive health. *Vaccine* **2016**, *34*, 3463–3468. [CrossRef] [PubMed]

33. Warholak, T.; Arya, V.; Hincapie, A.; Holdford, D.; West-Strum, D. Educating Pharmacists In Quality (EPIQ). Available online: http://pqaalliance.org/academic/epiq/welcome.asp (accessed on 20 March 2018).

34. Scott, S.; Albrecht, L.; O'Leary, K.; Ball, G.; Hartling, L.; Hofmeyer, A.; Jones, C.; Klassen, T.; Burns, K.; Newton, A.; et al. Systematic review of knowledge translation strategies in the allied health professions. *Implement. Sci.* **2012**, *7*, 70. [CrossRef] [PubMed]

35. Bacci, J.; McGrath, S. Implementation of targeted medication adherence interventions within a community chain pharmacy practice: The Pennsylvania project. *J. Am. Pharm. Assoc.* **2014**, *54*, 584–593. [CrossRef] [PubMed]

36. Houle, S.K.D.; Charrois, T.L.; Chowdury, F.F.; Tsuyuki, R.T.; Rosenthal, M. A randomized controlled study of practice facilitation to improve the provision of medication management services in Alberta community pharmacies. *Res. Soc. Adm. Pharm.* **2017**, *13*, 339–348. [CrossRef] [PubMed]

10

Pharmacists' Attitudes and Perceived Barriers to Human Papillomavirus (HPV) Vaccination Services

Tessa J. Hastings [1], Lindsey A. Hohmann [1], Stuart J. McFarland [2], Benjamin S. Teeter [3] and Salisa C. Westrick [1,*] 🆔

[1] Health Outcomes Research and Policy, Harrison School of Pharmacy Auburn University, 020 James E. Foy Hall, Auburn, AL 36849, USA; tjh0043@auburn.edu (T.J.H.); lah0036@auburn.edu (L.A.H.)

[2] College of Medicine, University of South Alabama, 307 N University Blvd, Mobile, AL 36688, USA; sjm1721@jagmail.southalabama.edu

[3] Department of Pharmacy Practice, College of Pharmacy, University of Arkansas for Medical Sciences, 4301 W Markham St, Little Rock, AR 72205, USA; BSTeeter@uams.edu

* Correspondence: westrsc@auburn.edu

Abstract: Use of non-traditional settings such as community pharmacies has been suggested to increase human papillomavirus (HPV) vaccination uptake and completion rates. The objectives of this study were to explore HPV vaccination services and strategies employed by pharmacies to increase HPV vaccine uptake, pharmacists' attitudes towards the HPV vaccine, and pharmacists' perceived barriers to providing HPV vaccination services in community pharmacies. A pre-piloted mail survey was sent to 350 randomly selected community pharmacies in Alabama in 2014. Measures included types of vaccines administered and marketing/recommendation strategies, pharmacists' attitudes towards the HPV vaccine, and perceived system and parental barriers. Data analysis largely took the form of descriptive statistics. 154 pharmacists completed the survey (response rate = 44%). The majority believed vaccination is the best protection against cervical cancer (85.3%), HPV is a serious threat to health for girls (78.8%) and boys (55.6%), and children should not wait until they are sexually active to be vaccinated (80.1%). Perceived system barriers included insufficient patient demand (56.5%), insurance plans not covering vaccination cost (54.8%), and vaccine expiration before use (54.1%). Respondents also perceived parents to have inadequate education and understanding about HPV infection (86.6%) and vaccine safety (78.7%). Pharmacists have positive perceptions regarding the HPV vaccine. Barriers related to system factors and perceived parental concerns must be overcome to increase pharmacist involvement in HPV vaccinations.

Keywords: human papillomavirus; community pharmacy; cervical cancer; adolescent vaccination

1. Introduction

Human papillomavirus (HPV) infection is an important public health issue. Almost 80 million people are infected with HPV in the United States, and most sexually active individuals will contract some form of HPV during their lifetime [1]. HPV strains 16 and 18 cause over 70% of cervical cancer cases [2]. Three types of HPV vaccine are currently approved in the U.S. to prevent infection with these HPV strains: Gardasil® (for girls and boys age 9–26 years), Gardasil 9® (for girls age 9–26 years and boys age 9–15 years), and Cervarix® (for girls age 9–25 years) [2]. In addition to strains 16 and 18, Gardasil® and Gardasil 9® protect against several additional less common cancer-causing strains [2]. Guidelines recommend administration of one of these vaccines as a three-dose series beginning at 11 years of age [2]. Despite this recommendation, adolescent HPV vaccination rates remain low. Globally, it is estimated that 59 million women (50.1%) receive at least one dose of HPV and 47 million (39.7%) complete the three-dose series [3]. In the United States in 2015, 4 out of 10 adolescent girls and

5 out of 10 adolescent boys had never received a single dose of the HPV vaccine [4]. Furthermore, completion of the three-dose series falls far below the 80% United States national objective, with only 41.9% of girls and 28.1% of boys vaccinated with three doses in 2015 [4]. This low vaccination rate is concerning for the prevention of cervical cancer in the United States, especially in southern states, where vaccination rates are disproportionately low but where vaccines are needed most, suggested by a higher than average incidence of cervical cancer [5,6]. In Alabama, 40.8% of girls and only 22.6% of boys completed the three dose series in 2015 [4].

Barriers to initiation and completion of the HPV vaccine series reported in existing literature include lack of recommendation by primary care providers, cost, insurance coverage, necessity of multiple visits to primary care providers, and parental concerns [7]. Also, about one-third of adolescents age 13–17 years old had no preventive care visits with their physicians, creating a lack of opportunity to recommend the HPV vaccine [8]. Innovative methods to overcome these barriers and to promote the HPV vaccine among hard-to-reach adolescents are needed to improve HPV vaccination and completion rates. One method that has been suggested is the use of non-traditional settings such as community pharmacies, as they are easily accessible with longer hours of operation and no need for appointments, unlike traditional settings such as a physician's office [9]. In addition to the convenience and accessibility offered by pharmacies, the literature shows that parents and adolescents support pharmacy-based provision of vaccinations [9–11].

Pharmacists are increasingly becoming accepted as immunization providers for adult vaccinations by patients, physicians, and national organizations in the United States [12], and globally [13–16]. Currently in the United States, all 50 states permit pharmacists to administer vaccines [17]. Many states include the HPV vaccine within this authority; however, the specific requirements and limitations vary widely by state [17]. Pharmacists in Alabama are permitted to administer any vaccine to patients with no age restrictions [18]. However, for some cases, such as the administration of the HPV vaccine, pharmacists are required to obtain a prescription from a licensed prescriber [18]. Despite wide acceptance among adults, little is known about adolescent vaccination services in US community pharmacies, especially for the HPV vaccine. The objectives of this study were to explore: (1) the extent to which HPV vaccination services are currently being offered in community pharmacies as well as strategies to increase the uptake of the HPV vaccine; (2) pharmacists' attitudes towards the HPV vaccine; and (3) perceived barriers to the provision of HPV vaccination services in community pharmacies.

2. Materials and Methods

2.1. Study Design and Sample

This study utilized a cross-sectional survey of community pharmacies in Alabama. The unit of analysis was at the pharmacy level. One key informant represented each pharmacy; they included pharmacy owners, managers, or staff pharmacists. All procedures were approved by the first author's Institutional Review Board as an expedited review.

The sampling frame used in this study to select community pharmacies was Hayes' Directory, a database of community pharmacies in the United States, which provided name, mailing address, county name, telephone number, and fax number for each community pharmacy. Pharmacies that did not serve the typical public (i.e., walk-in customers) or dispense medications were excluded from participation. Pharmacies were not required to provide HPV vaccination services in order to participate in this study. Of the 1176 community pharmacies in Alabama, 350 community pharmacies were randomly sampled. The decision to invite 350 pharmacies was made after careful consideration of the balance between survey costs and survey errors. Based on our previous survey studies with community pharmacies, we anticipated response rates to fall between 30% and 40%, which would result in an expected sample size of 105–140 [19,20]. Setting a confidence level of 95%, a sample size of 350 would yield a margin of error range between 7.4% and 8.8%, which was deemed acceptable.

The survey was administered from June to August 2014 based on a modified version of Dillman's Tailored Design Method [21]. To maximize the response rate and minimize the likelihood of non-response bias, four methods of contact were employed including a pre-notification postcard, a survey packet, a reminder postcard, and a replacement survey packet; all were delivered via first-class mail and addressed to the pharmacist. A web address was provided on all contacts that led to an online version of the survey for those who preferred to complete the survey electronically. To ensure that multiple pharmacists from one location did not complete the survey, a unique identifier was assigned to each pharmacy, which was required to access the electronic survey. Survey packets and replacement packets contained an invitation letter, information letter, survey, and pre-addressed, stamped return envelope. The invitation letter included in this packet briefly explained the purpose of this study, how to participate, and the completion deadline. Details regarding study participation were outlined in the information letter including risks, benefits, compensation, and confidentiality. Each respondent received a $20 incentive after receipt of their completed survey. To maintain confidentiality, the last page of the survey containing contact information for payment purposes was separated from the survey packet upon receipt. Respondents were made aware that findings would be reported in aggregated form and that identifiable data would be kept confidential and only accessed by the research team.

2.2. Survey Variables and Measures

The survey was comprised of 65 questions and required approximately 15 min to complete. Measures can be categorized into five sections: (1) key informant and pharmacy site demographic characteristics; (2) general vaccination services and strategies used to increase HPV vaccine uptake; (3) pharmacists' perceptions of HPV and the vaccine; (4) perceived system barriers to the provision of HPV vaccinations; and (5) perceived parental reasons for HPV vaccine hesitancy. The majority of questions were formatted as 5-point Likert-type rating scales. For example, *"How much do you agree or disagree with the following statements about the parents of teens and adolescents and their perceptions regarding HPV vaccine?"* with answer choices ranging from strongly disagree to strongly agree. Survey questions assessing vaccination services and strategies to increase uptake were informed by our prior research in vaccination services, while items measuring perceptions of HPV and the vaccine were modified from an existing instrument utilized by Khan and colleagues [22]. To assess system barriers, previous research informed the survey items [23–25]. Lastly, an existing measure developed by Luque and colleagues to assess perceived parental reasons for vaccine hesitancy was used [23].

2.3. Pre-Testing

The survey questions were written and refined by the research team. To ensure the content validity of survey questions, the research team consulted with a licensed pharmacist. After changes were made, the survey was pre-tested with 6 community pharmacists in Alabama in order to assess the face validity of the included measures. Based on their feedback, minor modifications to the formatting and answer choices were made to improve clarity. Due to their participation in pre-testing of the survey questions, these 6 pharmacists were excluded from the sampling frame prior to selecting the random sample.

2.4. Non-Response Bias Investigation

A non-response investigation was conducted after survey completion to determine if respondents' demographic characteristics and the vaccination services they offered differed significantly when compared to non-respondents. Community pharmacies that did not respond to survey requests were randomly selected and contacted via telephone. Using a five-minute structured telephone interview, scripted interview questions gathered information regarding key informant and pharmacy site demographics as well as general vaccination services provided. Non-respondents' data was aggregated and compared to that of respondents to assess any differences.

2.5. Data Analysis

All data analysis was performed using IBM SPSS Statistics version 22 software (IBM Corp., Armonk, NY, USA). Descriptive statistics were used to describe respondent characteristics, current vaccination practices, attitudes, and barriers. Comparison of non-respondents and respondents to investigate non-response bias was completed using one-way analysis of variance for continuous variables and chi-square for categorical variables. A significance level of 0.05 was used for all statistical analyses.

3. Results

3.1. Demographics and Non-Response Bias Investigation

A total of 154 pharmacies completed the survey (44% response rate). Table 1 displays the demographics of respondents and their pharmacies. The majority of key informants were female (57.5%), held a PharmD degree (50.6%), were employed as pharmacy managers (54.5%), and were trained in vaccine administration (80.8%). Thirty pharmacies were randomly sampled in the non-response bias investigation, of which 18 responded. There were no significant differences found between respondents and non-respondents in terms of individual and site demographics. Additionally, there were no significant differences found in the number of vaccine types offered in the past 12 months between respondents and non-respondents.

Table 1. Respondent and Pharmacy Characteristics.

Characteristics	Number (%)
Sex (N = 153)	
Male	65 (42.5)
Female	88 (57.5)
Education (N = 154)	
PharmD	78 (50.6)
B.S. Pharmacy	73 (47.4)
Residency	5 (3.2)
Masters	1 (0.6)
Other	3 (1.9)
Title (N = 154)	
Pharmacy Manager	84 (54.5)
Staff Pharmacist	45 (29.2)
Owner/Partner	33 (21.4)
Other	2 (1.3)
Trained in Vaccine Administration (N = 151)	
Yes	122 (80.8)
No	29 (19.2)
Type of Pharmacy (N = 153)	
Chain Pharmacy	81 (52.9)
Independently Owned Pharmacy	72 (47.1)
Hours Open per Week (N = 154)	
Less than 40 h	3 (1.9)
40–49 h	17 (11.0)
50–59 h	47 (30.5)
60–69 h	18 (11.7)
70–79 h	48 (31.2)
80 or more hours	21 (13.6)

Table 1. *Cont.*

Characteristics	Number (%)
Average Prescription Volume per Day (N = 153)	
Less than 100	15 (9.8)
100–199	58 (37.9)
200–299	39 (25.5)
300–399	19 (12.4)
400+	22 (14.4)
	Mean (SD)
Number of Years Practicing as a Pharmacist (N = 153)	16.8 (13.5)
Number of Years at Current Pharmacy (N = 151)	7.5 (7.6)
Number of Staff Pharmacists Employed (FTE) (N = 152)	2.1 (1.1)
Number of PharmD Staff Pharmacists Employed (FTE) (N = 146)	1.1 (.9)
Number of Technicians Employed (FTE) (N = 153)	3.8 (2.2)
Number of Pharmacists Trained in Vaccine Administration (N = 153)	1.8 (1.1)
Number of Pharmacists Actively Administering Vaccines (N = 153)	1.7 (1.2)
Number of Vaccine Types Available in the Past 12 Months (N = 113)	3.55 (3.5)

3.2. HPV Vaccination Services and Strategies Employed to Increase HPV Vaccine Uptake

Table 2 details the number of pharmacies providing vaccinations and the strategies employed to increase vaccine uptake. A total of 113 responding pharmacies (73.4%) reported offering at least one vaccination in the previous 12 months. Of these pharmacies, influenza was the most common vaccine provided (94.7%), followed by herpes zoster (83.2%), pneumococcal polysaccharide (PPSV23) (53.1%), and tetanus/diphtheria/pertussis (Tdap) (42.5%). Among those that provided at least one type of vaccine, most (82.6%) did not encounter any patients requesting information about the HPV vaccine. Further, 89% of pharmacies had not made any recommendations to male or female patients or parents of patients regarding the need for the HPV vaccine. Over 90% of pharmacies also indicated that they did not refer patients to places other than the pharmacy to obtain the HPV vaccine. Among the 9 pharmacies that did report referring patients to another location for the HPV vaccine, the most commonly mentioned site was a pediatrician's office.

Table 2. Vaccination Services and Strategies Utilized to Increase Human Papillomavirus Vaccinations.

Characteristics	No. (%)
Vaccination services offered in the past 12 months	
Influenza	107 (94.7)
Herpes zoster	94 (83.2)
Pneumococcal polysaccharide (PPSV23)	60 (53.1)
Tetanus/Diphtheria/Pertussis (Tdap)	48 (42.5)
Pneumococcal 13-valent conjugate (PCV13)	39 (34.5)
Hepatitis B	35 (31.1)
Meningococcal	33 (29.2)
Travel vaccines (yellow fever, typhoid, etc)	28 (24.8)
Hepatitis A	27 (23.9)
Measles, mumps, rubella (MMR)	23 (20.4)
Tetanus/Diphtheria (Td)	23 (20.4)
Human papillomavirus (HPV)	20 (17.7)
Varicella	11 (9.7)
Other	2 (1.8)
Patients requested information about the HPV vaccine in the past 12 months (N = 109)	
Yes	19 (17.4)
No	90 (82.6)

Table 2. *Cont.*

Characteristics	No. (%)
Recommended HPV vaccine to male and female patients or parents of male and female patients in the past 12 months (*N* = 110) [a]	
Male patients 11–12 years	3 (2.7)
Male patients 13–18 years	3 (2.7)
Male patients 19–26 years	2 (1.8)
Female patients 11–12 years	5 (4.5)
Female patients 13–18 years	3 (2.7)
Female patients 19–26 years	5 (4.5)
No recommendations have been made	98 (89)
Referred patients to other places for HPV vaccine in the past 12 months (*N* = 113)	
Yes	9 (8.0)
County Health Department	1 (11.1)
Physician in general	2 (22.2)
OBGYN specifically	1 (11.1)
PCP or gynecologist	1 (11.1)
Pediatrician	4 (44.4)
No	104 (92)
HPV vaccine administered in the past 12 months (*N* = 113)	
Yes	5 (4.4)
Per written protocol with physician	3 (60)
Patients obtain and bring in written prescription from physician	1 (20)
Pharmacy contacts other known physician/physician co-worker to obtain prescription	1 (20)
No	108 (95.6)
Plans to offer/continue offering HPV vaccine in the next 12 months (*N* = 113)	
Yes	36 (31.9)
No	77 (68.1)
	Mean (SD)
Number of HPV vaccine doses administered in the past 12 months (*N* = 5)	1.4 (0.55)

[a] Participants were instructed to choose all applicable categories.

Of the 18 pharmacies that reported having the HPV vaccine available in stock, only 5 pharmacies had actually administered the HPV vaccine, averaging less than 2 doses in the past year. Three of the five pharmacies that provided the vaccine in the past 12 months did so through a written protocol with a physician, while another stated that they contacted a physician they had worked with in the past in order to obtain a prescription for the patient allowing them to administer the HPV vaccine. The fifth pharmacy administered the HPV vaccine only after the patient obtained and delivered a written prescription from his or her physician. Although only 18 pharmacies reported having HPV vaccine in stock and only 5 had actually administered the vaccine in the past 12 months, 36 (31.9%) indicated that they planned to offer or continue offering the vaccine in the next 12 months.

It is worth noting the various marketing strategies the 5 pharmacies that administered the HPV vaccine in the past 12 months employed. Methods reported to market HPV vaccinations included: general flyers accompanying dispensed prescriptions, billboards, posters at the pharmacy, and generic telephone messages. When asked if they used a system to identify patients who were eligible for their first dose of HPV vaccine, 3 of 5 said no; they did not use any personalized methods to market their HPV vaccination services. When comparing general vaccination strategies used by those pharmacies that had administered the HPV vaccine in the past 12 months to those that had not, the proportion using flyers, generic telephone messages, billboards, and posters were similar (Table 3). Pharmacies that had not administered the HPV vaccine in the past 12 months reported employing additional strategies including newspapers (33.3%) and radio announcements (26.7%).

Table 3. Comparison of General Marketing Strategies Used by Pharmacies who had and had not Administered the HPV Vaccine in the Past 12 Months [a].

General Marketing Strategies	Pharmacies with HPV Vaccine in Stock ($N = 20$)	
	Administered HPV Vaccine in the Past 12 Months ($N = 5$)	Did not Administer HPV Vaccine in the Past 12 Months ($N = 15$)
Newspapers	0	5 (33.3%)
Radio announcements	0	4 (26.7%)
Flyers accompanying prescriptions dispensed	4 (80.0%)	12 (80.0%)
Generic telephone messages	3 (60.0%)	8 (53.3%)
Billboards	1 (20.0%)	4 (26.7%)
Posters at pharmacy	5 (100%)	14 (93.3%)
Other	0	3 (20.0%)
None	0	1 (6.7%)

[a] Strategies include those used for the marketing of any vaccine, not specific to the HPV vaccine.

3.3. Pharmacists' Attitudes towards HPV and the Vaccine

Table 4 shows pharmacists' attitudes towards HPV and the HPV vaccine. A large percentage (47.3%) of pharmacists strongly agreed that vaccination against HPV is the best protection against cervical cancer. Over 78% percent agreed that HPV infection is a serious threat to a girl's health, but a much lower proportion (55.6%) felt the same about HPV's threat to a boy's health. Over half of respondents (52.7%) agreed that the optimal age to have a child vaccinated against HPV is 11–12 years. Further, 43.7% agreed that vaccinated children will not practice riskier sexual behaviors. No differences were found in pharmacists' attitudes toward HPV/HPV vaccine based on demographic factors (gender, number of years practicing as a pharmacist, or vaccine administration training).

3.4. Barriers to Providing HPV Vaccinations

Pharmacists reported a number of perceived system barriers to providing HPV vaccination services (Table 5). Over half (56.5%) of respondents reported that a lack of patients who want the HPV vaccine was extremely or very likely to be a factor preventing their pharmacy from providing HPV vaccination services. Other factors perceived to be very/extremely likely to be barriers include: the failure of some insurance companies to cover the cost of the vaccination (54.8%); the vaccine expiring before use (54.1%); difficulty ensuring that patients complete the necessary three doses (39.9%); and lack of adequate reimbursement (38.4%).

Table 6 reports respondents' perceived parental reasons for HPV vaccine hesitancy. The majority of respondents believed that parents lack adequate education about the HPV infection (86.6% somewhat or strongly agree). Parental concerns about the safety (78.7%), reluctance to discuss sexuality/sexually transmitted infections (76%), concerns that the vaccine condones premarital sex (67.3%), beliefs that their child is not at risk (67.3%), beliefs that their child is too young (65.3%), concerns about efficacy (64.6%), concerns about children practicing riskier sex behaviors (58.7%), and cost (53.3%) were also found to be perceived barriers. No differences were found in pharmacists' perceived barriers to HPV vaccination based on demographic factors (gender, number of years practicing as a pharmacist, or vaccine administration training).

Table 4. Pharmacists' attitudes of Human Papillomavirus (HPV) and HPV vaccine, Number (%) [a,b].

Statement	Strongly Disagree	Somewhat Disagree	No Opinion/Unsure	Somewhat Agree	Strongly Agree
HPV vaccine is the best protection against cervical cancer. (N = 150)	2 (1.3)	5 (3.3)	15 (10.0)	57 (38.0)	**71 (47.3)**
HPV is a serious threat to a girl's health.	10 (6.6)	9 (6.0)	13 (8.6)	50 (33.1)	**69 (45.7)**
HPV is a serious threat to a boy's health.	12 (7.9)	15 (9.9)	40 (26.5)	**52 (34.4)**	32 (21.2)
I believe the optimal age to have a child vaccinated against HPV is age 11–12. (N = 150)	7 (4.7)	24 (16.0)	40 (26.7)	**49 (32.7)**	30 (20.0)
I believe the optimal age to have a child vaccinated against HPV is age 13–18. (N = 150)	13 (8.7)	19 (12.7)	41 (27.3)	**56 (37.3)**	21 (14.0)
Vaccinated children will not practice riskier sex behaviors.	29 (19.2)	24 (15.9)	32 (21.2)	**40 (26.5)**	26 (17.2)
HPV vaccine should be mandatory for all children age 11–12.	43 (28.5)	**49 (32.5)**	34 (22.5)	16 (10.6)	9 (6.0)
I have concerns about the safety of the HPV vaccine.	25 (16.6)	**43 (28.5)**	**43 (28.5)**	36 (24.8)	4 (2.6)
The side effects of HPV vaccine could outweigh the benefits.	25 (16.6)	**44 (29.1)**	33 (21.9)	36 (23.8)	13 (8.6)
I have concerns about the efficacy of the HPV vaccine. (N = 150)	32 (21.3)	**51 (34.0)**	35 (23.3)	23 (15.3)	9 (6.0)
I believe I would wait to encourage a child to be vaccinated against HPV until age 19–26.	**50 (33.1)**	49 (32.5)	40 (26.5)	9 (6.0)	3 (2.0)
I do not believe that children should be vaccinated against HPV until they are sexually active.	**64 (42.4)**	57 (37.7)	21 (13.9)	6 (4.0)	3 (2.0)
I do not believe in HPV vaccination because of religious or moral reasons.	**97 (64.2)**	26 (17.2)	25 (16.6)	3 (2.0)	0 (0)

[a] The most frequently chosen responses/answers are bold for each question; [b] N = 151 unless otherwise stated.

Table 5. Pharmacists' perceived system-related barriers to provision of HPV vaccine, Number (%) [a].

Statement on System Barriers [b]	Not at All	A Little	Moderate	Very	Extremely
There are too few patients who want the HPV vaccine. (N = 147)	15 (10.2)	23 (15.6)	26 (17.7)	**46 (31.3)**	37 (25.2)
The failure of some insurance companies to cover the cost of vaccination. (N = 146)	20 (13.7)	14 (9.6)	32 (21.9)	**46 (31.5)**	34 (23.3)
The vaccine expiring before use. (N = 148)	24 (16.2)	18 (12.2)	26 (17.6)	**43 (29.1)**	37 (25.0)
The difficulty ensuring patients are completing the necessary 3 doses of the HPV vaccine. (N = 148)	25 (16.9)	26 (17.6)	38 (25.7)	**39 (26.4)**	20 (13.5)
The lack of adequate reimbursement for the HPV vaccination. (N = 146)	31 (21.2)	26 (17.8)	33 (22.6)	**34 (23.3)**	22 (15.1)
The cost of stocking the HPV vaccine. (N = 147)	**42 (28.6)**	27 (18.4)	29 (19.7)	34 (23.1)	15 (20.2)
The need to acquire a prescription from a physician to administer the HPV vaccine. (N = 147)	**54 (36.7)**	25 (17.0)	35 (23.8)	24 (16.3)	9 (6.1)
The amount of time it takes to talk to patients and/or parents about the HPV vaccine. (N = 147)	**69 (46.9)**	27 (18.4)	29 (19.7)	18 (12.2)	4 (2.7)
The refrigerator space needed to store the HPV vaccine. (N = 147)	**90 (61.2)**	27 (18.4)	20 (13.6)	9 (6.1)	1 (0.7)

[a] The most frequently chosen responses/answers are bold for each question; [b] Respondents rated how likely each factor was to be a barrier in providing HPV vaccination services.

Table 6. Pharmacists' perceived parent-related barriers to provision of HPV vaccine ($N = 150$), Number (%) [a].

Statement on Parent-Related Barriers [b]	Strongly Disagree	Somewhat Disagree	Unsure	Somewhat Agree	Strongly Agree
Parents have concerns about the safety of the HPV vaccine.	0 (0)	6 (4.0)	26 (17.3)	**93 (62.0)**	25 (16.7)
Parents are concerned that by agreeing to have their children immunized, they are condoning premarital sex.	5 (3.3)	15 (10.0)	29 (19.3)	**83 (55.3)**	18 (12.0)
Parents have concerns about the efficacy of the HPV vaccine.	3 (2.0)	18 (12.0)	32 (21.3)	**83 (55.3)**	14 (9.3)
Parents lack adequate education / understanding about the HPV infection.	0 (0)	2 (1.3)	18 (12.0)	80 (53.3)	50 (33.3)
Parents believe their children are not at risk for HPV infection.	2 (1.3)	15 (10.0)	32 (21.3)	**80 (53.3)**	21 (14.0)
Parents are reluctant to discuss sexuality / sexually transmitted infections.	2 (1.3)	14 (9.3)	20 (13.3)	**76 (50.7)**	38 (25.3)
Parents believe their children are too young for the HPV vaccine.	2 (1.3)	8 (5.3)	42 (28.0)	**74 (49.3)**	24 (16.0)
Parents are concerned that their children will practice riskier sexual behaviors if they receive the HPV vaccine.	4 (2.7)	25 (16.7)	33 (22.0)	**73 (48.7)**	15 (10.0)
Parents believe the cost of the HPV vaccine is too high.	1 (0.7)	10 (6.7)	**59 (39.3)**	**59 (39.3)**	21 (14.0)
Parents will not consent to HPV vaccination.	4 (2.7)	23 (15.3)	**70 (46.7)**	51 (34.0)	2 (1.3)
Parents oppose HPV vaccination for moral or religious reasons.	5 (3.3)	27 (18.0)	**63 (42.0)**	48 (32.0)	7 (4.7)

[a] The most frequently chosen responses/answers are bold for each question; [b] Respondents rated how likely each factor was to be a barrier in providing HPV vaccination services.

4. Discussion

HPV vaccination rates are disproportionately low in the Southern United States, which is especially concerning due to the higher rate of cervical cancer in this region when compared to other regions of the U.S. [5]. Utilizing community pharmacies for the provision of the HPV vaccine may be a method to increase vaccination rates, especially in rural areas where access to vaccine providers is limited. However, this study shows that the HPV vaccine provision in community pharmacies is low. Of pharmacies providing vaccinations, we found that only 11.7% had the HPV vaccine in their inventory. This rate in Alabama is much lower than the national survey's results which reported that 37% of U.S. pharmacies provide the HPV vaccine [26]. This lower rate could be attributed to several system barriers such as perceived lack of patient interest, insufficient reimbursement, and perceived parental hesitancy. Results from the study show that marketing strategies did not differ markedly between pharmacies that administer the HPV vaccine and those that do not. As 68.1% of pharmacists reported that they do not plan to offer or continue offering the vaccine in the next year, future research should demonstrate successful HPV vaccine services in community pharmacies and outline strategies to overcome system barriers and parental hesitancy.

Pharmacists generally reported positive perceptions of the HPV vaccine; however, there were many perceived system barriers identified that could be limiting the provision of this vaccine in the community pharmacy setting. Some of these barriers are related to the vaccine itself while others are related to coverage and reimbursement for the vaccine. Lack of reimbursement has been identified in previous research as a barrier to general vaccine provision [27,28]. Countries such as the United Kingdom and Australia, which are able to overcome this reimbursement barrier due to differences in the structure of their health care system, have achieved much higher HPV vaccination uptake when compared to the United States. The United Kingdom and Australia reported HPV vaccination rates among girls to be 60.4% and 71.2% respectively [29]. Previous research has also identified the need to acquire a prescription from a physician to administer the vaccine as a challenge [17]. This did not appear to be a factor affecting the decision to offer the vaccine among the majority of pharmacists in this study, perhaps because other barriers overwhelm them.

Overall, the results of this study show that a greater proportion of pharmacists rated perceptions of parental concerns and hesitancy as likely barriers to a greater extent when compared to the system-related factors. This suggests that while system factors may hinder the provision of HPV vaccination services, pharmacists' perceptions of parental concerns and hesitancy may be more of a factor in impeding pharmacists' from making recommendations to parents. This is not surprising, as many system-related barriers may have already been addressed in the development of immunization services for other vaccinations. Looking specifically at parental concerns, the majority of pharmacists believe that parents lack adequate understanding regarding the HPV infection in general. This perception may be valid, as studies in southern regions have reported that parents have limited knowledge and awareness of the HPV infection and HPV vaccine [30,31]. Overall, the majority of pharmacists believed that parents' perceptions of the HPV infection and vaccine were barriers to teens and adolescents receiving this vaccine. Additionally, the majority of responders believe that the optimal age to be vaccinated against HPV is 11–12. Because of the young age of vaccine recipients, pharmacists may perceive that parents would not be ready for pharmacists to provide the HPV vaccine to their adolescent children; this belief is consistent with the findings reported by Westrick and colleagues [9]. Hence, addressing system factors may be helpful but will likely be unsuccessful unless pharmacists' perceived parental barriers are overcome. One method to overcome these barriers may include training pharmacy staff to be confident and proactive in educating and recommending the HPV vaccine to parents. Receiving positive responses from parents could help improve their perceptions of parental concerns and motivate them to recommend the vaccine to the parents of adolescents.

Research has shown that provider recommendations are a key factor influencing vaccine uptake [7]. However, we found that pharmacists in this study did not recommend the HPV vaccine. Such missed opportunities have been successfully reduced via the use of provider reminder systems [32]. Thus, to bring about change in community pharmacies, pharmacists' recommendations may be facilitated by installation of reminder systems in pharmacy dispensing software to aid in identifying vaccine-eligible patients. Potential reminder strategies may include posters in the pharmacy, immunization registry-based reminders and age-based "flags" in patients' prescription bags to alert pharmacists to vaccination opportunities, or ready-made forms to quickly allow pharmacists or technicians to make personalized recommendations while counseling patients or at prescription drop-off, respectively [32–35]. Two of the five pharmacies administering the HPV vaccine in this study had implemented systems such as these to identify eligible patients. These strategies require minimum time-commitment from the pharmacist and pharmacy staff, and have been shown to increase patients' commitment to receive vaccination services at a community pharmacy [33]. Buy-in and referrals from local physicians are also important and may be achieved through letters to physicians' offices highlighting pharmacy vaccination services [32]. Buy-in could also be established through collaborative practice agreements; three of the five pharmacies administering the HPV vaccine in this study did have a written protocol. These physicians may partner with pharmacies such that the first dose of the HPV vaccine is administered at the physician's office and the physician writes a prescription for the second and third doses to be obtained at a community pharmacy [32]. This strategy may ultimately save physicians' and nurses' time, maximize pharmacies' profitability, and increase convenience for the patient due to pharmacies' extended hours of operation.

This study has several limitations that must be considered. First, although the overall response rate was 44% (154 pharmacies out of 350 sampled), only 5 respondents (3.2%) reported administering the HPV vaccine in the past 12 months, which might limit meaningful interpretation of pharmacies' marketing strategies to increase HPV vaccinations. HPV vaccine specific marketing strategies used by respondents who had not administered the HPV vaccine in the past 12 months were not assessed. It is possible that these pharmacies were using HPV vaccine specific marketing strategies but that they were not successful. Future research should further examine marketing strategies in greater detail, including variations in success for specific vaccines. Furthermore, identification of potential vaccine recipients is the first step. As such, future research should assess how pharmacists identify potential recipients and their confidence in doing so. While this study assessed pharmacists' attitudes toward the HPV vaccine, pharmacists' confidence in speaking to parents and patients about the vaccine was not addressed. This is an area of future study that will be necessary for the development of suggested educational training programs. Additionally, a greater proportion of key informants were female (57.5%) and employed as pharmacy managers (54.5%). Thus, the study's findings may not be generalizable to all pharmacists in Alabama. Also, the study's population of interest was community pharmacies in Alabama, and therefore results may not be generalizable to community pharmacies in other countries and areas of the United States. As this study collected self-reported attitudes and behaviors, social-desirability and recall bias may be a concern. Finally, individuals who responded to the survey may differ from non-respondents. However, no statistically significant differences were found in the non-response bias investigation.

5. Conclusions

Pharmacists have positive attitudes regarding provision of the HPV vaccine to teens and adolescents. However, system factors and perceived parental concerns may prevent pharmacists from engaging in the provision of the HPV vaccination in community pharmacies. Overcoming these barriers is necessary to increase pharmacist involvement in HPV vaccinations. Strategies to do so may include pharmacy staff training, reminder systems, and physician partnerships among others.

Acknowledgments: The authors wish to acknowledge Auburn University Research Initiative in Cancer (AURIC) for their role in funding this study. This sponsor played no role in manuscript preparation.

Author Contributions: Tessa J. Hastings contributed to data analysis and lead the manuscript preparation. Lindsey A. Hohmann contributed to data analysis and manuscript preparation. Stuart J. McFarland and Benjamin S. Teeter contributed to study planning, data collection, and manuscript editing. Salisa C. Westrick contributed to all aspects of the study, leading the study design and data collection as well as serving as the corresponding author.

Disclaimer: Poster presentation at the National Immunization Conference held 13–15 September 2016 in Atlanta, GA, USA.

Funding Sources: The authors wish to acknowledge Auburn University Research Initiative in Cancer (AURIC) for their role in funding this study.

References

1. Centers for Disease Control and Prevention. STD Facts—Human papillomavirus (HPV). 2014. Available online: http://www.cdc.gov/std/HPV/STDFact-HPV.htm#a7 (accessed on 24 March 2016).

2. National Cancer Institute. Human Papillomavirus (HPV) Vaccines. 2015. Available online: http://www.cancer.gov/about-cancer/causes-prevention/risk/infectious-agents/hpv-vaccine-fact-sheet (accessed on 26 August 2016).

3. Bruni, L.; Diaz, M.; Barrionuevo-Rosas, L.; Herrero, R.; Bray, F.; Bosch, F.X.; de Sanjosé, S.; Castellsagué, X. Global estimates of human papillomavirus vaccination coverage by region and income level: A pooled analysis. *Lancet Glob. Health* **2016**, *4*, e453–e463. [CrossRef]

4. Reagan-Steiner, S.; Yankey, D.; Jeyarajah, J.; Elam-Evans, L.D.; Curtis, C.R.; MacNeil, J.; Markowitz, L.E.; Singleton, J.A. National, Regional, State, and Selected Local Area Vaccination Coverage Among Adolescents Aged 13–17 Years—United States, 2015. *Morb. Mortal. Wkly. Rep.* **2016**, *65*, 850–858. [CrossRef] [PubMed]

5. Rahman, M.; Islam, M.; Berenson, A.B. Differences in HPV Immunization Levels Among Young Adults in Various Regions of the United States. *J. Commun. Health* **2015**, *40*, 404–408. [CrossRef] [PubMed]

6. Centers for Disease Control and Prevention. Human Papillomavirus (HPV). 2015. Available online: http://www.cdc.gov/std/HPV/STDFact-HPV.htm#a7 (accessed on 1 July 2015).

7. Brewer, N.T.; Fazekas, K.I. Predictors of HPV vaccine acceptability: A theory-informed, systematic review. *Prev. Med.* **2007**, *45*, 107–114. [CrossRef] [PubMed]

8. Nordin, J.D.; Solberg, L.I.; Parker, E.D. Adolescent primary care visit patterns. *Ann. Fam. Med.* **2010**, *8*, 511–516. [CrossRef] [PubMed]

9. Westrick, S.C.; Hohmann, L.A.; McFarland, S.J.; Teeter, B.S.; White, K.K.; Hastings, T.J. Parental acceptance of human papillomavirus vaccinations and community pharmacies as vaccination settings: A qualitative study in Alabama. *Papillomavirus Res.* **2017**, *3*, 24–29. [CrossRef] [PubMed]

10. Reiter, P.L.; Brewer, N.T.; Gottlieb, S.L.; McRee, A.L.; Smith, J.S. Parents' health beliefs and HPV vaccination of their adolescent daughters. *Soc. Sci. Med.* **2009**, *69*, 475–480. [CrossRef] [PubMed]

11. McRee, A.-L.; Reiter, P.L.; Pepper, J.K.; Brewer, N.T. Correlates of comfort with alternative settings for HPV vaccine delivery. *Hum. Vaccines Immunother.* **2013**, *9*, 306–313. [CrossRef]

12. Centers for Disease Control and Prevention. *Letter to Pharmacists and Community Vaccinators*; Centers for Disease Control and Prevention: Atlanta, GA, USA, 2012.

13. Evans, A.M.; Wood, F.C.; Carter, B. National community pharmacy NHS influenza vaccination service in Wales: A primary care mixed methods study. *Br. J. Gen. Pract.* **2016**, *66*, e248–e257. [CrossRef] [PubMed]

14. Hattingh, H.L.; Sim, T.F.; Parsons, R.; Czarniak, P.; Vickery, A.; Ayadurai, S. Evaluation of the first pharmacist-administered vaccinations in Western Australia: A mixed-methods study. *BMJ Open* **2016**, *6*, e011948. [CrossRef] [PubMed]

15. Kirkdale, C.L.; Nebout, G.; Megerlin, F.; Thornley, T. Benefits of pharmacist-led flu vaccination services in community pharmacy. *Ann. Pharm. Fr.* **2017**, *75*, 3–8. [CrossRef] [PubMed]

16. Warner, J.G.; Portlock, J.; Smith, J.; Rutter, P. Increasing seasonal influenza vaccination uptake using community pharmacies: Experience from the Isle of Wight, England. *Int. J. Pharm. Pract.* **2013**, *21*, 362–367. [CrossRef] [PubMed]

17. Brewer, N.T.; Chung, J.K.; Baker, H.M.; Rothholz, M.C.; Smith, J.S. Pharmacist authority to provide HPV vaccine: Novel partners in cervical cancer prevention. *Gynecol. Oncol.* **2014**, *132* (Suppl. S1), S3–S8. [CrossRef] [PubMed]

18. APhA; NASPA. *Survey of State Immunization Laws/Rules*; APhA: Washington, DC, USA, 2015.

19. Westrick, S.C.; Breland, M.L. Sustainability of pharmacy-based innovations: The case of in-house immunization services. *J. Am. Pharm. Assoc.* **2009**, *49*, 500–508. [CrossRef] [PubMed]

20. Westrick, S.C.; Mount, J.K. Impact of perceived innovation characteristics on adoption of pharmacy-based in-house immunization services. *Int. J. Pharm. Pract.* **2009**, *17*, 39–46. [CrossRef] [PubMed]

21. Dillman, D.A. *Mail and Internet Surveys: The Tailored Design Method*, 2nd ed.; Wiley & Sons: New York, NY, USA, 1999.

22. Kahn, J.A.; Ding, L.; Huang, B.; Zimet, G.D.; Rosenthal, S.L.; Frazier, A.L. Mothers' intention for their daughters and themselves to receive the human papillomavirus vaccine: A national study of nurses. *Pediatrics* **2009**, *123*, 1439–1445. [CrossRef] [PubMed]

23. Luque, J.S.; Tarasenko, Y.N.; Dixon, B.T.; Vogel, R.L.; Tedders, S.H. Recommendations and administration of the HPV vaccine to 11- to 12-year-old girls and boys: A statewide survey of Georgia vaccines for children provider practices. *J. Lower Genit. Tract Dis.* **2014**, *18*, 298–303. [CrossRef] [PubMed]

24. Keating, K.M.; Brewer, N.T.; Gottlieb, S.L.; Liddon, N.; Ludema, C.; Smith, J.S. Potential barriers to HPV vaccine provision among medical practices in an area with high rates of cervical cancer. *J. Adolesc. Health* **2008**, *43*, S61–S67. [CrossRef] [PubMed]

25. Kahn, J.A.; Cooper, H.P.; Vadaparampil, S.T.; Pence, B.C.; Weinberg, A.D.; LoCoco, S.J.; Rosenthal, S.L. Human papillomavirus vaccine recommendations and agreement with mandated human papillomavirus vaccination for 11-to-12-year-old girls: A statewide survey of Texas physicians. *Cancer Epidemiol. Biomark. Prev.* **2009**, *18*, 2325–2332. [CrossRef] [PubMed]

26. U.S. Department of Health and Human Services. *Annual Pharmacy-Based Influenza and Adult Immunization Survey*; U.S. Department of Health and Human Services: Washington, DC, USA, 2013.

27. Ko, K.J.; Wade, R.L.; Yu, H.-T.; Miller, R.M.; Sherman, B.; Goad, J. Implementation of a pharmacy-based adult vaccine benefit: Recommendations for a commercial health plan benefit. *J. Manag. Care Pharm.* **2014**, *20*, 273–282. [CrossRef] [PubMed]

28. Johnson, D.R.; Nichol, K.L.; Lipczynski, K. Barriers to adult immunization. *Am. J. Med.* **2008**, *121*, S28–S35. [CrossRef] [PubMed]

29. Rimer, B.; Harper, H.; Witte, O. *Accelerating HPV Vaccine Uptake: Urgency For Action To Prevent Cancer*; A Report to the President of the United States from the President's Cancer Panel; National Cancer Institute: Bethesda, MD, USA, 2014.

30. Fazekas, K.I.; Brewer, N.T.; Smith, J.S. HPV vaccine acceptability in a rural Southern area. *J. Women's Health* **2008**, *17*, 539–548. [CrossRef] [PubMed]

31. Cates, J.R.; Brewer, N.T.; Fazekas, K.I.; Mitchell, C.E.; Smith, J.S. Racial differences in HPV knowledge, HPV vaccine acceptability, and related beliefs among rural, southern women. *J. Rural Health* **2009**, *25*, 93–97. [CrossRef] [PubMed]

32. Weitzel, K.W.; Goode, J.V. Implementation of a pharmacy-based immunization program in a supermarket chain. *J. Am. Pharm. Assoc.* **2000**, *40*, 252–256. [CrossRef]

33. Bryan, A.R.; Liu, Y.; Kuehl, P.G. Advocating zoster vaccination in a community pharmacy through use of personal selling. *J. Am. Pharm. Assoc.* **2013**, *53*, 70–77. [CrossRef]

34. Ernst, M.E.; Chalstrom, C.V.; Currie, J.D.; Sorofman, B. Implementation of a community pharmacy-based influenza vaccination program. *J. Am. Pharm. Assoc.* **1997**, *Ns37*, 570–580. [CrossRef]

35. Rothholz, M.; Tan, L. Promoting the immunization neighborhood: Benefits and challenges of pharmacies as additional locations for HPV vaccination. *Hum. Vaccines Immunother.* **2016**, *12*, 1646–1648. [CrossRef] [PubMed]

11

Are We Ready to Implement Competence-Based Teaching in Pharmacy Education in Poland?

Agnieszka Skowron *, Justyna Dymek, Anna Gołda and Wioletta Polak

Faculty of Pharmacy, Jagiellonian University Medical College, Krakow 30-699, Poland;
jdymek@cm-uj.krakow.pl (J.D.); annagolda@cm-uj.krakow.pl (A.G.); wpolak@cm-uj.krakow.pl (W.P.)
* Correspondence: agnieszka.skowron@uj.edu.pl

Academic Editor: Jeffrey Atkinson

Abstract: Pharmacists in Poland are responsible for the dispensing and quality control of pharmaceuticals. The education process in pharmacy is regulated and monitored at the national level. Pharmacy education at Jagiellonian University is organized in a traditional way based on input and content teaching. The aim of the study was to determinate whether the Jagiellonian University curriculum in the Pharmacy program meets the criteria of the European Competence Framework. The mapping of the *intended curriculum* was done by four academic teachers. The qualitative and quantitative analysis of the distribution of the European Competence Framework among a group of courses and study years was done. We observed that most of the *personal competencies* are offered to students in their senior years, while *the patient care competencies* are distributed equally during the cycle of the study, and only some of them are overrepresented at the senior years. We need a legislation change at the national level as well as organizational and mental change at the university level to move from learning outcome-based pharmacy education to competence-based.

Keywords: learning outcomes; pharmacy; competence framework; higher education institution

1. Introduction

The Pharmacist designation in Poland is recognized in the Polish Health System as a profession responsible for the dispensing and quality control of pharmaceuticals [1]. According to the Constitution of the Republic of Poland, the pharmacist is considered as a "profession in which the public repose confidence, (. . .) and self-governments shall concern themselves with the proper practice of such professions in accordance with, and for the purpose of protecting, the public interest" [2]. It also constitutes pharmacists as a "regulated profession", which is in accordance with the European Directive [3].

The pharmacist profession in Poland is still seen as a stable and well-paid. Analysis of the labor market showed that pharmacy graduates need only about 2–4 weeks to be employed, and during the first two years after graduation, their salaries are higher than any other medical graduates [4]. Due to the European Directive, the Master Diploma in Pharmacy (MDPharm) awarded in Poland is recognized in EU states, which improves the mobility among pharmacists and determines the competitiveness of the profession compared to other graduates [4,5]. Therefore, the main determinant which influenced the decision of young adults in choosing the pharmacy school in Poland is the confidence that in the future they will be able to find a well-paid position in Poland or in EU states [6].

Pharmaceutical education in Poland is based on the Bologna process, which regulation was implemented into the Higher Education System in Poland at the beginning of the XXI century [7,8]. As a regulated profession, the pharmacist is one of the health professions for which education is based on national standards established by law act amended by the Ministry of Science and Higher Education (MSHE) [9].

The National Standards for Pharmacy Education Act consists of five parts: (1) general requirements for pharmacy program, (2) general learning outcomes (gLO), (3) specific learning outcomes (sLO), (4) organization of the process of education, and (5) methods recommended to be used in the assessment process. The minimal requirements for the MDPharm program are the following: 11 semesters with no less than 5300 contact hours at courses and internships and 330 ECTS (European Credit Transfer System) in total. The general and specific learning outcomes are described as learning outcomes in knowledge, professional, and social skills. The specific learning outcomes are grouped into five main dimensions of sciences, such as (A) biomedical and humanistic sciences; (B) physics and chemistry; (C) analysis, synthesis, and technology; (D) biopharmacy and pharmacotherapy outcomes; (E) pharmacy practice; and (F) student's scientific project. In Table 1, the distribution of contact hours and ECTS credits established in the national standard for pharmacy is presented in detail. The learning outcomes in the Polish National Standard for Pharmacy are described separately for knowledge and professional or social skills [9].

Table 1. The National Standard for Pharmacy—distribution of contact hours and credits in the main scientific and internship dimensions [9].

Area	Topic Group Name	Contact Hours for Student (in Total)	ECTS
Basic sciences	(A) biomedical and humanistic sciences	660	98
	(B) physics and chemistry	765	
Pharmaceutical Sciences	(C) analysis, synthesis, and technology	840	140
	(D) biopharmacy and pharmacotherapy outcomes	480	
	(E) pharmacy practice	410	
	(F) scientific project	375	
Internships	(I) holiday internships	320	10
	(IS) senior students internship (6-month)	960	40

Despite the regulation described above, the autonomy of universities empowers academics to develop, plan, and organize the specific MDPharm program as well as to use teaching methods which ensure that student will achieve the learning outcomes established in the national standard [9].

Nowadays, among the ten Faculties of Pharmacy located in the main medical universities in Poland, approximately 1500 students graduate each year, who mainly start their professional work as pharmacists in the community and in hospital pharmacies [4,5]. In the last twenty years in pharmacy education, we observed the tendency to switch from chemistry-based pharmacy which was focused on the medicinal product, to medicine-based pharmacy which is more patient-oriented [10].

Jagiellonian University established a quality control system which aims to analyze and improve the education process to ensure that it fulfills the national standards. The Faculty of Pharmacy at Jagiellonian University Medical College (FP-JUCM) with a 250-year tradition in pharmacy teaching is one of the oldest schools of pharmacy in Central-Eastern Europe and the oldest in Poland; for the last few years, it has also been recognized as the best one in Poland [11].

The education process in the MDPharm at FP-JUCM is organized in a traditional way based on input and content teaching; this means that the student has to participate and pass the final exams of obligatory and optional courses and internships. The course syllabus contains the description of the learning outcomes and information about the teaching and evaluation methods, which are used to ensure that the student will achieve all learning outcomes. The FP-UJCM offers pharmacy students about one hundred separate courses, and half of them are obligatory. Despite obligatory courses, the student is obliged to pass at least twenty-two optional courses. Each of the obligatory courses should cover sLO described in the national standard for pharmacy. In Table 2, detailed information about the distribution of the sLO in the obligatory courses in pharmacy is shown. According to the Polish National Standard for Pharmacy, the MDPharm program covers 5.5 years of courses and internships, including six months of internship in community or hospital pharmacy [9].

Table 2. The quantitative analysis of the distribution of the specific learning outcomes (sLO) into the courses in the Master Diploma in Pharmacy (MDPharm) program at the Faculty of Pharmacy at Jagiellonian University Medical College (FP-JUCM) [9].

Courses in Specific Topic Group	Learning Outcomes (n *)		
	Knowledge	Professional Skills	Social Skills
(A) Biology/Genetics, Anatomy, Physiology, Pathophysiology, Biochemistry, Immunology, Molecular Biology, Microbiology, Botanics, First Aid, Philosophy, Psychology	32	22	3
(B) Biophysics, Inorganic and Organic Chemistry, Analytical Chemistry, Maths, Statistic, IT technology	27	17	3
(C) Medicinal Chemistry, Medicinal synthesis, Biotechnology, Pharmacognosis, Pharmaceutical Technology	41	17	-
(D) Biopharmacy, Pharmacokinetics, Pharmacology, Toxicology, Bromatology, Herbal drugs	47	69	-
(E) Pharmaceutical care, Clinical Pharmacy, Law and Ethics, Pharmacoeconomics, Epidemiology, Drug Information, Pharmacy Practice	55	55	-
(F) Scientific project	2	6	-

* number of learning outcomes in specific category.

A "set of competencies for pharmacists" was presented as one of the results of "Pharmacy Education in Europe—PHARMINE project" Afterwards, The PHAR-QA consortium together with the European Association of Faculties of Pharmacies extended the PHARMINE results to "produce a harmonized model for quality assurance in pharmacy education" [12]. The European Competence Framework (ECF) is one of core results of PHAR-QA project, which could be used in "setting up and/or modifying curricula in European pharmacy departments" [12]. ECF is a list of competencies for pharmacists. They consist of the two major categories—*personal competence* and *patient care competences*, which are divided into four and seven subcategories, respectively [13].

The aim of our study was to determine whether the FP-JUCM curriculum program in the MDPharm meets the criteria of the European Competence Framework [13] and to recognize the gaps and areas which need to be improved if we want our graduates to be a competent and well-educated pharmacist in the future.

2. Materials and Methods

The mapping process was based on "intended curriculum" of the MDPharm program designed and developed at the FP-UJCM. The MDPharm program documents consist of the *courses syllabuses* and the *program matrix table*. The *program matrix table* shows which of the obligatory courses reflect the sLO. The matrix table contains in the horizontal dimension the list of all obligatory courses and in the vertical dimension the list of sLO. The matrix is completed separately every year, and is used in quality control process to ensure that all sLO are presented in MDPharm program content.

The group of four academic teachers from FP-UJCM was involved in the mapping process. All of them were pharmacists who were awarded their Diploma in Pharmacy at Jagiellonian University. Two of the teachers were experienced academics (AS and AG) with at least ten years of experience in research and teaching in pharmaceutical sciences, and two were less-experienced (JD and WP). All teachers worked as community pharmacists in the past. Additionally, one of them (AS) was also employed in the regional office of National Fund of Health, which was a legislative and financial institution.

The mapping process consisted of two steps. In the first step, each academic fulfilled the matrix of competencies (in the vertical dimension) and sLO (in the horizontal dimension). So, the academics had to decide whether the sLO reflects the specific competence (from the European Competence

Framework). In the second step, the matrix of competencies and sLO were translated to courses (from the MDPharm program). We use the *program matrix table* to attribute each competence to a specific obligatory course. A schedule of the mapping process is presented in Figure 1.

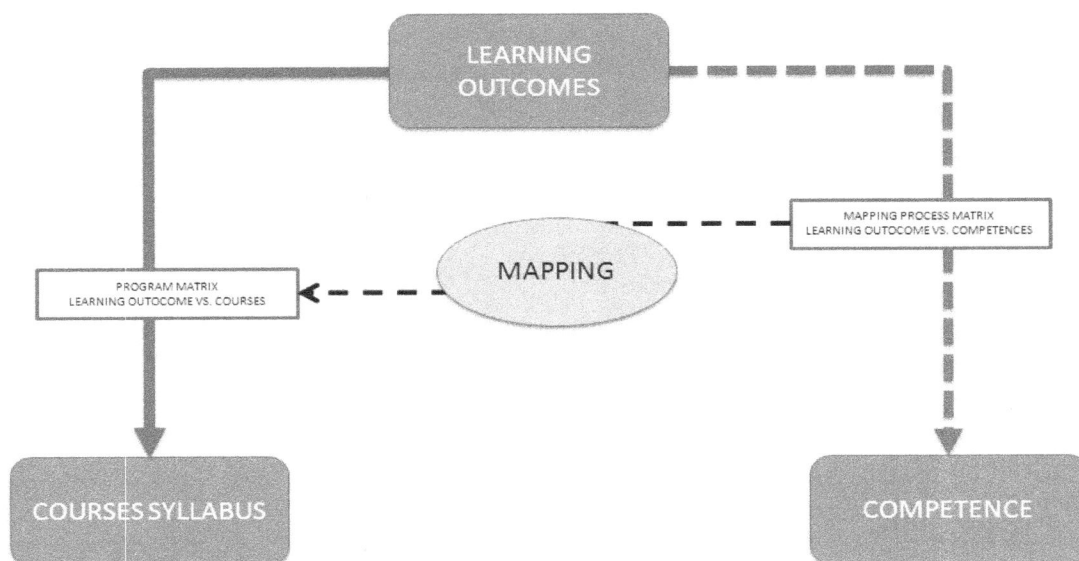

Figure 1. A schedule of the mapping process of the MDPharm program at FP-UJCM.

Finally, a quantitative analysis was done to identify gaps in the existing program. We summarize the number of courses in which learning outcomes in knowledge and skills reflect the specific competence. We also subjectively categorize the required level of the competence using the Dutch Competence Standard Framework, which consists of five levels. The gradation of students' knowledge, skills, and professional behavior starts from level one, where the student demonstrates knowledge and basic professional behavior and ends on level five, where student "independently performs the professional activity" [14].

3. Results

3.1. Matrix of Learning Outcomes versus Competence

We assumed that a specific competence was reflected by a specific learning outcome if it was marked by at least two of the academics. The qualitative analysis of the competence vs. learning outcomes matrix showed the following:

– each competence was reflected by 23 sLO on average (the median value = 20), the maximum number of sLO reflecting the separate competence was 72, and there were two competencies which was not reflected by any of sLO; on average, competencies were reflected by 13 knowledge sLO (the median value = 10) and 10 skills sLO (the median value = 9)
– each sLO reflected three competencies on average (the median value = 2), most sLO reflected two competencies (mode)

The detailed data of some knowledge and skills sLO covering the group of competencies is presented in Table 3.

Table 3. Qualitative and quantitative analysis of the distribution of the learning outcomes in the European Competence Framework (ECF) [9,12].

		Learning outcomes	
		Knowledge	Skills
1. Personal competences: learning and knowledge	1.1. Ability to identify learning needs and to learn independently (including continuous professional development (CPD)).	1	1
	1.2. Ability to apply logic to problem solving.	0	0
	1.3. Ability to critically appraise relevant knowledge and to summarise the key points.	1	1
	1.4. Ability to evaluate scientific data in line with current scientific and technological knowledge.	3	12
	1.5. Ability to apply preclinical and clinical evidence-based medical science to pharmaceutical practice.	10	14
	1.6. Ability to apply current knowledge of relevant legislation and codes of pharmacy practice.	15	9
2. Personal competences: values	2.1. A professional approach to tasks and human relations.	3	2
	2.2. Ability to maintain confidentiality.	4	2
	2.3. Ability to take full responsibility for patient care.	7	1
	2.4. Ability to inspire the confidence of others in one's actions and advice.	8	1
	2.5. Knowledge of appropriate legislation and of ethics.	24	10
3. Personal competences: communication and organisational skills.	3.1. Ability to communicate effectively—both oral and written—in the locally relevant language.	2	4
	3.2. Ability to effectively use information technology.	3	7
	3.3. Ability to work effectively as part of a team.	5	6
	3.4. Ability to implement general legal requirements that impact upon the practice of pharmacy (e.g., health and safety legislation, employment law).	8	1
	3.5. Ability to contribute to the training of staff.	4	1
	3.6. Ability to manage risk and quality of service issues.	1	1
	3.7. Ability to identify the need for new services.	0	0
	3.8. Ability to understand a business environment and develop entrepreneurship.	2	1
4. Personal competences: research and industrial pharmacy.	4.1. Knowledge of design, synthesis, isolation, characterisation and biological evaluation of active substances.	56	15
	4.2. Knowledge of good manufacturing practice and of good laboratory practice.	29	34
	4.3. Knowledge of European directives on qualified persons.	3	3
	4.4. Knowledge of drug registration, licensing and marketing.	11	9
	4.5. Knowledge of the importance of research in pharmaceutical development and practice.	24	16
5. Patient care competences—patient consultation and assessment.	5.1. Ability to interpret basic medical laboratory tests.	6	13
	5.2. Ability to perform appropriate diagnostic tests e.g., measurement of blood pressure or blood sugar.	4	7
	5.3. Ability to recognise when referral to another member of the healthcare team is needed.	8	0
6. Patient care competences—need for drug treatment.	6.1. Ability to retrieve and interpret information on the patient's clinical background.	25	2
	6.2. Ability to compile and interpret a comprehensive drug history for an individual patient.	5	2
	6.3. Ability to identify non-adherence to medicine therapy and make an appropriate intervention.	3	0
	6.4. Ability to advise physicians on the appropriateness of prescribed medicines and—in some cases—to prescribe medication.	17	23

Table 3. *Cont.*

		Learning outcomes	
		Knowledge	Skills
7. Patient care competences–drug interactions.	7.1. Ability to identify and prioritise drug-drug interactions and advise appropriate changes to medication.	23	14
	7.2. Ability to identify and prioritise drug-patient interactions, including those that prevent or require the use of a specific drug, based on pharmaco-genetics, and advise on appropriate changes to medication.	29	13
	7.3. Ability to identify and prioritise drug-disease interactions (e.g., NSAIDs in heart failure) and advise on appropriate changes to medication.	11	14
8. Patient care competences: drug dose and formulation.	8.1. Knowledge of the bio-pharmaceutical, pharmacodynamic and pharmacokinetic activity of a substance in the body.	42	30
	8.2. Ability to recommend interchangeability of drugs based on in-depth understanding and knowledge of bioequivalence, bio-similarity and therapeutic equivalence of drugs.	24	21
	8.3. Ability to undertake a critical evaluation of a prescription ensuring that it is clinically appropriate and legally valid.	15	5
	8.4. Knowledge of the supply chain of medicines thus ensuring timely flow of quality drug products to the patient.	3	0
	8.5. Ability to manufacture medicinal products that are not commercially available.	17	7
9. Patient care competences–patient education.	9.1. Ability to promote public health in collaboration with other professionals within the healthcare system.	9	9
	9.2. Ability to provide appropriate lifestyle advice to improve patient outcomes (e.g., advice on smoking, obesity, etc.).	24	12
	9.3. Ability to use pharmaceutical knowledge and provide evidence-based advice on public health issues involving medicines.	30	8
10. Patient care competences–provision of information and service.	10.1. Ability to use effective consultations to identify the patient's need for information.	18	9
	10.2. Ability to provide accurate and appropriate information on prescription medicines.	22	34
	10.3. Ability to provide evidence-based support for patients in selection and use of non-prescription medicines.	24	30
11. Patient care competences–monitoring of drug therapy.	11.1. Ability to identify and prioritise problems in the management of medicines in a timely and effective manner and so ensure patient safety.	12	22
	11.2. Ability to monitor and report Adverse Drug Events and Adverse Drug Reactions (ADEs and ADRs) to all concerned, in a timely manner, and in accordance with current regulatory guidelines on Good Pharmacovigilance Practices (GVPs).	21	17
	11.3. Ability to undertake a critical evaluation of prescribed medicines to confirm that current clinical guidelines are appropriately applied.	19	14
	11.4. Ability to monitor patient care outcomes to optimise treatment in collaboration with the prescriber.	18	20
	11.5. Ability to contribute to the cost effectiveness of treatment by collection and analysis of data on medicines use.	10	19

3.2. Matrix of Competencies versus Courses

The courses were grouped according to the scientific fields (as described in Table 3) and to the year of the study; we also included the scientific project, holiday, and final internships.

Most of the *Personal competencies in learning and knowledge* are covered by the courses in group C, which are offered mostly at final years of the study. The *Personal competencies: Values* are covered by the first and senior years of study, which offer ethics courses on the one hand, and on the other the senior internship, where the student has an opportunity to observe "real life" and to develop their attitude toward the ethical dilemma. The *Personal competencies such as communication and organization skills and research and industrial pharmacy* seem to be balanced between all groups of courses and all study years. The details of the distribution of *personal competencies* between topic groups and the years of the MDPharm are shown in Table 4.

The *Patient Care Competencies* are less covered by courses from the group B (physics and chemistry), which are mainly offered to the second year students. FP-UJCM students may achieve most of the *Patient Care Competencies* at the senior years of their MDPharm (fourth to sixth years). The details of the distribution of *Patient Care Competencies* between topic groups and years of the MDPharm are shown in Table 5.

Table 4. Quantitative analysis of the distribution of the *Personal competencies* into the group of courses or the study year at FP-UJ CM [12].

PERSONAL COMPETENCE		GROUP A (n = 13)	GROUP B (n = 8)	GROUP A (n = 13)	GROUP D (N = 6)	GROUP E (N = 10)	YEAR 1 (N = 13)	YEAR 2 (N = 6)	YEAR 3 (N = 8)	YEAR 4 (N = 10)	YEAR 5+6 (N = 9)
		n	n	n	n	n	n	n	n	n	n
LEARNING AND KNOWLEDGE	1.1. Ability to identify learning needs and to learn independently (including continuous professional development (CPD)).						1				1
	1.2. Ability to apply logic to problem solving.										
	1.3. Ability to critically appraise relevant knowledge and to summarise the key points.						1			1	1
	1.4. Ability to evaluate scientific data in line with current scientific and technological knowledge.	4	1			4	4		1	2	2
	1.5. Ability to apply preclinical and clinical evidence-based medical science to pharmaceutical practice.		1		3	5	1			4	4
	1.6. Ability to apply current knowledge of relevant legislation and codes of pharmacy practice.	1				7	1			2	5
VALUES	2.1. A professional approach to tasks and human relations.	3				4	1	1	1		4
	2.2. Ability to maintain confidentiality.	2			1	2	1		1	1	2
	2.3. Ability to take full responsibility for patient care.	1				3			1		3
	2.4. Ability to inspire the confidence of others in one's actions and advice.	2				5	1		1		5
	2.5. Knowledge of appropriate legislation and of ethics.	1			1	6	1			2	5
COMMUNICATION AND ORGANISATIONAL SKILLS	3.1. Ability to communicate effectively–both oral and written–in the locally relevant language.	1	2	1	2	2	2		2	2	2
	3.2. Ability to effectively use information technology.		4			2	3	1			2
	3.3. Ability to work effectively as part of a team.	1	3		1	3	2	1	1	2	2
	3.4. Ability to implement general legal requirements that impact upon the practice of pharmacy (e.g., health and safety legislation, employment law).					4					4
	3.5. Ability to contribute to the training of staff.	3					1		1	1	
	3.6. Ability to manage risk and quality of service issues.	1	2				1			1	1
	3.7. Ability to identify the need for new services.										
	3.8. Ability to understand a business environment and develop entrepreneurship.						1				1
RESEARCH AND INDUSTRIAL PHARMACY	4.1. Knowledge of design, synthesis, isolation, characterisation and biological evaluation of active substances.	2	7	5	4		5	4	2	3	3
	4.2. Knowledge of good manufacturing practice and of good laboratory practice.	8	3	7	4		5	4	5	4	3
	4.3. Knowledge of European directives on qualified persons.			4	2				2	1	2
	4.4. Knowledge of drug registration, licensing and marketing.			6	1	7			2	3	8
	4.5. Knowledge of the importance of research in pharmaceutical development and practice.	1	4	7	2	1	4	1	2	4	3

N–total number of courses in the group or study year, n–number of courses reflecting the specific competence.

Table 5. Quantitative analysis of the distribution of the *Patient care competencies* into the topic groups or the year of the pharmacy course at FP-UJ CM [12].

	PATIENT CARE COMPETENCE	GROUP A (n=13)	GROUP B (n=8)	GROUP A (n=13)	GROUP D (n=6)	GROUP E (n=10)	YEAR 1 (N=13)	YEAR 2 (N=6)	YEAR 3 (N=8)	YEAR 4 (N=10)	YEAR 5+6 (N=9)
		n	n	n	n	n	n	n	n	n	n
PATIENT CONSULTATION AND ASSESSMENT	5.1. Ability to interpret basic medical laboratory tests.	5	1	1		1	2	2	3		1
	5.2. Ability to perform appropriate diagnostic tests e.g., measurement of blood pressure or blood sugar.	4	1	1			2	2	2		
	5.3. Ability to recognize when referral to another member of the healthcare team is needed.	1			2	4			1	2	4
NEED FOR DRUG TREATMENT	6.1. Ability to retrieve and interpret information on the patient's clinical background.	9		2		2	3	3	3	1	2
	6.2. Ability to compile and interpret a comprehensive drug history for an individual patient.	1		1	1	2			1	2	2
	6.3. Ability to identify non-adherence to medicine therapy and make an appropriate intervention.					2					2
	6.4. Ability to advise physicians on the appropriateness of prescribed medicines and–in some cases–to prescribe medication.	1	1	5	5	6	1		3	5	8
DRUG INTERACTIONS	7.1. Ability to identify and prioritise drug-drug interactions and advise appropriate changes to medication.	7		1	5	2	3	2	4	3	3
	7.2. Ability to identify and prioritise drug-patient interactions, including those that prevent or require the use of a specific drug, based on pharmaco-genetics, and advise on appropriate changes to medication.	6		3	5	2	2	2	4	3	4
	7.3. Ability to identify and prioritise drug-disease interactions (e.g., NSAIDs in heart failure) and advise on appropriate changes to medication.			3	5	2			2	3	4
DRUG DOSE AND FORMULATION	8.1. Knowledge of the bio-pharmaceutical, pharmacodynamic and pharmacokinetic activity of a substance in the body.	9	1	6	5	2	4	3	6	5	4
	8.2. Ability to recommend interchangeability of drugs based on in-depth understanding and knowledge of bioequivalence, bio-similarity and therapeutic equivalence of drugs.			6	6				3	5	3
	8.3. Ability to undertake a critical evaluation of a prescription ensuring that it is clinically appropriate and legally valid.			5	4	2			3	3	4
	8.4. Knowledge of the supply chain of medicines thus ensuring timely flow of quality drug products to the patient.					2					2
	8.5. Ability to manufacture medicinal products that are not commercially available.	1		5	3	1	1		3	2	3
PATIENT EDUCATION	9.1. Ability to promote public health in collaboration with other professionals within the healthcare system.	4			2	2		1	3	1	3
	9.2. Ability to provide appropriate lifestyle advice to improve patient outcomes (e.g., advice on smoking, obesity, etc.).	9			2	1	3	3	3	2	1
	9.3. Ability to use pharmaceutical knowledge and provide evidence-based advice on public health issues involving medicines.	6			3	4	2	2	2	4	3
PROVISION OF INFORMATION AND SERVICE	10.1. Ability to use effective consultations to identify the patient's need for information.	5			2	5	3		2	3	4
	10.2. Ability to provide accurate and appropriate information on prescription medicines.	2		5	5	5	1		3	5	7
	10.3. Ability to provide evidence-based support for patients in selection and use of non-prescription medicines.	2		5	5	5	1		3	4	8
MONITORING OF DRUG THERAPY	11.1. Ability to identify and prioritise problems in the management of medicines in a timely and effective manner and so ensure patient safety.	1		3	4	4	1		2	3	6
	11.2. Ability to monitor and report Adverse Drug Events and Adverse Drug Reactions (ADEs and ADRs) to all concerned, in a timely manner, and in accordance with current regulatory guidelines on Good Pharmacovigilance Practices (GVPs).			4	4	4			1	6	5
	11.3. Ability to undertake a critical evaluation of prescribed medicines to confirm that current clinical guidelines are appropriately applied.		2	5	6	7	2		3	7	8
	11.4. Ability to monitor patient care outcomes to optimize treatment in collaboration with the prescriber.	1	1	5	5	6	2		2	6	8
	11.5. Ability to contribute to the cost effectiveness of treatment by collection and analysis of data on medicines use.		4	4	2	4	3	1	2	4	4

N–total number of courses in the group or study year, n–number of courses reflecting the specific competence.

3.3. Analysis of the Level of Competencies

We based our subjective analysis (which reflects the levels of the *Dutch Competence Standard Framework*) on the document on the one hand, and our personal experience as a pharmacist and a teacher on the other. Two of our colleagues (JD and WP) could also use their experience as a pharmacy student because at least half of their courses were established basing on Bologna process. We also took into account the composition of knowledge sLO and skills sLO covering the specific competence as well as a teaching and assessing methods described in the course syllabus. The results of our discussion are presented in Table 6. In the brackets, we listed the numbers of the competencies (according to the Tables 4 and 5) which could be achieved on the specific level at the end of the MDPharm program.

Table 6. A desk analysis of the level of competence achieved by a student at the MDPharm program at FP-UJCM [14].

		Level *
Personal Competencies	learning and knowledge	1a (1,3,4); 1c (5,6)
	values	2 (3,4); 3 (5); 4 (1,2)
	communication and organisational skills	1a (1,3); 1c (4); 2 (6); 3 (7,8); 4 (2)
	research and industrial pharmacy	1c (3,5); 3 (2,4); 5 (1)
Patient Care Competencies	patient consultation and assessment	1a (1,3)
	need for drug treatment	1a (2,3); 1c (1,4)
	drug interactions	1a (1); 2 (2,3)
	drug dose and formulation	1c (2); 2 (5); 3 (1,4); 4 (3)
	patient education	1c (2); 2 (3); 3 (1)
	provision of information and service	1c (1); 2 (2,3)
	monitoring of drug therapy	1a (3,5); 2 (1); 4 (2,4)

* the level of Dutch Competence Standard Framework; in the brackets, we used the numbers of the specific competencies from Tables 4 and 5.

Most of the competencies (n = 12) seem to be possible to be achieved by students on the level 1 (1a to 1 c), which is a basic level and means that a student can present the knowledge and demonstrate professional behavior only in a test situation.

4. Discussion

The mapping process of the curriculum at the FP-UJCM was a part of the cooperation of the partners of the PHAR-QA Consortium [12], and by the discussion between partners, it was limited to "intended curriculum" mapping. We mapped the "intended curriculum" based only on official documents of the MDPharm program at our faculty, which means that the results of our analysis did not reflect the opinion of the students or another teacher. We hope it can be used to identify the gaps and to see what could be improved in future [15].

The MDPharm program at Jagiellonian University is based on learning outcomes defined at the national level [9]. It educates students to be future professional staff in a community and hospital pharmacy, so the patient-oriented European Competence Framework [13] should be widely represented and recognized in the curriculum documents.

In the first step of our analysis, we had to "translate" the sLO created for knowledge, professional, and social skills into the competencies. We observed a high inconsistency among the total number of sLO, which could be recognized as reflecting the specific *Personal competencies*. For example, we found:

–   71 sLO (56 in knowledge and 15 in skills) which we matched to competence: *Knowledge of design, synthesis, isolation, characterization and biological evaluation of active substances* (4.1 in Table 3)

–   only two sLO (one in knowledge and one in skills) for competencies:

  ○   *ability to identify learning needs and to learn independently (including continuous professional development (CPD)-1.1 in Table 3);*

○   *ability to critically appraise relevant knowledge and to summarize the key points (1.3 in Table 3);*
○   *ability to manage risk and quality of service issues (see 3.6 in Table 3).*

–   two Personal competence: *ability to apply logic to problem-solving* (1.2 in Table 3) and *ability to identify the need for new services* (3.7 in Table 3), which we could not recognize as directly represented by sLO, and consequently, delivered by any obligatory course.

A similar situation was recognized in the group of *Patient care competencies*, where:

–   72 sLO (42 in knowledge and 30 in skills) reflected the competence *Knowledge of the bio-pharmaceutical, pharmacodynamic and pharmacokinetic activity of a substance in the body* (8.1 in Table 3)
–   only three sLO (in knowledge) reflected the competence *Ability to identify non-adherence to medicine therapy and make an appropriate intervention* (6.3 in Table 3) and *Knowledge of the supply chain of medicines thus ensuring timely flow of quality drug products to the patient* (8.4 in Table 3).

The analysis of the distribution of competences among the study years (Tables 4 and 5) showed that a student has an opportunity to achieve *personal competencies* mostly during the senior years of the study (5th and 6th year). Only competencies in *research and industrial pharmacy* are distributed equally at the junior and senior years of the study. Students achieve the *patient care competencies* at the 3rd, 4th, 5th, and 6th years of the study. However, most of them—especially in the group *provision of information and services*—are distributed among the courses of the last three years (4th to 6th).

Based on the Dutch Competence Standard Framework [14], we also tried to subjectively assess the level of competencies achieved by the student [14]. In general, we assumed (Table 6) that most competencies are achieved at a level 1 or 2. There is a limited group of competencies among *Personal competencies* and *patient care competencies* which could be considered as achieved at the 4th level, and only one—*knowledge of design, synthesis, isolation, characterization and biological evaluation of active substances*—which could be achieved at a level 5. We can conclude that despite wide reflection of the *need for drug treatment* or *provision of information and service* competencies in the sLO, the subjective assessment showed that it is highly possible that a student can only present the knowledge about the specific competence and demonstrate the skills only in a test situation. This means that she is not "able to adequately carry out professional activities in an authentic professional situation under the supervision of an experienced practitioner" [14].

A major limitation of the mapping process based on "intended curriculum" is the fact that it is based on documents only, so we could not be sure that the ideas described in documents are implemented into the daily teaching activity. This means that even those competencies which we recognized as "well" reflected by the sLO might not be achieved by all students. To verify the results of our study, we plan to extend the analysis, and we are planning the study of the student's perception about their competencies.

Because the results of our analysis already showed gaps and lack of balance between competencies and learning outcomes, we will recommend Dean's office to start the discussion with the teachers at FP-UJ CM to encourage them to switch to competence-based learning.

The main conclusion of our analysis is that the education system for pharmacy in Poland based on learning outcomes does not directly reflect the competencies. This means that to start with competence-based pharmacy education, we need to change the legal regulation at the national level and redefine our teaching at the university level. Despite the changes in the national regulations in the pharmacy field, academics should remember that their main obligation is to ensure that their graduates will be able to work independently and responsibly to improve the health of the society and to ensure the safe and effective use of drugs. As academics who are experienced in teaching, we have to be aware of our responsibility for creating the professional attitude and competencies of our students. As pharmacists and academics, we are also responsible for developing the professional education system to let our students become the professionals of the future.

Author Contributions: A.S. conceived and designed the experiments; A.S., J.D., A.G., and W.P prepared the tools and performed the mapping process; A.S. analyzed the data and wrote the paper.

References

1. The Pharmaceutical Law of 6th September 2001. Available online: http://isap.sejm.gov.pl/DetailsServlet?id=WDU20011261381 (accessed on 7 January 2017). (In Polish)

2. The Constitution of The Republic of Poland of 2nd April 1997 as published in Dziennik Ustaw No. 78, item 483. Available online: http://www.sejm.gov.pl/prawo/konst/angielski/konse.htm (accessed on 10 January 2017).

3. Directive 2005/36/EC of the European Parliament and of the Council of 7th September 2005 on the recognition of professional qualifications. *Off. J. Eur. Union* **2005**, *48*, 22–142. Available online: http://eur-lex.europa.eu/legal-content/EN/TXT/?uri=OJ:L:2005:255:TOC (accessed on 20 January 2017).

4. The Professional Career of the Graduates of the Faculty of Pharmacy of the Jagiellonian University Medical College in the academic year 2014/2015—report. Available online: http://www.sdka.cm.uj.edu.pl/documents/13606729/32429686/Raport%20losy%20absolwent%C3%B3w%20-%20Wydzia%C5%82%20Farmaceutyczny%2014_15.pdf (accessed on 10 January 2017). (In Polish)

5. Report on economic aspects of the career of the graduates of the Faculty of Pharmacy of the Jagiellonian University Medical College. Available online: http://absolwenci.nauka.gov.pl/reports/UJK_6446.pdf (accessed on 23 January 2017).

6. Schulz, A. Motivation for Pursuing a Career in Pharmacy. In *Economic Notes. Selected Economic and Social Problems within the Economies of Poland and the World*; Grzywacz, J., Kowalski, S., Eds.; PWSZ: Płock, Poland, 2014; Volume 20, pp. 135–143. Available online: http://www.wydawnictwo.pwszplock.pl/Ekonomia/nauki_ekonomiczne_20.pdf (accessed on 10 January 2017).

7. Law Act of 27th July 2005 on Higher Education Law as published in Dziennik Ustaw 2016, item 1842. Available online: http://isap.sejm.gov.pl/DetailsServlet?id=WDU20160001842 (accessed on 10 January 2017).

8. Joint declaration of the European Ministers of Education—The Bologna Declaration of 19 June 1999. Available online: http://www.ehea.info/cid100210/ministerial-conference-bologna-1999.html (accessed on 23 January 2017).

9. Regulation of the Minister of Science and Higher Education of 9th May 2012 on education standards for fields of study: Medicine, dentistry, pharmacy, nursing and midwifery as published in Dziennik Ustaw 2012, item 631. Available online: http://isap.sejm.gov.pl/DetailsServlet?id=WDU20120000631 (accessed on 8 January 2017).

10. Atkinson, J. Heterogeneity of Pharmacy Education in Europe. *Pharmacy* **2014**, *2*, 231–243. [CrossRef]

11. Ranking of the Faculties of Pharmacy in Poland in the year 2016. Available online: http://www.perspektywy.pl/RSW2016/ranking-kierunkow-studiow/kierunki-medyczne-i-o-zdrowiu/farmacja (accessed on 20 January 2017).

12. Atkinson, J.; Rombaut, B.; Sánchez Pozo, A.; Rekkas, D.; Veeski, P.; Hirvonen, J.; Bozic, B.; Skowron, A.; Mircioiu, C. A description of the European Pharmacy Education and Training Quality Assurance Project. *Pharmacy* **2013**, *1*, 3–7. [CrossRef]

13. Atkinson, J.; de Paepe, K.; Sánchez Pozo, A.; Rekkas, D.; Volmer, D.; Hirvonen, J.; Bozic, B.; Skowron, A.; Mircioiu, C.; Marcincal, A.; et al. The PHAR-QA project: Competency framework for pharmacy practice—First steps, the results of the European network Delphi round 1. *Pharmacy* **2015**, *3*, 307–329. [CrossRef]

14. 2016 Pharmacist Competency Framework and Domain-Specific Frame of Reference for Netherlands. Available online: https://www.knmp.nl/downloads/pharmacist-competency-frameworkandDSFR-Netherlands.pdf (accessed on 20 January 2017).

15. Kelley, K.A.; Demb, A. Instrumentation for Comparing Student and Faculty Perceptions of Competency-based Assessment. *Am. J. Pharm. Educ.* **2006**, *70*, 134. [CrossRef] [PubMed]

12

Improving Pharmacists' Targeting of Patients for Medication

Vanessa Marvin [1,2,*], **Emily Ward** [1,2], **Barry Jubraj** [2,3], **Mark Bower** [4] and **Iñaki Bovill** [5]

[1] Department of Pharmacy, Chelsea and Westminster Hospital NHS Foundation Trust, London SW10 9NH, UK; emily.ward@chelwest.nhs.uk

[2] Medicines Optimisation, NIHR CLAHRC NW London, London SW10 9NH, UK; barry.jubraj@kcl.ac.uk

[3] Institute of Pharmaceutical Science, King's College London, London SE1 9NH, UK; barry.jubraj@kcl.ac.uk

[4] Department of Oncology, Chelsea and Westminster Hospital NHS Foundation Trust, London SW10 9NH, UK; m.bower@imperial.ac.uk

[5] Department of Elderly Medicine, Chelsea and Westminster Hospital NHS Foundation Trust, London SW10 9NH, UK; inaki.bovill@chelwest.nhs.uk

* Correspondence: vanessa.marvin@chelwest.nhs.uk

Abstract: Background: In an acute hospital setting, a multi-disciplinary approach to medication review can improve prescribing and medicine selection in patients with frailty. There is a need for a clear understanding of the roles and responsibilities of pharmacists to ensure that interventions have the greatest impact on patient care. **Aim:** To use a consensus building process to produce guidance for pharmacists to support the identification of patients at risk from their medicines, and to articulate expected actions and escalation processes. **Methods:** A literature search was conducted and evidence used to establish a set of ten scenarios often encountered in hospitalised patients, with six or more possible actions. Four consultant physicians and four senior pharmacists ranked their levels of agreement with the listed actions. The process was redrafted and repeated until consensus was reached and interventions were defined. **Outcome:** Generalised guidance for reviewing older adults' medicines was developed, alongside escalation processes that should be followed in a specific set of clinical situations. The panel agreed that both pharmacists and physicians have an active role to play in medication review, and face-to-face communication is always preferable to facilitate informed decision making. Only prescribers should deprescribe, however pharmacists who are not also trained as prescribers may temporarily "hold" medications in the best interests of the patient with appropriate documentation and a follow up discussion with the prescribing team. The consensus was that a combination of age, problematic polypharmacy, and the presence of medication-related problems, were the most important factors in the identification of patients who would benefit most from a comprehensive medication review. **Conclusions:** Guidance on the identification of patients on inappropriate medicines, and subsequent pharmacist-led intervention to prompt and promote deprescribing, has been developed for implementation in an acute hospital.

Keywords: deprescribing; medication review; pharmaceutical care; polypharmacy; hospitalisation; frailty; older adults

1. Introduction

A medicines optimisation project hosted at a 400 bed acute hospital in London began in January 2015 to improve prescribing and adherence in patients with frailty. Interventions included educational updates and medicine safety sessions for doctors and pharmacists in training. The overall aim was to recognise and reduce potentially inappropriate prescriptions (PIPs) in acute hospital settings, and to produce a tool to promote safe deprescribing through targeted review [1–3].

Prescribing medicines for in-patients is a routine responsibility held by the majority of medically qualified doctors in the UK, and is a very significant part of the daily duties of junior physicians in particular. In addition, pharmacists, nurses and other allied health professionals may obtain a post-graduate qualification in order to prescribe medicines independently. Independent Prescribing Pharmacists (IPs) are qualified to prescribe in addition to the checking, dispensing, reviewing and advising role of all hospital pharmacists in the UK. Often IPs work within a specialism (e.g., microbiology, neurology, respiratory), as do their senior medical colleagues.

All prescribed medicines, for most UK acute hospital in-patients, are checked for accuracy, reviewed for appropriateness, and reconciled with the patient's medication history by a pharmacist as soon as possible after admission. The process should start at first contact between the pharmacist and the patient, as suggested by the Royal Pharmaceutical Society [4]. During hospitalisation, medications are reviewed frequently, either (a.) acutely, in response to illness and recovery, or (b.) in a more planned and structured manner, for example during a comprehensive geriatric assessment.

Standards for comprehensive and interim medication reviews were defined at the project initiation (see Box 1), as described in our previous medication review studies [5,6], and used throughout the current work.

Box 1. Types of Medication Review.

Comprehensive medication review (adapted from NICE [7]) ▸ A structured critical examination by a senior clinician of all current medication, with the objective of reaching an agreement with the patient about optimising treatment and minimising medicines-related problems. With the patient, the reviewer systematically considers the benefits and risks of all medicines, stops or reduces any that are inappropriate, and starts others, taking into account their views and concerns (as well as those of their family members or carers where appropriate).
Interim medication review ▸ In the acute hospital setting, reviews leading to short-term medication changes frequently take place. Medicines are reviewed when a patient presents acutely unwell at hospital, or when their condition deteriorates or improves. Individual medicines may be changed or held because they are considered 'non-essential', or currently 'unnecessary', or as preparation for a surgical operation. In addition, in these settings, individual medicines are stopped if they are identified as directly contributing to morbidity.

Similarly, our local PIP list was updated from the STOPP criteria of 2015 [8] and those from the NHS Scotland Polypharmacy Guidance in the same year [9]. Additional lines came from other nationally available sources, as cited in our final iteration [1].

Local audit revealed a high prevalence of PIPs in falls-risk patients, and at least one inappropriate or unnecessary medicine was found in 19% of inpatients over 70 years old who were assessed as 'frail' [6]. Furthermore, nearly a third were taking ten or more regular medicines (a number that appears in our cohort to be associated with more problematic polypharmacy) [10,11].

We have previously demonstrated that pharmacists are efficient at recognising PIPs, but less so in timely intervention [6]. For example, alerting the junior doctor to an inappropriate anticholinergic medicine in a patient at risk of falls, can be a misdirected intervention, as our junior doctors are not confident or comfortable at making changes to medication started by a more senior colleague [12]. The process of deprescribing needs a step-wise approach with shared decision-making between clinicians and patients [13], including input from pharmacists. In a review of their impact in medication reviews, it was shown that pharmacists have a positive effect on patient safety through their interventions, although more data is needed [14].

We recognised the need to embed more pro-active pharmacy actions into medication reviews in our hospital practices. For this, we wanted to improve the understanding of roles and shared responsibilities within the multidisciplinary team in targeting vulnerable patients for remedial action, such as dose reduction, holding medication temporarily (hereafter described as 'HOLD') and deprescribing.

2. Aim

The aim of this phase of our medicines optimisation project was to improve the process of identification by pharmacists of frail patients at risk from their medicines, and to produce guidance on expected actions and escalation processes.

3. Objectives

To establish lists of hazardous medicines and combinations to be avoided or reduced in frail individuals.

To formulate a definitive list of actions for pharmacists when a patient is admitted with, or is at risk of, acquiring a medicines-related problem (MRP).

4. Method

An expert panel was convened, comprising four consultant physicians and four senior pharmacists based at acute North West London hospitals, to consider a multidisciplinary approach to reducing inappropriate prescribing in elderly patients. The panel were chosen from colleagues working currently with inpatients and with many years' experience of the effects of prescription medicines in older adults.

The first consideration was the target age group. Older adults, according to the STOPP/START criteria, [8] are those aged 65 years or older; we have previously used 70 years for our local application of a tool in falls-risk patients [6]. NHS Scotland suggest targeting patients 75 years and older for deprescribing interventions if resources are limited [9]. The panel were asked to consider these target ages i.e., 65, 70 and 75 years; we also tested 85 years and above as a separate older age group. A Medline literature search was carried out, looking for research evidence of who, other than the chronologically 'old', are most at risk of medicines related problems (MRPs), and from which medicines. Patients with frailty [15,16], multimorbidity [16,17], polypharmacy [10,11,16,18], on high risk medicines [19–21], and high risk combinations [8,9], are described in many of the publications found. Also noted was the increase in risk of adverse drug reactions if a pharmacist had not seen and screened a patient's medicines on admission, or when there was no system in place for medicines reconciliation [14,16,19].

The team met in person to discuss possible ways of identifying frailty through the local electronic prescribing and medicines administration (EPMA) system alerts. Falls risk assessments are documented here and patients are flagged automatically if criteria for falls risk are met. Other 'alerts' on the EPMA system, such as dementia and learning disability, were similarly considered by the panel for their usefulness in identifying patients at risk.

PDSA (Plan Do Study Act) cycles were completed in October 2015 and February 2016, yielding a set of ten scenarios that reflect the common situations that pharmacists may encounter with medicines. For each scenario, a choice of six or more actions were described.

These scenarios were emailed, and in addition printed and sent to the panel members for their consideration. They were each asked independently to rank their agreement with each of the possible actions on a scale from zero to nine, with zero as 'fully disagree', and 9 as 'fully agree'. The numerical results were analysed, and where all participants scored zero, 1 or 2, these scenarios were rejected. Through further PDSA cycles and a second face to face meeting of the panel where there was variation and therefore no consensus, the scenarios and actions were redrafted.

The panel were asked to rescore the resulting draft, and this was to be repeated until an agreed list of actions was reached.

5. Results

A set of scenarios covering common clinical situations and medicine combinations were finalised through an iterative process and a series of PDSA cycles. From the original ten scenarios, the wording and age limits for intervention were revised and grouped so that guidelines for pharmacists in identifying and following-up patients at risk in four different situations were produced.

Consensus was reached in the first round on the following guiding principles:

- Only prescribers can deprescribe. Pharmacists who are not also trained as prescribers* can 'hold' medicines acutely, if in the best interest of the patient. In all cases, the reason for holding a medicine must be documented on the prescription, whether on paper or the EPMA; immediate verbal contact should be made with the prescriber or senior colleague.
- The 'Falls Risk flag' is not to be used as a target or marker for frailty, as it is too broad and includes many young patients in trauma and recovering from orthopaedic procedures. It was originally suggested as a suitable screening tool for frailty. It was later agreed that it would be more sensitive to screen through age plus a PIP, MRPs or polypharmacy.
- Any inpatient who has a learning disability, hearing or visual impairment, or has a limited ability to speak English, may be at additional risk of harm from medicines, and steps should be taken to ensure these risks are minimised and interventions made with these factors in mind.

*In the UK, registered pharmacists can train and qualify as independent prescribers (IPs). All registered pharmacists, with or without the IP qualification, may perform clinical duties including altering prescriptions for clarification (e.g., formulation change, timing of a dose) and withholding medicines for safety reasons.

Rejected scenarios from round one were:

1. Patient over 64 but less than 85 years old with falls risk.
2. Patient 85 years old or older with falls risk.
3. Patient over 69 but less than 85 years old on six or more medicines.
4. Patient over 69 years old on 10 or more medicines.

Rejected actions from round one were:
"No action needed" was removed as an option.
"Pharmacist should deprescribe or change any inappropriate medicine and leave a note for the doctor" was removed, leaving the favoured action 'hold' and 'alert' (see final scenarios below).

Consensus was reached in the second round on the remaining six statements:

- Seventy-five years was selected as the age at which elderly care 'interventions' should be made on PIPs.
- Polypharmacy was agreed as six or more regular medicines.
- Sixty-five was selected as the age at which intervention is needed for a patient with a current medication-related problem, including confirmed or potential for non-adherence.
- Sixty-five years was agreed as the age at which intervention is needed for a patient on a hazardous combination; the 'triple whammy' or 'sick day' medicines [9].

Re-worded and merged scenarios from round two were (originally):

1.   Patient over 69 years but less than 85 years old on six or more regular medicines.
2.   Patient 85 years old or older on 6 or more regular medicines.
3.   Patient over 69 years old but less than 85 on a PIP.
4.   Patient 85 years old or older on a PIP.

The following guidance on the pharmacist's role in prompting medication review was then produced:

1.   When a patient is identified as at-risk from their medicines by the pharmacy team (often during medicines reconciliation on admission to hospital), the pharmacist should contact the prescriber immediately to discuss next steps and document actions in the patient's medical record.
2.   In all cases where a junior doctor is the prescriber, the pharmacist should communicate directly with them face-to-face, or immediately by telephone, to inform them of 'holds' or to prompt them to take appropriate action. A message can be written in addition to, but not instead of, this dialogue, so that there is an opportunity for learning and improving prescribing practice.
3.   In complex cases, junior pharmacists should refer to their senior colleagues for advice. If working outside their area of expertise, pharmacists are encouraged to escalate appropriately to specialists.
4.   Details of any medication reviews should be included appropriately in the discharge summary written by the doctor, added to and countersigned by the screening/reconciling pharmacist, whether or not any changes were made prior to the patient leaving hospital.
5.   Pharmacist actions are recommended in specific situations given below:

N.B. These lists are not intended to be exhaustive. Screening and checking of all prescribed medicines, combinations and interactions in their clinical settings in all age groups, is expected as a standard for clinical pharmacy; this standard underpins our own current work. Please see Box 2 for key terms and definitions.

Box 2. Key to Terms Used in Scenarios.

Complex	No strict definition, but includes patients with multimorbidity and on medication for long term conditions where polypharmacy may be necessary. Intervention by the pharmacist depends on his/her own level of competence; changes may require input from other professionals and referral to specialists.
Deprescribe	The process of safely stopping regular medicines long term through shared decision making. This is an active systematic process of identifying and discontinuing those medicines with unfavourable risk-benefit trade-offs in the context of illness severity, advanced age, agreed care goals and personal preferences. Deprescribing also involves titrating, changing and switching medicines, but is not about denying effective treatments in eligible patients [22]. Hazardous combinations Medicines prescribed together that adversely interact or compound a clinical condition such as acute kidney injury. See the Triple Whammy and Sick Day Guidance specifically [9].
Polypharmacy	For the purposes of this study: six or more medicines taken currently and regularly i.e., not including any 'as required' in the count.
Hold	The temporary cessation of a medicine with a view to further monitoring and review.
MRP	Medicine-related problem, encompassing all adverse drug events and reactions, adherence and supply issues (e.g., medicines, or their omission, contributing to bleeding, falls, confusion, metabolic disturbance, constipation).

5.1. Scenario 1

Patient is 75 years old or older on 6 or more regular medicines (polypharmacy) or on a PIP [1].
Pharmacist should prompt the junior doctor to review medicines and HOLD or DEPRESCRIBE any unnecessary (i.e., no longer indicated).

Where there is a risk of acute harm, pharmacist should HOLD any inappropriate medicine immediately and alert the doctor at the first opportunity.

Complex cases should be brought to the multidisciplinary team (MDT) lead clinician, or the pharmacist should otherwise alert the registrar or consultant concerned, to the need for them to arrange a comprehensive medication review (See Box 1).

5.2. Scenario 2

Patient is 65 years old or older and presents with a medicine-related problem (MRP)

Pharmacist should HOLD or reduce any medicine causing harm immediately and highlight the situation to the prescriber at the first opportunity.

Pharmacist should prompt the junior doctor to review the patient and make appropriate changes to the prescription, including starting alternatives to the culprit medicine where needed (e.g., paracetamol in place of codeine for analgesia if constipated).

Pharmacist should notify the MDT, the registrar, or the consultant, of the need for a comprehensive medication review.

5.3. Scenario 3

Patient is 65 years old or older on the 'Triple Whammy' [9]; a combination of an angiotensin -converting enzyme inhibitor (ACEi) or an angiotensin-II receptor antagonist (ARB,) plus a diuretic, plus a non-steroidal anti-inflammatory drug (NSAID).

Pharmacist should HOLD the NSAID immediately and alert the prescriber at the first opportunity.

Pharmacist should prompt the junior doctor to review and HOLD or DEPRESCRIBE appropriately.

Pharmacist should notify the MDT, the registrar, or the consultant, of the need for a comprehensive medicines review.

5.4. Scenario 4

Patient is 65 years old or older with dehydration or signs of acute kidney injury (AKI), and is on metformin, or an ACEi, an ARB, a diuretic, or an NSAID (Sick Day Guidance) [9].

Pharmacist should HOLD all 'sick day' medicines [19] immediately and alert prescriber at the first opportunity.

Pharmacist should prompt junior doctor to review all medicines and HOLD 'sick day' medicine(s) if he/she has not already done so.

Complex cases should be brought to the MDT, or the pharmacist should otherwise alert the registrar or consultant to the need for a comprehensive medication review.

6. Discussion

This improvement work was undertaken as part of a wider project, in which we found there was a need to be more active in the acute setting in reducing inappropriate and harmful prescribing for vulnerable adults. We have developed multi-disciplinary agreed guidance for appropriate positive action in order to tackle problematic polypharmacy. These actions include and encourage safe, targeted deprescribing.

It is recognised that pharmacists have an important role in decreasing medication related problems (MRPs), but as suggested by O'Mahoney [23], agreement is often difficult to reach between doctors, pharmacists, nurses and patients, about *how* it should be done and by whom [23]. We have formed our consensus statements to tackle this area of indecision. We encourage clinical pharmacists to be active participants in MDTs in all areas where medications are reviewed for appropriateness, continuation, or deprescription. Deprescribing is ultimately the responsibility of a qualified prescriber, but in addition to this, our expert panel considers that it needs to be undertaken as an integral part of a comprehensive review. To do the task safely there is a need to include the patient and to consider other medications and interactions.

It is clear that specialist clinicians (including independent prescribing pharmacists) must lead the review in their area of expertise, but this should be supported with more active highlighting of medicines eligible for deprescription by general pharmacists [14,18,23–25]. We have addressed this in our suggested actions for pharmacists: that is to 'hold' culprit medicines and alert the appropriate clinician to review and take further action.

The pharmacist should also be challenging unjustified prescriptions and performing regular reviews, whilst engaging with patients in conversations about their medicines, including discussions around medication adherence [26,27]. There is a need for this to be done routinely and systematically—as with optimising drug use in line with kidney and liver function [19]—perhaps by applying screening criteria. Several established tools have been successfully applied in practice, such as STOPP [23,25], and the Good Palliative-Geriatric Practice algorithm [28]. Others have been locally developed utilising an EPMA system for communications [24,29]. A 2013 review of the application of such tools suggests that STOPP identified more medications associated with adverse drug events than the Beers criteria [30]. We reviewed current literature and drew on the clinical experience of senior clinicians to produce the list of clinical criteria and medication combinations that are known to cause harm in aged individuals.

In a systematic review of the risk prediction models available for adverse drug reactions in older adults (over 65 years), evidence was found for the efficacy of having systems in place to ensure reliable medicines reconciliation [19]. The Medication Safety Thermometer (Harmfreecare) http://www.safetythermometer.nhs.uk lists fundamentals for safety as: allergy status documented; medicines reconciliation for all medicines by the pharmacy team (started) within 24 hours of admission; no omission of prescribed medicines without valid reason accurately documented [31]. Omitted and delayed medicines were also the subject of a National Patient Safety Alert in the UK [21]. We are reminded that patients are at risk from unintentional omissions, as well as commissions.

These publications all suggest that a clinical pharmacy medicines' screening service with allergy and interaction checks and pharmacist-led reliable reconciliation is fundamental to the safety of hospitalised patients. All are locally integrated into the daily ward pharmacy service at the host hospital, to the standard set out by the Royal Pharmaceutical Society [4], and subject to quality improvement initiatives prior to the current project [32].

However, reconciliation and allergy checks do not identify or prevent all inappropriate prescribing [7].

As described by The British Geriatrics Society (BGS), chronological age is a poor predictor of susceptibility to adverse outcomes; biological age is reflected in the degree of frailty. Frailty identifies older adults who are at increased risk of poor outcomes such as cognitive decline, falls and hospitalization [15]. Medicines are poorly tolerated in frail individuals (even more so when individuals are dehydrated [9,33]), where those over 65 years of age are at particular risk of acute kidney injury [33]. Although there are checklists available, frailty is difficult to assess in practice. We have falls and thrombosis risk checklists, but no Frailty checklist in routine use locally. A recent study suggests they, in any case, these may not be a reliable way of identifying patients who are at risk from their medicines [34].

Singled out by the BGS as associated with most adverse outcomes in frailty are anticholinergics, long acting benzodiazepines, NSAIDs and polypharmacy [15]. Those most often associated with problems leading to hospitalisation include antiplatelets, anticoagulants, diuretics and ACE inhibitors [35]. The sets of scenarios and the PIP list we used included reference to these.

Medicines in many situations are known to be unsuitable or hazardous for those over 65 [8,9,19], especially if the patient has a long-term condition; yet there is more likelihood of co-morbidity in the elderly [17]. Those with frailty or cognitive decline are more likely to be on a PIP [36].

Where a MRP is the reason for hospitalisation, documentation of the cause in the patient's record is vital for safe continuity of care. Graabaek and colleagues describe a successful system where MRPs are communicated to the physician via the medical notes on the EPMA in a Denmark hospital [29].

Our expert panel favoured direct verbal communications followed by clear documentation in the patient's medical notes. This was agreed as the appropriate action, as it allows for continual learning about safe prescribing and medicines use. There is, at present, a paper medical record and an electronic documentation system linked with the EPMA locally. In practice, pharmacists use the EPMA to record actions required and interventions made. Importantly, these actions and notes regarding medication review and changes to medicines must be transcribed onto the discharge summary letter to the General Practitioner and copied to the patient (and community pharmacist in many cases), to ensure continuity of care.

A decade ago, preventable MRPs were identified as accounting for 3.7% of admissions in one study, and antiplatelets, diuretics and NSAIDs accounted for 50% of these [37]. There is no evidence to suggest this is very different currently.

We have compiled from our work a description of patients at greatest risk from their medicines for particular focus by clinical pharmacists, and a list of culprit medicines and combinations most often implicated. From this, we produced the preferred actions, having reached consensus between eight senior clinicians on what those actions should be. Some patients are at immediate risk; others would benefit from a comprehensive review at some point during their hospital stay. We have put systems in place to enable the most appropriate communication to the prescribing team in common clinical situations. This is expected to lead to more comprehensive reviews and deprescribing, as described with our STOPIT work [2,3] and falls patients previously [6].

7. Limitations

We selected six or more regular medicines as Polypharmacy. There are many other limits and definitions; therefore, this may not be universally applicable.

We recruited eight participants to our expert panel. As they were selected by the project team from clinicians we know and work with closely, there is likely bias, and the possibility that the consensus is based on local custom and practice rather than real expertise.

The hospital's electronic prescribing system is unique, with in-built decision support (again, developed locally), and may not be applicable to areas with paper prescription charts for inpatients or other EPMA support.

8. Conclusions

An iterative, scenario-led ranking process achieved consensus on clinical parameters to target at-risk inpatients for medicines optimisation. This targeting strategy was combined with the development of pharmacist-led intervention guidance, including who should review medication, and how urgent actions should be escalated. These interventions are to be embedded into local clinical pharmacy practice. We believe there is scope for a wider application to include care homes, outpatients and other non-acute settings.

Acknowledgments: Alan J. Poots, Formerly the Principal Information Analyst, NIHR CLAHRC NWL and Imperial College London. Colin Mitchell, Consultant Physician and Geriatrician, Department of Elderly Medicine, St. Mary's Hospital, London W2. NW London Training Program Director for General Internal Medicine. Laurel Issen, Formerly Improvement Science Manager NIHR CLAHRC NWL. Peter Kroker, Consultant Physician and Geriatrician, Department of Elderly Medicine, Chelsea & Westminster Hospital. Sheena Patel, Lead Anticoagulation Pharmacist. Chelsea and Westminster Hospital NHS Foundation Trust. Susan Barber Improvement Science Manager NIHR CLAHRC NWL.

Author Contributions: For research articles with several authors, a short paragraph specifying their individual contributions: Vanessa Marvin, Project design and prepared the manuscript for publication. Emily Ward, Project manager and assisted in preparing the manuscript for publication. Barry Jubraj, Contributed to the project design, assisted in the analysis and in preparing the manuscript for publication. Mark Bower, Contributed to the project design, assisted in the analysis and in preparing the manuscript for publication. Iñaki Bovill, Oversaw original project, assisted in the analysis and in preparing the manuscript for publication.

References

1.   List of Potentially Inappropriate Prescriptions (PIPs). Available online: http://clahrc-northwestlondon.nihr. ac.uk/resources/PIP (accessed on 6 April 2018).
2.   Abdul-Saheb, M.; Jubraj, B.; Bovill, I.; Kuo, S.; Marvin, V. Intermediate Care: An optimal setting for review of inappropriate medication in elderly patients? *Geriatr. Med.* **2014**, *44*, 13–17.
3.   Duraisingham, S.; Jubraj, B.; Marvin, V.; Kuo, S.; Bovill, I.; Poots, A.J. Stopping Inappropriate medicines in the Outpatient Setting. *Geriatr. Med.* **2015**, *45*, 35–41.
4.   Royal Pharmaceutical Society. Professional Standards for Hospital pharmacy Services: Version 3. December 2017. Available online: https://www.rpharms.com/Portals/0/RPS%20document%20library/ Open%20access/Professional%20standards/Professional%20standards%20for%20Hospital%20pharmacy/ Hospital%20Standards-2017.pdf?ver=2017-12-21-132808-697 (accessed on 6 April 2018).
5.   Szymanski, T.; Marvin, V.; Emily, W.; Jubraj, B. Deprescribing following medication review in acute care: The ReMAC project. Abstract and presentation at the Pharmaceutical Care Network Europe, Hillerød, Denmark. *Int. J. Clin. Pharm.* 2016. [CrossRef]
6.   Marvin, V.; Ward, E.; Poots, A.J.; Heard, K.; Rajagopalan, A.; Jubraj, B. Deprescribing medicines in the acute setting to reduce the risk of falls. *Eur. J. Hosp. Pharm.* **2017**, *24*, 10–15. [CrossRef] [PubMed]
7.   NICE Guidance 2015. Medicines Optimisation: The Safe and Effective Use of Medicines to Enable Best Possible Outcomes. 4 March 2015. Available online: http://nice.org/guidance/ng5 (accessed on 6 April 2018).
8.   O'Mahony, D.; O'Sullivan, D.; Byrne, S.; O'Connor, M.N.; Ryan, C.; Gallagher, P. STOPP/START Criteria for potentially inappropriate prescribing in older people: Version 2. *Age Ageing* **2015**, *44*, 213–218. [CrossRef] [PubMed]
9.   NHS Scotland. Polypharmacy Guidance. March 2015. Available online: http://www.polypharmacy.scot. nhs.uk/ (accessed on 6 April 2018).
10. The Kings Fund. Polypharmacy and Medicines Optimisation: Making it Safe and Sound. Available online: https://www.kingsfund.org.uk/publications/polypharmacy-and-medicines-optimisation (accessed on 6 April 2018).
11. Barnett, N.; Oboh, L. When less is more: the challenge of polypharmacy. *Eur. J. Hosp. Pharm.* **2014**, *21*, 63–64. [CrossRef]
12. Jubraj, B.; Marvin, V.; Poots, A.J.; Patel, S.; Bovill, I.; Barnett, N.; Issen, L.; Bell, D. A pilot survey of junior doctors' attitudes and awareness around medication review and deprescribing: Time to change our educational approach? *Eur. J. Hosp. Pharm.* **2015**. [CrossRef] [PubMed]
13. Jansen, J.; Natganathan, V.; Carter, S.M.; NcLachlan, A.J.; Nickel, B.; Irwig, L.; Bonner, C.; Doust, G.; Colvin, J.; Heaney, A.; et al. Too much medicine in older people? Deprescribing through shared decision making. *BMJ* **2016**, *353*, i2893. [CrossRef] [PubMed]
14. Graabaek, T.; Kjeldsen, L.J. Medication Reviews by Clinical Pharmacists at Hospitals Lead to Improved Patient Outcomes: A Systematic Review. *Basic Clin. Pharm. Toxicol.* **2013**, *112*, 359–373. [CrossRef] [PubMed]
15. British Geriatrics Society. Fit for Frailty. Consensus Best Practice Guidance for the Care of Older People Living with Frailty in Community and Outpatient Settings. 2014. Available online: www.bgs.org.uk/ campaigns/fff/fff_full.pdf (accessed on 6 April 2018).
16. Warren, A. Pharmacist involvement in tackling polypharmacy in frail adults. *Pharmacoepidemiol. Drug Saf.* **2013**. [CrossRef]
17. NICE Guidance. Multimorbidity: Clinical Assessment and Management. 2016. Available online: http://nice.org. uk/guidance/ng56 (accessed on 21 September 2016).
18. Scott, I.A.; Hilmer, S.N.; Reeve, E.; Potter, K.; Le Couteur, D.; Rigby, D.; Gnjidic, D.; Del Mar, C.B.; Roughead, E.E.; Page, A.; et al. Reducing Inappropriate Polypharmacy. The process of deprescribing. *JAMA* **2015**, *175*, 827–834. [CrossRef]

19. Stevenson, J.M.; Williams, J.L.; Burnham, T.G.; Provost, A.T.; Schiff, R.; Erskine, S.D.; Davies, J.G. Predicting adverse drug reactions in older adults; a systematic review of the risk prediction models. *Clin. Interv. Ageing* **2014**, *9*, 1581–1593. [CrossRef] [PubMed]

20. Wilmer, C.M.; Huiskes, V.J.B.; Natsch, S.; Rennings, A.J.M.; van den Bemt, B.J.F.; Bos, J.M. Drug related problems in a clinical setting: A literature review and cross-sectional study evaluating factors to identify patients at risk. *EJ Hosp. Pharm.* **2015**, *22*, 229–235. [CrossRef]

21. National Patient Safety Agency. Rapid Response Alert 009 on 24/2/10: Reducing Harm from Omitted and Delayed Medicines in Hospital. Available online: http://www.nrls.npsa.nhs.uk/resources/?entryid45=130397 (accessed on 6 April 2018).

22. Scott, I.A.; Anderson, K.; Freeman, C. Evidence-based deprescribing: Reversing the tide of potentially inappropriate polypharmacy. *J. Clin. Outcome Manag.* **2016**, *23*, 359–369.

23. O'Mahoney, D. Pharmacists and prevention of inappropriate prescribing in hospital. *Age Aging* **2016**, *45*, 181–183. [CrossRef] [PubMed]

24. Cottrell, R.; Caldwell, M.; Jardine, G. Developing and Implementing a Pharmacy Risk Screening Tool. Available online: http://www.hospitalpharmacyeurope.com/featured-articles/developing-and-implementing-pharmacy-risk-screening-tool (accessed on 6 April 2018).

25. Delgado-Silveira, E.; Albinana-Perez, M.S.; Munoz-Garcia, M.; Garcia-Mina, F.M.; Fernandez-Villalba, E.M. Pharmacist comprehensive review of treatment compared with STOP-START criteria to detect potentially inappropriate prescription in older complex patients. *Eur. J. Hosp. Pharm.* **2018**, *25*, 16–20. [CrossRef]

26. Zarkali, A. More is not always better: Stop overtreating patients. *Pharm. J.* **2015**, *295*, 16–17.

27. Barnett, N.L. Medication adherence: Where are we now? A UK perspective. *Eur. J. Hosp.* **2014**, *21*, 181–184. [CrossRef]

28. Garfinkel, D.; Mangin, D. Feasibility study of a systematic approach for discontinuation of multiple medications in older people. *Arch. Int. Med.* **2010**, *170*, 1648–1654. [CrossRef] [PubMed]

29. Graabaek, T.; Krogsgaard Bonnerup, D.; Kjeldsen, L. Pharmacist led medication review in an acute admissions unit: A systematic procedure description. *Eur. J. Hosp. Pharm.* **2015**, *22*, 202–206. [CrossRef]

30. Hill-Taylor, B.; Sketris, I.; Hayden, J.; Byrne, S.; O'Sullivan, D.; Christie, R. Application of the STOPP/START criteria: A systematic review of the prevalence of potentially inappropriate prescribing in older adults, and evidence of clinical, humanistic and economic impact. *J. Clin. Pharm. Ther.* **2013**, *38*, 360–372. [CrossRef] [PubMed]

31. The Medication Safety Thermometer (Harmfreecare): NHS Improvement. 2013. Available online: http://www.safetythermometer.nhs.uk (accessed on 13 March 2017).

32. Marvin, V.; Kuo, S.; Poots, A.J.; Woodcock, T.; Vaughan, L.; Bell, D. Applying Quality Improvement methods to address gaps in medicines reconciliation at transfers of care from an acute UK hospital. *BMJ Open* **2016**, *6*, e010230. [CrossRef] [PubMed]

33. NICE 2016. Acute Kidney Injury (AKI): Use of Medicines in People with or at Increased Risk of AKI. Key Therapeutic Topic. 26 February 2016. Available online: http://nice.org.uk/guidance/ktt17 (accessed on 6 April 2018).

34. Papoutsi, C.; Poots, A.; Clements, J.; Wyrko, Z.; Offord, N.; Reed, J.E. Improving patient safety for older people in acute admissions: Implementation of the Frailsafe checklist in 12 hospitals across the UK. *Age Ageing* **2018**, *47*, 311–317. [CrossRef] [PubMed]

35. Kongkaew, C.; Hann, M.; Mandal, J.; Williams, S.D.; Metcalfe, D.; Noyce, P.; Ashcroft, D. Risk Factors for Hospital Admissions Associated with Adverse Drug Events. *Pharmacotherapy* **2013**, *33*, 827–837. [CrossRef] [PubMed]

36. Poudel, A.; Peel, N.M.; Nissen, L.; Mitchell, C.; Gray, L.C.; Hubbard, R.E. PIP in older patients discharged from acute care hospitals to residential aged care facilities. *Ann Pharm.* **2014**, *11*, 1425–1433.

37. Howard, R.L.; Avery, A.J.; Slavenburg, S.; Pipe, G.; Lucassen, P.; Pirmohamed, M. Which drugs cause preventable admissions to hospital? A systematic review. *B. J. Pharmacol.* **2007**, *63*, 136–147. [CrossRef] [PubMed]

13

Prevalence of Self-Medication among Students of Pharmacy and Medicine Colleges of a Public Sector University

Fatimah Ali Albusalih [1], Atta Abbas Naqvi [2,*], Rizwan Ahmad [3] (iD) and Niyaz Ahmad [4]

[1] College of Clinical Pharmacy, Imam Abdulrahman Bin Faisal University (University of Dammam), Dammam 31441, Saudi Arabia; ph.fatimahali582@gmail.com

[2] Department of Pharmacy Practice, College of Clinical Pharmacy, Imam Abdulrahman Bin Faisal University (University of Dammam), Dammam 31441, Saudi Arabia

[3] Natural Products and Alternative Medicines, College of Clinical Pharmacy, Imam Abdulrahman Bin Faisal University (University of Dammam), Dammam 31441, Saudi Arabia; rizvistar_36@yahoo.com

[4] Department of Pharmaceutics, College of Clinical Pharmacy, Imam Abdulrahman Bin Faisal University (University of Dammam), Dammam 31441, Saudi Arabia; niyazpharma@gmail.com

* Correspondence: aaghulam@uod.edu.sa or bg33bd@student.sunderland.ac.uk

Abstract: Pharmacy and medical students are expected to be more knowledgeable regarding rational use of medications as compared to the general public. A cross-sectional study was conducted among students of pharmacy and medicine colleges of Imam Abdulrahman Bin Faisal University in Dammam, Saudi Arabia using a survey questionnaire. The duration of the study was six months. The aim was to report self-medication prevalence of prescription and non-prescription drugs among pharmacy and medical students. The prevalence of self-medication in the pharmacy college was reported at 19.61%. Prevalence of self-medication at the medical college was documented at 49.3%. The prevalence of multivitamin use was reported at 30.53%, analgesics; 72.35%, antihistamines; 39.16%, and antibiotic use at 16.59%. The prevalence of anti-diarrheal medicines and antacids use among students was found to be 8.63% and 6.64%, respectively. The variable of college and study year was statistically associated with the nature of the medicines. The most common justifications given by students indulging in self-medication were 'mild problems' and 'previous experience with medicines'. Our study reported that prevalence of self-medication in the College of Clinical Pharmacy was low, i.e., 19.61%. The figure has been reported for the first time. Students were mostly observed self-medicating with OTC drugs, however, some reported using corticosteroids and isotretenoin, which are quite dangerous if self-medicated. Students have a positive outlook towards pharmacists as drug information experts.

Keywords: self-medication; pharmacy students; medical students; prevalence; epidemiology; Saudi Arabia

1. Introduction

Self-medication (SM) is a global phenomenon. It is prevalent in every age group, though its extent differs among individuals and regions. Previously, it was considered as unnecessary, however, responsible self-medication is regarded as an important aspect of self-care nowadays [1]. On the contrary, irresponsible or irrational SM is discouraged as it may not only harm the patient in the form of adverse drug reactions (ADRs) or medication-related problems (MRPs), but may also increase the direct costs, including the cost of treatment and hospital admission [2–4].

SM is defined as the use of medicines by a person for self-treatment based on self-diagnosed symptoms without consulting a physician and/or without a valid prescription [5]. It may incorporate over the counter (OTC) medications that are dispensed without prescription, as well as prescription-only medications (POM) which require a valid prescription, such as antibiotics. Though self-medication with POM is not advisable, the latter is common in those countries which do not have strict regulations on the sale of pharmaceuticals [6–8]. Self-medication practice offers ease of access to OTC medications at a lower cost, which serves as an alternative to the costly and time-consuming clinical consultations. Safety issues are a major concern as many diseases have similar symptoms. Additionally, the risk of self-medication is increased if the individual does not have knowledge and understanding of the disease. Additionally, this practice is associated with an increased risk of misdiagnosis, ADRs, drug abuse and misuse [9].

One of the reasons to indulge in this practice is the financial condition of the patient. This is common in those countries where the individual has to pay direct cost for treating the condition. As a result, patients may prefer self-treatment over costly consultation. Another possible reason can be the non-regulated practices concerning sale of prescription drugs. This may result in the availability of POM without a valid prescription and, hence, patient may skip consultation and directly purchase prescription medications [10]. Evidence indicates that self-medication is practiced by teenagers, adults, parents, and students in Saudi Arabia [11]. Familial practice may also render individuals to indulge in self-medication as it lowers their stigma towards SM. This highlights the need to educate parents about the problem as well. A pharmacist or a doctor at the community level can play an important role in this situation. This brings the discussion to the point of evaluating Saudi pharmacy and medical student's outlooks toward this issue.

Pharmacy and medical students are expected to be more knowledgeable regarding rational use of medications as compared to general public. The curriculum of pharmacy and medicine teaches them about rational use of medicines and consequences of irrational use. Hence, this population is well aware of the phenomenon and issues related to this practice. Additionally, students of medicine would assume portfolio of a prescriber in future and may prescribe medicines. Similarly, pharmacy students would become future pharmacists and may find themselves counseling patients on safe use of medicines. Thus, both of these professionals play a significant role in patient care especially regarding this practice. Hence, understanding the practice and self-beliefs related to self-medication in this population is of paramount importance.

However, previous studies have reported that this population is also affected by the same practice [12,13]. A number of studies have been conducted in Saudi academia pertaining to the matter that reported a varying prevalence of SM. However, there were some limitations observed as those studies did not investigate the determinants, such as beliefs of students who either indulge or refrain from practice. Data regarding self-medication has not been reported from this academia before. Our study aimed to document this practice in pharmacy and medicine students at the university. It also had the objective of reporting prevalence of both POM and OTC medicines currently used by students at the campus.

2. Methods

A cross-sectional study was conducted among students of pharmacy and medicine colleges of Imam Abdulrahman Bin Faisal University (formerly known as University of Dammam) located in the city of Dammam in Eastern Province of Saudi Arabia. It was designed in the form of survey. The duration of study was four months, i.e., December 2016–April 2017.

2.1. Participants and Eligibility Criteria

The study included students of pharmacy and medicine colleges. This segment was identified as the target population of the study. Students of other colleges were not included. Additionally, students who did not consent to participate and incomplete questionnaires were also excluded from the study.

2.2. Sample Size and Sampling Procedure

The study employed purposive sampling to gather responses from students. The questionnaire was distributed among consenting participants. Students were approached in their free time (10 min) between their lectures and at prayer/lunch break. Additionally, students were allowed to take questionnaires to their homes and return them to the investigator at their time of convenience. The sample size was calculated online (Raosoft Inc., Seattle, WA, USA) [14]. According to official figures, the number of students enrolled in pharmacy and medical institutions in the country were 6242 and 15,559, respectively [15]. The sum of both figures was assumed as the total population, the confidence level was set at 95%, and the alpha margin of error kept at 5%. The sample size was found to be 378. The study was completed after gathering a total response from 450 students.

2.3. Research Instrument

A questionnaire was designed by reviewing the available research literature. It was designed in the English language, since it was the language of instruction at university colleges. Some of the research questions were incorporated from the research instrument developed by Naqvi et al. with permission [13]. The questionnaire was divided into two sections and consisted of 16 close-ended and four open-ended questions. The categories of variables identified were demographics of students that included age, gender, college affiliation, year of study, residence status, marital status, number of children, siblings, and past illness. All of these were included in Section 1 of questionnaire. Section 2 was concerned with self-medication information and included questions related to students' beliefs about self-medication practice, indulgence in the practice, frequency of self-medication per month, source of information regarding the same, type and nature of medicines used, and place of obtaining medications, as well as common symptoms experienced prompting self-medication.

2.4. Piloting and Validation Process

The questionnaire was first presented to a panel of experts including college professors, health practitioners, and pharmacists. Based on their recommendations, the demographic variable of residence status was added in Section 1 of the questionnaire. Further to this, the panel recommended documenting the prevalence of self-medication in this population. For this purpose, two separate items related to indulgence in SM and frequency of SM per month, were added in Section 2. The questionnaire was then piloted in 180 students in pharmacy and medical colleges all over the Saudi Arabia to check for any errors. Some questions had spelling and grammatical errors which were rectified. It was observed that the categories for demographic variable of 'number of children' lacked the option of 'not applicable' for un-married respondents. This prompted confusion among respondents who selected the option 'single' in the marital information. This was identified and rectified by adding the required option. Furthermore, the two categories (df) of the demographic variable of 'number of children', i.e., 'Between 3 and 5' and 'More than 5' were merged together to increase data reliability.

The questionnaire was also statistically validated by employing reliability testing that revealed a Chronbach's alpha value of 0.781. The exploratory factor analysis (EFA) using principle component analysis extraction and direct oblimin rotation with Kaiser Normalization was also employed, which extracted five components. The Kaiser Mayer Olkin (KMO) measure of sampling adequacy and Bartlett's test for sphericity was also employed, which reported a value of 0.6 and a significant p value less than 0.001, respectively. Based on the statistical data, the questionnaire was distributed into five sections, namely: demographic information; prevalence information; common illness prompting SM; commonly used medications for self-use; reasons for/against SM and advice to others regarding SM practice. At this point, the questionnaire was deemed validated. The correlation matrix is presented in Table 1 and pattern matrix in Table 2.

The components with eigenvalues above 1.0 are graphically represented in Figure 1.

Table 1. Correlation matrix.

		V1	V2	V3	V4	V5	V6	V7	V8	V9	V10	V11
Correlation	V1	1.000	−0.433	−0.056	−0.012	−0.009	−0.071	0.039	0.169	0.203	−0.029	0.130
	V2	−0.533	1.000	0.032	0.075	0.124	0.111	−0.042	−0.240	−0.179	−0.014	−0.237
	V3	−0.056	0.032	1.000	0.124	0.111	0.073	0.097	−0.028	0.024	0.151	−0.043
	V4	−0.012	0.075	0.124	1.000	0.139	0.280	0.022	−0.103	−0.084	−0.032	−0.094
	V5	−0.009	0.124	0.111	0.139	1.000	0.207	0.003	−0.110	−0.108	0.062	0.020
	V6	−0.071	0.111	0.073	0.280	0.207	1.000	−0.004	−0.121	−0.075	0.121	−0.127
	V7	0.039	−0.042	0.097	0.022	0.003	−0.004	1.000	0.017	0.001	0.044	−0.018
	V8	0.169	−0.240	−0.028	−0.103	−0.110	−0.121	0.017	1.000	0.445	−0.194	0.308
	V9	0.203	−0.179	0.024	−0.084	−0.108	−0.075	0.001	0.445	1.000	0.088	0.188
	V10	−0.029	−0.014	0.151	−0.032	0.062	0.121	0.044	−0.194	0.088	1.000	−0.029
	V11	0.130	−0.237	−0.043	−0.094	0.020	−0.127	−0.018	0.308	0.188	−0.029	1.000
Sig. (1-tailed)	V1		0.000	0.120	0.402	0.424	0.068	0.207	0.000	0.000	0.268	0.003
	V2	0.000		0.250	0.055	0.004	0.009	0.186	0.000	0.000	0.387	0.000
	V3	0.120	0.250		0.004	0.009	0.060	0.020	0.279	0.302	0.001	0.181
	V4	0.402	0.055	0.004		0.002	0.000	0.319	0.015	0.038	0.247	0.023
	V5	0.424	0.004	0.009	0.002		0.000	0.472	0.010	0.011	0.093	0.338
	V6	0.068	0.009	0.060	0.000	0.000		0.463	0.005	0.057	0.005	0.003
	V7	0.207	0.186	0.020	0.319	0.472	0.463		0.356	0.488	0.174	0.354
	V8	0.000	0.000	0.279	0.015	0.010	0.005	0.356		0.000	0.000	0.000
	V9	0.000	0.000	0.302	0.038	0.011	0.057	0.488	0.000		0.031	0.000
	V10	0.268	0.387	0.001	0.247	0.093	0.005	0.174	0.000	0.031		0.269
	V11	0.003	0.000	0.181	0.023	0.338	0.003	0.354	0.000	0.000	0.269	

a. Determinant = 0.359

Table 2. Pattern matrix.

Variable	Component				
	1	2	3	4	5
V1	0.814	−0.050	−0.289	0.010	0.071
V2	0.748	−0.056	0.165	−0.018	0.065
V3	0.564	0.018	−0.010	−0.130	−0.174
V4	−0.062	0.707	−0.292	−0.059	0.186
V5	−0.054	0.706	0.077	0.008	−0.046
V6	0.026	0.620	0.103	0.018	−0.125
V7	−0.089	−0.003	0.916	−0.083	0.028
V8	0.007	0.095	0.011	−0.854	0.022
V9	−0.094	0.064	−0.082	0.796	−0.046
V10	−0.105	−0.127	−0.069	−0.133	0.854
V11	0.189	0.208	0.309	0.186	0.518

2.5. Data Coding and Analysis

The responses were analyzed using version 22 of SPSS (Statistical Package for Social Sciences) (IBM Corp., Armonk, NY, USA). The data was analyzed for frequency counts, and cross-tabulation was performed on associations. The chi square (X^2) test was used to identify and report statistically significant associations. Prevalence was calculated by Medcalc® and reported in terms of 95% confidence interval values [16,17]. An alpha margin of error (α) was identified at 0.05.

2.6. Ethical Approval and Participant Consent

The study was submitted for ethical approval to the ethics committee of the university. It was granted exemption from review (ID #2130001853). A verbal consent was sought from the respondents before handing the questionnaire. The participation was voluntary and without any incentive or pressure from investigators.

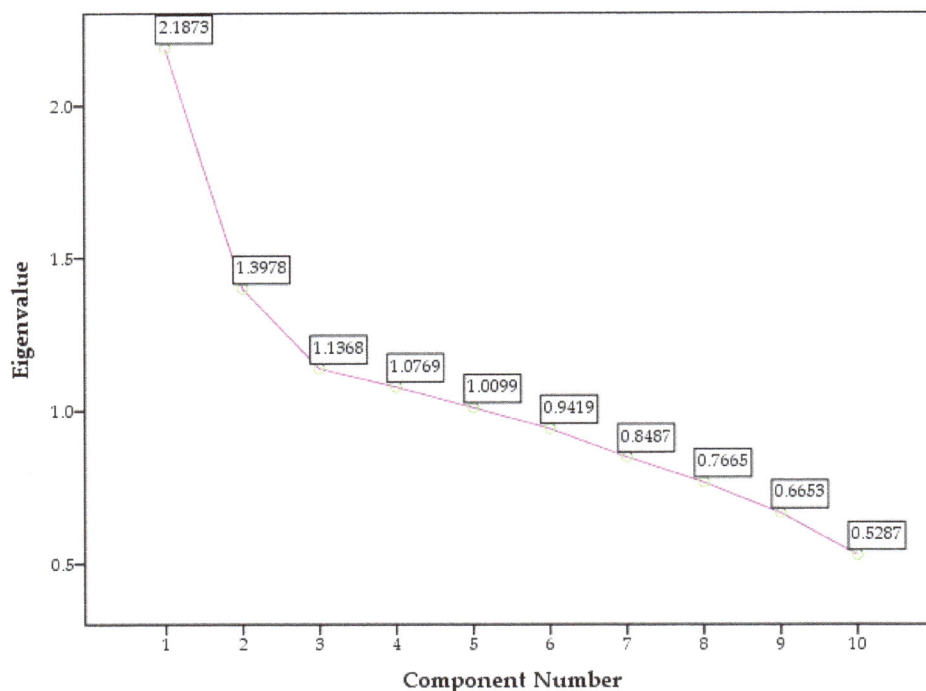

Figure 1. Scree plot.

3. Results

3.1. Response Rate

The study incorporated students from pharmacy and medicine colleges. Out of N = 478 students, a total of 450 responses were received, giving a cumulative response rate (RR) of 94.12%. In terms of a college-wise response, a response rate of 96.8% was obtained from College of Clinical Pharmacy as 158 survey questionnaires were handed over to the pharmacy students and 153 were received. Similarly, a total of 320 surveys were handed to the medical students and 297 were received, giving a response rate of 92.81% for the College of Medicine.

3.2. Demographic Information

The majority of students were aged between 18 and 23 years (N = 427, 94.9%). In terms of gender, slightly more than half were males (N = 249, 55.3%). Most of the students (N = 297, 66%) were from College of Medicine. Study year-wise breakdown revealed that most students (N = 138, 30.7%) were from 3rd Professional year, followed by 5th Professional year students (N = 103, 22.9%). The majority of students (N = 385, 85.6%) were single and did not have children (N = 385, 85.6%). A small segment of students were married without children (N = 43, 9.6%). Furthermore, the bulk of students (N = 375, 83.3%) lived with their families. Most of them (N = 195, 43%) had 3–5 siblings, followed by slightly more than a quarter of students (N = 124, 27.6%) who had 6–8 siblings. Amongst them, an overwhelming majority of students (N = 400, 88.9%) considered themselves healthy, while some (N = 10, 2.2%) had glucose 6–phosphate dehydrogenase (G6PD) deficiency and asthma (N = 8, 1.8%). The demographic information is tabulated in Table 3.

Table 3. Demographic information.

Demographic Information (N = 450)	Sample (N)	Percentage (%)
Age		
Less than 18 years	5	1.1
Between 18 and 23 years	427	94.9
Between 24 and 30 years	18	4
Gender		
Male	249	55.3
Female	201	44.7
College		
Clinical Pharmacy	153	34
Medicine	297	66
Study year		
Preparatory year	8	1.7
2nd year	98	21.8
3rd Year	138	30.7
4th Year	89	19.8
5th Year	103	22.9
6th year	14	3.1
Marital status		
Single	385	85.6
Married	61	13.6
Other	4	0.8
Number of children		
1 to 2	20	4.4
3 or more	2	0.4
Married without children	43	9.6
I am Single/not applicable	385	85.6
Resident status		
Living with family	375	83.3
Living alone (University accommodation)	75	16.7
Siblings		
Between 1 and 2 siblings	40	8.9
Between 3 and 5 siblings	195	43.3
Between 6 and 8 siblings	124	27.6
More than 8 siblings	63	14
No sibling	28	6.2
Illness		
Diabetes Mellitus (DM)	7	1.6
Hypertension (HTN)	7	1.6
Thyroid disorders	4	0.9
Anemia	7	1.6
Asthma	8	1.8
Glucose 6–phosphate dehydrogenase (G6PD)	10	2.2
Skin Diseases	1	0.2
Depression	6	1.3
No disease (healthy)	400	88.8

3.3. Self-Medication Information

The respondents were asked if they indulge in self-medication. More than half of students (N = 248, 55.1%) responded positively. The majority of students (N = 290, 64.4%) rarely indulged (once a month) in the practice, followed by a small segment (N = 54, 12%) that frequently (once every two weeks) indulged in SM. The overall prevalence of self-medication in the whole sample, i.e., among pharmacy and medicine students combined, was 26% (22.01–30.31% for a 95% confidence interval). The prevalence of self-medication among pharmacy students alone was reported at 19.61% (13.64–26.79% for 95% CI) and was 49.3% (44.84–53.77% for 95% CI) for medical students.

Most of the students (N = 124, 27.6%) obtained information from pharmacists followed by a quarter segment (N = 116, 25.8%) using the internet as well as obtaining information from physicians (N = 106, 23.6%). Almost half of students (N = 216, 48%) used non-prescription drugs, followed by a third (N = 152, 33.8%) using both OTC and POMs. An overwhelming majority obtained medications for self-use from a pharmacy store (N = 306, 68%), followed by a third proportion indicating availability of medicines in homes (N = 139, 30.9%). The most common symptoms experienced by students that prompted SM were headache, fever, pain, and dysmenorrhea (N = 64, 14.2%), followed by allergy and cold/flu (N = 16, 3.6%). The majority of students (N = 293, 65.1%) highlighted more than one symptom and few (N = 57, 12.7%) did not experience any symptom that prompted them to self-medicate. Further to this, majority of the students (N = 102, 22.7%) self-medicated with analgesics and antipyretics (paracetamol and NSAIDs), followed by cold and flu medicines (N = 10, 2.2%). A small segment (N = 6, 1.3%) self-medicated with antibiotics.

The prevalence of multivitamins use was reported at 30.53% (26.31–35% for 95% CI). The term 'dietary supplement' included only multivitamins. The prevalence of analgesics use, which included paracetamol and NSAIDs, was reported at 72.35% (67.97–76.4%); antihistamines and cold/flu products was 39.16% (34.63–43.83%). The prevalence of antibiotics and anti-diarrheal use among students was found to be 16.59% (13.28–20.35%) and 8.63% (6.21–11.61%), respectively. For antacids use, the prevalence was documented at 6.64% (4.52–9.34%). The detailed summary of self-medication information is graphically represented in Figure 2 and tabulated in Table 4.

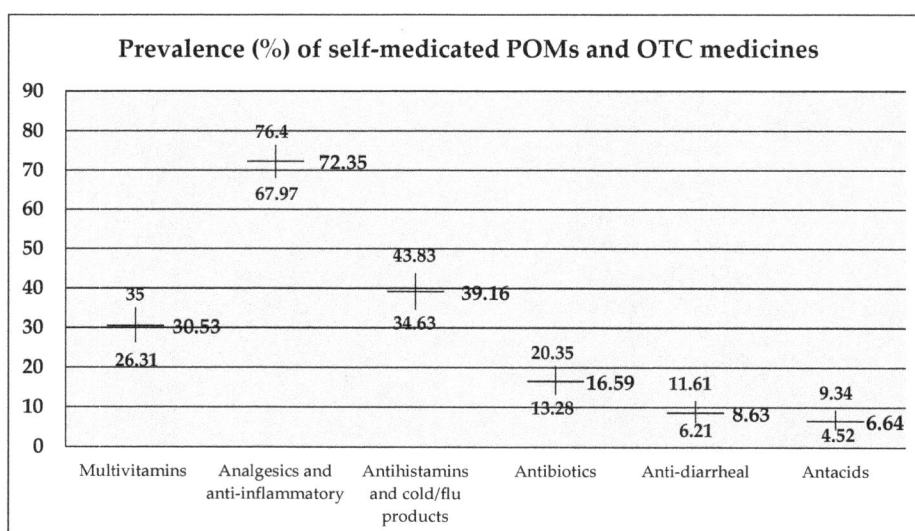

Figure 2. Prevalence of self-medicated POMs and OTC medicines.

Table 4. Self-medication information.

Self-Medication Information (N = 450)	Sample (N)	Percentage (%)
Did you practice self-medication during the last month?		
Yes	248	55.1
No	202	44.9
Frequency of practice?		
No SM	87	19.3
Rarely (Once a month)	290	64.5
Frequently (Once every two week)	54	12
Very frequently (Once a week)	19	4.2
Source of Information		
Pharmacist	124	27.6
Physician	106	23.6
Medical professionals	43	9.5
Family and Friends	61	13.6
Internet	116	25.7
Nature of the medication used		
Prescription only medicines (POMs)	82	18.2
Non-prescription (OTC) drugs	216	48
Both	152	33.8
Place of obtaining medications for self use		
Pharmacy store	306	68
Friends	5	1.1
Available in house	139	30.9
Symptoms experienced		
Headache, fever and pain, dysmenorrhea	64	14.2
Cold and Flu Allergy	16	3.6
Gastric symptoms (Diarrhea/constipation/ indigestion)	11	2.4
Throat, RTI and skin infection	9	2
None	57	12.7
More the one	293	65.1
Types of medications used for SM		
Analgesics/Antipyretics (Paracetamol/NSAIDs)	102	22.7
Antibiotics (Amoxicillin, Cefexime)	6	1.3
Cough and Flu (Psuedoephedrine)	10	2.3
Anti-diarrheal/Laxatives (Lactulose)	2	0.4
Anti-histamines (Loratadine, Citirizine)	5	1.1
Multivitamins	13	2.9
CNS stimulants (Amphetamines, Methylphenidate)	1	0.2
I do not remember	53	11.8
More than one medication used	258	57.3

3.4. Attitudes Towards Self-Medication Practice

The study documented students' attitude towards self-medication practice. More than a third of students (N = 158, 35.1%) responded positively to SM practice by mentioning 'mild problems' that could be treated by SM. Few students (N = 64, 14.2%) indicated that they had 'previous experience with such medicines', hence, they felt more poised to self-medicate. Similarly, those who had a negative attitude towards SM practice believed that consultation with a physician was essential to stay healthy (N = 119, 26.4%). A small segment of students (N = 68, 15.2%) was concerned with ADRs and did not self-medicate. Most students (N = 366, 81.3%) highlighted that they were against SM practice in principle, but agreed that it may be used in rare situations. A small segment of students (N = 57, 12.7%) favored SM practice at all times. The details are tabulated in Table 5.

Table 5. Student attitudes towards self-medication practice.

Attitudes towards Self-Medication (N = 450)	Sample (N)	Percentage (%)
Reasons in favor of self-medication practice		
Mild problems	158	35.1
Previous experience	64	14.2
I find SM practice as taking active role in managing my health	23	5.1
Waiting in queues and time issues	25	5.6
Lack of trust on prescribers	9	2
Self-knowledge is enough to self-medicate rationally	14	3.1
Informed by elders/family members and friends	8	1.8
I am not sure	114	25.3
Combination of above mentioned reasons	35	7.8
Reasons against self-medication practice		
Consultation with physician is essential	119	26.4
Risk of adverse drug reactions (ADRs)	68	15.1
Practitioner can diagnose an illness	48	10.7
A patient cannot rationalize SM	18	4
Prescribing a medication is the job of a prescriber	18	4
I am not sure	130	28.9
Combination of above mentioned reasons	49	10.9
Advice to others regarding self-medication		
I am always in favor of SM practice	57	12.7
I am against SM but it can be used in rare situations	366	81.3
I am always against SM practice	27	6

The association between gender and the source of information regarding SM was statistically significant with the chi square (X^2) value reported at 22.302 and p value less than 0.0001, with a low to moderate effect size, i.e., a phi value reported at 0.223. The association between demographic variable of college and source of information regarding SM was also statistically significant with X^2 values reported at 13.390 and p value less than 0.05, with a weak effect size, i.e., a phi value reported at 0.172. The association of the variable of college was also significant with nature of medications used by students. The value of X^2 was reported at 6.669 and p value was less than 0.05, with a weak effect size, i.e., a phi value reported at 0.122. Moreover, cross-tabulation for the abovementioned three associations had no cell with minimum expected count less than five; therefore, the results are reliable.

Furthermore, cross-tabulation of study year with nature of medications used by students was significant as X^2 value was reported at 30.421 and p value was less than 0.01, with a weak to moderate effect size, i.e., a phi reported at 0.260. Only five cells (27.8%) had a minimum expected count less than five; therefore, the results may be considered reliable. The association between number of siblings and advice regarding SM practice was found to be statistically significant with the X^2 value reported at 16.079 and p value less than 0.05, with a weak effect size, i.e., a phi value reported at 0.189. Only four cells (26.7%) had an expected count less than five; therefore, the results may be considered reliable. The summary of cross-tabulation is presented in Table 6.

Table 6. Cross-tabulation between demographic and dependent variables.

Demographic Variable	Source of Information					p Value
Gender	**Pharmacist**	**Physician**	**Medical professionals**	**Family and Friends**	**Internet**	
Male	89 (68.6)	53 (58.7)	16 (23.8)	34 (33.8)	57 (64.2)	0.0001
Female	35 (55.4)	53 (47.3)	27 (19.2)	27 (27.2)	59 (51.8)	
College	**Pharmacist**	**Physician**	**Medical professionals**	**Family and Friends**	**Internet**	
Clinical Pharmacy	54 (42.2)	23 (36)	12 (14.6)	21 (20.7)	43 (39.4)	0.01
Medicine	70 (81.8)	83 (70)	31 (28.4)	40 (40.3)	73 (76.6)	
Nature of medications used by students						
College	**(Prescription) Rx drugs**		**(Over-the-counter) OTC drugs**		**Both**	
Clinical Pharmacy	19 (27.9)		84 (73.4)		50 (51.7)	0.036
Medicine	63 (54.1)		132 (142.6)		102 (100.3)	
Study year	**Rx drugs**		**OTC drugs**		**Both**	
Preparatory year	3 (1.5)		1 (3.8)		4 (2.7)	0.01
2nd Year	33 (17.9)		35 (47)		30 (33)	
3rd Year	23 (25.1)		70 (66.2)		45 (46.6)	
4th Year	7 (16.2)		46 (42.7)		36 (30.1)	
5th Year	14 (18.8)		57 (49.4)		32 (34.8)	
6th Year	2 (2.6)		7 (6.7)		5 (4.7)	
Advice regarding self-medication practice						
Siblings	**Always in favor**		**Against SM but can be used when necessary**		**Always against the practice**	
Between 1 and 2 siblings	9 (5.1)		28 (32.5)		3 (2.4)	0.041
Between 3 and 5 siblings	25 (24.7)		159 (158.6)		11 (11.7)	
Between 6 and 8 siblings	12 (15.7)		109 (100.9)		3 (7.4)	
More than 8 siblings	7 (8)		47 (51.2)		9 (3.8)	
No sibling	4 (3.5)		23 (22.8)		1 (1.7)	

4. Discussion

This study was conducted among students of pharmacy and medicine colleges at a public sector university in Dammam, Saudi Arabia. The age and marital status of the students represents the characteristic student enrollment in Saudi academia [18,19]. The prevalence of self-medication in both medicine and pharmacy colleges, combined was reported at 26%. This is quite low compared to the prevalence of SM previously reported in allied health students of other public sector universities of Saudi Arabia [18,19]. Furthermore, the prevalence of SM in College of Clinical Pharmacy alone was reported at 19.61%. This figure has been reported for the first time in this population as there is a lack of data pertaining to self-medication practice prevailing among Saudi pharmacy students. A study conducted in pharmacy students of a university in Saudi Arabia reported SM prevalence of 77%, however; the figure is not specific for pharmacy students as it was obtained from students of pharmacy, nursing, and dentistry, combined [20,21]. In regional context, study conducted in the pharmacy college of a university in the UAE and Pakistan reported SM prevalence of 86% and 67.2%, respectively [22,23].

The prevalence of SM in College of Medicine was found to be 49.3%. Studies have reported varying prevalence in medicine colleges from 66% to 87% among Saudi universities [18,19,21,23–25]. Our study has reported lowest SM prevalence in a medical college of Saudi university as of now. In regional context, the difference in prevalence between pharmacy and medicine colleges within universities can be attributed to the fact that students of medicines are deemed to become future prescribers. Hence, they find themselves more confident in indulging in self-medication. On the other hand, pharmacy students have more knowledge about drugs and their toxicology which may increase reluctance to indulge in the practice [18,25]. Further investigation is warranted.

There was a surge in the use of multivitamins as our study reported a prevalence of 30.53% which is quite high as compared to previously-reported prevalence of 3–5% [18,19,25,26]. In the region, prevalence of multivitamins use in university students of the UAE was reported at 39% [27]. The use of analgesics, such as paracetamol and NSAIDs, was quite high. Our study reported the prevalence at 72.35% which is the second highest figure reported among Saudi universities currently. The prevalence for the same was reported in previous literature in ranges of 28.7% to 80% among other Saudi universities [18,19,22,25]. Our study also reported the prevalence of antibiotics use among students which was documented at 16.59%. This was second to the lowest figure, i.e., 5% previously reported from King Saud University [19]. High prevalence of antibiotic use was previously reported in the range of 30% to 32% from Taibah and Qassim University, respectively [18,21,25]. Additionally, prevalence of antihistamines and cold/flu products use was comparatively higher than figures reported from other universities of the country. Our study reported a prevalence of antihistamines use at 39.16% which was far higher than figures reported from Taibah University (1.1%) and King Saud University (5%) [18,19]. It was second to highest prevalence reported i.e. from Qassim University, (41%) [25]. The prevalence of anti-diarrheals and antacids was reported for the first time from this population.

Self-medication with anti-fungal (N = 1), corticosteroids (N = 2), anti-acne, i.e., Isotretenoin (N = 1), and anti-emetic i.e., ondansetron (N = 2), CNS stimulants i.e., methylphenidate (N = 1) and anti-spasmodic, i.e., mebavarine (N = 1) was also reported. The prevalence of depression and psychoactive stimulants use in pharmacy students of Pakistan was reported at 1.31% [12,28]. Previous studies conducted in Saudi Arabia found a number of students indulged in substance abuse, especially abuse of such products. Studies have reported the growing substance abuse among students of Saudi universities [24,25,29]. In our study, only a single student acknowledged self-medicating with methylphenidate.

The most common source of information regarding SM were pharmacists, as well as physicians. This finding was also statistically associated with gender and colleges. Pharmacists were the preferred choice for males to seek SM-related information. Females were more inclined towards physicians. Pharmacy students sought information regarding SM from pharmacists. Similarly, students from the College of Medicine highlighted their preference of a physician for such information. Since students of medical college were taught by physicians, it may have promoted confidence in seeking such information from physicians [19,20]. The same principle may apply to pharmacy students.

The majority of the students self medicated with OTC medicines, however, a third proportion of the students used both OTC and POMs. This finding was statistically associated with college and year of study. Medical students and those studying in the 2nd Professional year self-medicated with POM, more than their counterparts. One possible explanation regarding this association could be the fact that physicians in this part of the globe have sole prescribing rights and are deemed by society to prescribe medicines. Medical students who were taught by physicians may find themselves in a much more comfortable position to use POMs as compared to pharmacy students since they are ingrained with a prescribing authority. They may be more inclined towards this practice. Students appeared self-medicating with POM in the 2nd year in higher numbers compared to any other study year. The professional education in pharmacy and medicine at the university starts when the students have progressed from the preparatory year into 2nd year. As the students progress in their educational career, they become more educated and informed about the phenomenon. Professional education may influence their perception towards SM practice and use of POMs. As a result, they may develop reluctance in self-medicating with POM progressively. Hence, our study found that the number of students self-medicating with POMs decreased as they progressed in their educational career.

The most common reasons given as a justification to indulge in SM were 'mild problem' and 'previous experience with medicine'. This finding was congruent with previous literature reported from the country, as well as the region [18]. The importance of physician consultation was stated the most common reason against this practice, which was also reported from university students of Pakistan [13]. Contrastingly, an overwhelming majority of students highlighted their stance that they were against SM practice, in principle, but clarified that SM could be used in rare situations. This was a novel finding as previous studies conducted among the same population reported that most of the students of Jazan University (52.6%) and Taibah University (87%) appeared totally against the practice [18,23]. It can be deduced from this finding that students at Imam Abdulrahman Bin Faisal University understand importance of responsible self-medication.

5. Conclusions

The prevalence of self-medication in pharmacy students was quite low and has been reported for the first time. The prevalence of self-medication in medical students was the second lowest reported from a Saudi university, currently. Students mostly self-medicated with OTC drugs however, the use of antibiotics was also observed. The prevalence of antibiotics use was the second lowest among Saudi universities, however, and some students reported using corticosteroids and isotretenoin, which are quite dangerous if self-medicated. Students had a positive outlook towards pharmacists as drug information experts. Our study reported an increased use of multivitamins. Full-scale studies are needed to document the prevalence of multivitamins use in this population. The most common reasons to self-medicate were 'mild problems' and 'previous experience with medicine'. Students of medicine and pharmacy colleges at IAU understand importance of responsible self-medication.

Acknowledgments: This research paper is based on the undergraduate research project undertaken as a bachelor thesis for partial fulfillment of Doctor of Pharmacy (Pharm.D) degree program by Fatima Ali Albusalih (ID 2130001853) at the College of Clinical Pharmacy, Imam Abdulrahman Bin Faisal University (formerly University of Dammam), Dammam 31441, Saudi Arabia.

Author Contributions: F.A.A. conceived the idea jointly with A.A.N. A.A.N. designed the methodology and research questionnaire in collaboration with R.A. and N.A. F.A.A. conducted the pilot study and modified the research instrument according to pilot results. A.A.N. conducted statistical analysis of the research tool and finalized the questionnaire. F.A.A. and N.A. collected the data and entered in S.P.S.S. with R.A. and A.A.N. A.A.N. analyzed the data and conducted statistical analysis. A.A.N. wrote the introduction and methodology section. R.A. and N.A. formulated the tables and wrote the results section and collaborated in discussion with A.A.N. and F.A.A. F.A.A. wrote the abstract and conclusion. The whole manuscript was edited and finalized by A.A.N. and R.A. The response to reviewers' comments was jointly addressed by F.A.A., A.A.N., R.A. and N.A. All authors read and approved the final version of the manuscript.

References

1. Garofalo, L.; Giuseppe, G.D.; Angelillo, I.F. Self-Medication Practices among Parents in Italy. *BioMed. Res. Int.* **2015**, *2015*. [CrossRef] [PubMed]

2. Shah, A.; Naqvi, A.A.; Ahmad, R. The need for providing pharmaceutical care in geriatrics: A case study of diagnostic errors leading to medication-related problems in a patient treatment plan. *Arch. Pharm. Pract.* **2016**, *7*, 87–94.

3. Naqvi, A.A.; Naqvi, S.B.; Zehra, F.; Ahmad, R.; Ahmad, N. The cost of poliomyelitis: Lack of cost-of-illness studies on poliomyelitis rehabilitation in Pakistan. *Arch. Pharm. Pract.* **2016**, *7*, 182–184. [CrossRef]

4. Hussaim, M.; Naqvi, S.B.S.; Khan, M.A.; Rizvi, M.; Alam, S.; Abbas, A.; Akram, M. Direct cost of treatment of diabetes mellitus type 2 in Pakistan. *Int. J. Pharm. Sci.* **2014**, *6*, 261–264.

5. Ruiz, M.E. Risks of Self-Medication Practices. *Curr. Drug Saf.* **2010**, *5*, 315–323. [CrossRef] [PubMed]

6. Sarahroodi, S.; Arzi, A.; Sawalha, A.F.; Ashtarinezhad, A. Antibiotics self-medication among southern Iranian university students. *Int. J. Pharmacol.* **2010**, *6*, 48–52. [CrossRef]

7. Abay, S.M.; Amelo, W. Assessment of self-medication practices among medical, pharmacy, and health science students in Gondar University Ethiopia. *J. Young Pharm.* **2010**, *2*, 306–310. [CrossRef] [PubMed]

8. Abbas, A.; Ahmed, F.R.; Rizvi, M.; Khan, M.H.; Kachela, B. Evaluation of drug dispensing practices by pharmaceutical drug retailers in Pakistan. *World J. Pharm. Res.* **2015**, *4*, 189–197.

9. Gellman, M.D.; Turner, J.R. "Self-medication". In *Encyclopedia of Behavioral Medicine*; Springer: New York, NY, USA, 2013.

10. Aljadhey, H.; Assiri, G.; Mahmoud, M.; Al-Aqeel, S.; Murray, M. Self-medication in Central Saudi Arabia. Community pharmacy consumers' perspectives. *Saudi Med. J.* **2015**, *36*, 328–334. [CrossRef] [PubMed]

11. Bawazir, S.A. Prescribing pattern at community pharmacies in Saudi Arabia. *Int. Pharm. J.* **1992**, *6*, 5.

12. Abbas, A.; Ahmed, F.R.; Yousuf, R.; Khan, N.; Nisa, Z.N.; Ali, S.I.; Rizvi, M.; Sabah, A.; Tanwir, S. Prevalence of Self-Medication of Psychoactive Stimulants and Antidepressants among Undergraduate Pharmacy Students in Twelve Pakistani Cities. *Trop. J. Pharm. Res.* **2015**, *14*, 527–532. [CrossRef]

13. Naqvi, A.A.; Ahmad, R.; Qadeer, O.; Khan, M.H.; Nadir, M.N.; Alim, M. The Prevalence of Self Medication and the Factors influencing its Practice in Pharmacy Students of Karachi, Pakistan: A mix mode study. *J. Young Pharm.* **2016**, *8*, 230–238. [CrossRef]

14. Sample Size Calculator. Raosoft, Inc. Available online: http://www.raosoft.com/samplesize.html (accessed on 18 July 2017).

15. Health Statistics Annual Book. Ministry of Health: Riyadh, Saudi Arabia, 2014–2015. Available online: http://www.moh.gov.sa/en/ministry/statistics/book/documents/1433.pdf (accessed on 27 July 2017).

16. Prevalence Rate Calculator. Medcalc Easy to Use Software. Available online: https://www.medcalc.org/calc/diagnostic_test.php (accessed on 28 July 2017).

17. IBM Corp. *Released 2013: IBM SPSS Statistics for Windows*; Version 22.0; IBM Corp: Armonk, NY, USA.

18. Aljaouni, M.E.; Hafiz, A.A.; Alalawi, H.H.; Alahmadi, G.A.; AlKhawaja, I. Self-medication practice among medical and non-medical students at Taibah University, Madinah, Saudi Arabia. *Int. J. Acad. Sci. Res.* **2015**, *3*, 54–65.

19. Eissa, A. Knowledge, Attitudes and Practices towards Medication Use among Health Care Students in King Saud University. *Int. J. Med. Stud.* **2013**, *1*, 66–69.

20. Adnan, S.; Tanwir, S.; Abbas, A.; Beg, A.E.; Sabah, A.; Safdar, H.; Moin, M.; Fatima, R.; Mobeen, K.; Shams, M. Perception of physicians regarding patient counselling by pharmacist: A blend of quantitative and qualitative insight. *Int. J. Pharm. Ther.* **2014**, *5*, 117–121.

21. Adnan, M.; Karim, S.; Khan, S.; Sabir, A.; Lafi Al-Banagi, A.R.; Sajid Jamal, Q.M.; Al Wabel, N. Evaluation of Self-Medication Practices and Awareness among Students in Al Qassim Region of Saudi Arabia. *Clin. Pharmacol. Biopharm.* **2015**, *4*. [CrossRef]

22. Sharif, S.I.; Mohamed Ibrahim, O.H.; Mouslli, L.; Waisi, R. Evaluation of self medication among pharmacy students. *Am. J. Pharmacol. Toxicol.* **2012**, *7*, 135–140. [CrossRef]

23. Albasheer, O.B.; Mahfouz, M.S.; Masmali, B.M.; Ageeli, R.A.; Majrashi, A.M.; Hakami, A.N.; Hakami, Z.H.; Hakami, A.A.; Douf, T.A. Self-medication practice among undergraduate medical students of a Saudi tertiary institution. *Trop. J. Pharm. Res.* **2016**, *15*, 2253–2259. [CrossRef]

24. Ibrahim, N.K.; Alamoudi, B.M.; Baamer, W.O.; Al-Raddadi, R.M. Self-medication with analgesics among medical students and interns in King Abdulaziz University, Jeddah, Saudi Arabia. *Pak. J. Med. Sci.* **2015**, *31*, 14–18. [CrossRef] [PubMed]

25. Al-Worafi, Y.A.; Long, C.; Saeed, M.; Alkhoshaiban, A. Perception of self-medication among university students in Saudi Arabia. *Arch. Pharm. Pract.* **2014**, *5*, 149–152. [CrossRef]

26. Almalaka, H.; Albluwia, A.I.; Alkhelba, D.A.; Alsaleha, H.M.; Khan, T.M.; Ahmad Hassali, M.A.; Aljadhey, H. Students' attitude toward use of over the counter medicines during exams in Saudi Arabia. *Saudi Pharm. J.* **2014**, *22*, 107–112. [CrossRef] [PubMed]

27. Alhomoud, F.K.; Basil, M.; Bondarev, A. Knowledge, Attitudes and Practices (KAP) Relating to Dietary Supplements among Health Sciences and Non-Health Sciences Students in One of the Universities of United Arab Emirates (UAE). *J. Clin. Diagn. Res.* **2016**, *10*, JC05–JC09. [CrossRef] [PubMed]

28. Abbas, A.; Rizvi, S.A.; Hassan, R.; Aqeel, N.; Khan, M.; Bhutto, A.; Khan, Z.; Mannan, Z. The prevalence of depression and its perceptions among undergraduate pharmacy students. *Pharm. Educ.* **2015**, *15*, 57–63.

29. Al-Haqwi, A.I. Perception among medical students in Riyadh, Saudi Arabia, regarding alcohol and substance abuse in the community: A cross-sectional survey. *Subst. Abuse Treat. Prev. Policy* **2010**, *5*. [CrossRef] [PubMed]

14

The Country Profiles of the PHARMINE Survey of European Higher Educational Institutions Delivering Pharmacy Education and Training

Jeffrey Atkinson

Pharmacolor Consultants Nancy, Villers 54600, France; jeffrey.atkinson@univ-lorraine.fr

Academic Editor: Antonio Sanchez-Pozo

Abstract: The PHARMINE (Pharmacy Education in Europe) consortium surveyed pharmacy education and practice in 2012. Surveys were updated in 2017 for publication. The PHARMINE consortium was especially interested in specialization in pharmacy education and practice (for community, hospital, and industrial pharmacy), and in the impact of the Bologna agreement and the directive of the European Commission on education and training for the sectoral profession of pharmacy on European degree courses. The surveys underline the varying attitudes of the different European countries to these various aspects. The surveys will now be published in *Pharmacy*. They will be useful to researchers in education, and to staff and students interested in mobility amongst different European and/or non-European countries. In order to assure a full understanding of the country profiles to be published in the journal *Pharmacy*, this introductory article describes the general format of the survey questionnaire used.

Keywords: pharmacy; education; practice; Europe

1. Introduction

In the 21st century, the role of pharmacists is changing. For instance, community and hospital pharmacists play an increasingly important role individually (monitoring of chronic diseases, vaccinations, etc.), and as partners, in the efficient use of health care resources [1]. Industrial pharmacists are major players in the developmental transition of the pharmaceutical industry [2] as it undergoes a transformation from a chemical, small molecule industry to a biotechnological, peptide industry. For all pharmacists, such new functions will require new competences.

The PHAR-QA (Quality Assurance in Pharmacy Education and Training) [3] consortium investigated such competences. However, before proposing a framework of new competences, it was necessary to survey the present state of pharmacy education and training (PET) in Europe in order to establish capacity in European PET. This was done by the PHARMINE (Pharmacy Education in Europe) consortium [4] which prefigured the PHAR-QA consortium.

The PHARMINE project brought together the academic members of the European Association of Faculties of Pharmacy (EAFP) [5], and EU partner associations representing pharmaceutical practitioners: community (PGEU) [6], hospital (EAHP) [7], and industrial pharmacy (EIPG) [8]. The European Pharmacy Students' Association [9] was also an important partner.

The PHARMINE consortium produced profiles for the countries in the European Higher Education Area [10] by surveying pharmacy practice and resources, management, and curricula of pharmacy degree courses. Resources and curricula were surveyed at the fundamental, general practice level and at the advanced specialization level (i.e., community, hospital, and industrial pharmacy elective courses).

Finally, the consortium examined the opportunities in different countries for the introduction into PET of the principles of the Bologna declaration [11] on European university degree courses (not only pharmacy) including the potential separation of a tunnel-structured five-year degree course such as that for pharmacy, into a basic three-year bachelor course followed by an advanced five-year master course. It should be noted that the Bologna declaration, and its subsequent amendments, are the fruit of the collaboration of the ministers of education of the different European countries. This does not represent European Union (EU) law.

In parallel, the consortium examined to what extent different countries abide by the proposals in the European Commission's (EC) directive on education and training for the sectoral professions such as pharmacy, concerning management of the degree course (pharmacy being a five-year tunnel course in the eyes of the EC) and subject area content of the course [12]. Subject area content will have a direct impact on the competences to be taught. It should be noted that an EC directive is an instrument of the law of the European Union, and as such is to be adopted by the different member states into their national legislation.

2. Methodology

The PHARMINE questionnaire was based on that used in a first survey of pharmacy departments carried out by the EAFP in the 1990s [13].

The project ran from spring 2009 through summer 2011. All country profiles were updated in the spring of 2017 for publication.

The survey form was sent out to at least one department in each country of the European Higher Education Area. Data for the survey were collected by electronic means [14]. This was backed up by telephone calls and/or by on-site visits to help and encourage respondents to fill out the form.

3. Results and Discussion

3.1. Survey Chapters

The survey document had eight chapters:

1. Personal details of respondent
2. Organization of the activities of pharmacists, professional bodies
3. Pharmacy higher education institutions (HEIs), students, and courses
4. Teaching and learning methods
5. Subject areas
6. Impact of the Bologna principles
7. Impact of EC directive
8. Quality assurance or pharmacy education and training (E&T)

3.2. Personal Details of the HEI Respondent

The survey asked for contact details (name, address, telephone, email, and website) of at least one person from each HEI. The contact person implicitly agreed to act as contact for enquires from students, staff, researchers, and/or practitioners once the survey had been published.

PHARMINE also asked respondents to provide useful website addresses (for mobility . . .) and supporting material such as texts of national law.

Respondents were then asked to give information on the following chapters.

3.3. Organization of the Activities of Pharmacists, Professional Bodies

The aim was to produce sufficient data (numbers, descriptions . . .) to draw a realistic and relevant picture of the practice of community, hospital, industrial pharmacists, and pharmacists working in other professions, as well as pharmacy technicians. A final section dealt with the role of the professional bodies in legal and ethical matters.

Questions were asked on the following topics.

Pharmacy practice

1. Community pharmacy practice

   a. Numbers of community pharmacies and pharmacists
   b. Competences and roles of community pharmacists
   c. Whether the ownership of community pharmacies is limited to pharmacists
   d. The rules governing the geographical distribution of community pharmacies
   e. The availability of drugs and other healthcare products by channels other than pharmacies

2. Pharmacy technicians

   a. Their titles and number(s)
   b. Their qualifications

      i. Organizations providing and validating their E&T
      ii. Duration of studies
      iii. Subject areas

   c. Their competences and roles

3. Hospital pharmacy practice

   a. Whether such a function exists. PHARMINE was interested in whether "hospital pharmacy practice" could be defined by work place or duties, i.e., is a hospital pharmacist a pharmacist who works in a hospital or a pharmacist with specific, legally defined tasks related to practice with hospitalized patients?
   b. Number of hospital pharmacists
   c. Number of hospital pharmacies

4. Industrial pharmacy

   a. Pharmaceutical and related industries

      i. Number of companies with production, R&D, and/or distribution
      ii. Number of companies producing generic drugs only

   b. Industrial pharmacists

      i. Number of pharmacists working in industry
      ii. Competences and roles of industrial pharmacists

5. Pharmacists working in other sectors

   a. Number of pharmacists working in other sectors
   b. Sectors in which pharmacists are employed
   c. Competences and roles of pharmacists employed in other sectors

   Professional associations: roles.

1. Registration of pharmacists
2. Creation of community pharmacies and control of territorial distribution
3. Ethics and professional conduct
4. Quality assurance and validation of HEI courses for pharmacists

In this and other sections numerical data for individual countries was compared to those for Europe [15].

3.4. Pharmacy HEIs, Students, and Courses

The aim was to produce sufficient data (numbers, descriptions . . .) to draw a realistic and relevant picture of PET. A final section concerned the past and future changes in PET.

Questions were asked on the following topics.

1. HEIs

    a. Total number of pharmacy HEIs in your country, public and private
    b. Independent department or attached to a science or medical faculty
    c. B + M degree structure

        i.   Availability
        ii. M open to students with a non-pharmacy B degree

2. Staff (at the level of the country and at that of the responding HEI)

    a. Number of teaching staff (nationals)
    b. Number of international teaching staff—European and non-European
    c. Number professionals (pharmacists and others) from outside the HEI, involved in pharmacy E&T

3. Students (at the level of the country and at that of the responding HEI)

    a. Number of places at traditional entry (beginning of S1/B1, following secondary school)
    b. Number of applicants for entry
    c. Number of graduates that become professional pharmacists.
    d. Number of international students—European (Erasmus) [16] and non-European
    e. Specific pharmacy-related (national or HEI) entrance examination
    f. National numerus clausus
    g. Advanced entry (>S1/B1)

        i.   Which level
        ii. Requirements

    h. Fees for home, European, and non-European students

4. Specialization

    i.   Which years
    ii.   Which topics (industry, hospital . . .)
    iii. Student numbers in each specialization

5. Changes in PET: past and future

3.5. Teaching and Learning Methods

The aim was to produce sufficient data (numbers, descriptions . . .) to draw a realistic and relevant picture of the methods used in teaching and learning.

Questions were asked on the following topics.

1. Course organization

    a. Student hours in each year for lectures, tutorials, practicums, independent project work

b.   Traineeship (community, hospital, industry)

c.   Electives

d.   Validation of courses, etc.

3.6. Subject Areas

The aim was to produce sufficient data (numbers, descriptions . . .) to draw a realistic and relevant picture of the methods used in teaching and learning.

Questions were asked on the number of hours per year in each of the following seven subject areas (slightly modified version of definition of subject areas used in first EAFP survey cited above).

1.   Chemical sciences (CHEMSCI)

   a.   General, organic, and inorganic chemistry
   b.   Analytical chemistry
   c.   Pharmaceutical chemistry and pharmacopeial analysis
   d.   Medicinal physico-chemistry/structure-activity/drug design

2.   Physical and mathematical sciences (PHYSMATH)

   a.   Physics
   b.   Mathematics, pharmaceutical calculations
   c.   Information technology, information technology applied to community pharmacy, information technology applied to national health-care
   d.   Statistics
   e.   Experimental design and analysis

3.   Biological sciences (BIOLSCI)

   a.   Foundation biology
   b.   Cell biology
   c.   Botany
   d.   Mycology
   e.   Zoology
   f.   Biochemistry
   g.   Molecular biology
   h.   Genetics

4.   Pharmaceutical technology (PHARMTECH)

   a.   Formulation
   b.   Drug disposition and metabolism/pharmacokinetics
   c.   Novel drug delivery systems
   d.   Drug design
   e.   Pharmaceutical R&D
   f.   Drug production
   g.   Quality assurance in production
   h.   Drug/new chemical entity registration and regularization
   i.   Common technical document (quality (pharmaceutical), safety (safety pharmacology and toxicology), efficacy (preclinical and clinical studies))
   j.   Ophthalmic preparations
   k.   Medical gases
   l.   Cosmetics

m. Management strategy in industry
n. Economics of the pharmaceutical industry and R&D

5. Medicinal sciences (MEDISCI)

a. Human anatomy and physiology
b. Medical terminology
c. Pharmacology
d. Pharmacognosy
e. Pharmacotherapy/therapeutics
f. Toxicology
g. Pathology, histology
h. Microbiology
i. Nutrition, non-pharmacological treatment
j. Hematology
k. Immunology
l. Parasitology
m. Hygiene
n. Emergency therapy
o. Clinical chemistry/bioanalysis (of body fluids)
p. Radiochemistry
q. Dispensing process, drug prescription, prescription analysis (detection of adverse effects and drug interactions)
r. Generic drugs
s. Planning, running, and interpretation of the data of clinical trials
t. Medical devices
u. Orthopedics
v. OTC medicines, complementary therapy
w. At-home support and care
x. Skin illness and treatment
y. Homeopathy
z. Phytotherapy

aa. Drugs in veterinary medicine
bb. Pharmaceutical care, pharmaceutical therapy of illness and disease

6. Law and social sciences (LAWSOC)

a. Legislation, law relating to pharmacy
b. Social sciences
c. Forensic science
d. Professional ethics
e. Philosophy
f. Economics, financial affairs, book keeping, economic planning, and management
g. Public health/health promotion
h. Quality management
i. Epidemiology of drug use (pharmaco-epidemiology)
j. Economics of drug use (pharmaco-economics)
k. History of pharmacy

7.   Generic competences (GENERIC)

    a.   General knowledge
    b.   Academic literacy
    c.   Languages
    d.   First aid
    e.   Communication
    f.   Management
    g.   Practical skills

3.7. Impact of the Bologna Principles

Respondents were asked how the principles outlined in the Bologna declaration on degree comparability and student and staff mobility, cited above, affect PET in their HEI:

1.   Easily readable and comparable degrees? Issue of a Diploma Supplement?
2.   Courses divided into two main cycles: three-year B and two-year M?
3.   Relevance of B degree to the European labor market
4.   Possibility for students with a three-year B degree from an HEI other than pharmacy (natural sciences, chemistry ...) and/or from another country to enroll into the pharmacy M
5.   Use of the European system of credits (ECTS) [17] to promote student mobility and/or lifelong learning
6.   Efforts made to remove obstacles to student and staff mobility (with language courses ...)
7.   Numbers of Erasmus exchange staff and students.
8.   Involvement in European co-operative programs on quality assurance with attempts to develop comparable criteria and methodologies?
9.   European dimensions in higher education regarding curriculum development, general inter-institutional co-operation and integrated programs of study, training and research

3.8. Impact of EC Directive

Questions were asked as to what extent HEIs followed the EC directive on the sectoral profession of pharmacy, especially concerning the five-year, 'tunnel' degree structure imposed by the directive that is in opposition to the Bologna recommendations.

Questions were asked on the three main elements of directive:

1.   Course length
2.   Course content
3.   Traineeship

4. Conclusions

Country profiles for European PET will be published in 'pharmacy'. This article serves as an introduction to these surveys and as a vade mecum for the reader of such articles. The information contained in the country profile articles is of a descriptive nature; it will serve as a tool for those wishing to do educational research on European PET and/or promote student and staff mobility.

Data for individual countries are compared with European averages already published [15]. For such comparisons we used a European linear regression estimation. Data were taken from the 25 EU members of the EHEA that had at least one pharmacy department. The calculation was as follows: estimations of numbers of pharmacies, etc. (X, dependent variable) were calculated from the linear regression equation with the country population as the independent (Y) variable. It was assumed in this calculation that when $X = 0$, then $Y = 0$. The reported number for the country was then expressed as a ratio of the estimated number. This will be illustrated by an example using community pharmacies in France. The global EU data for X = country population (in millions $\times 10^{-6}$) and Y = number of community pharmacies, gave a slope of 298 $\pm$ 18 (n = 25 countries). Thus the EU linear regression estimation of the number of pharmacies in France = 64.7 million $\times$ 298 = 19,280. The reported number of pharmacies in France is 23,133, thus giving a ratio compared to the estimate of 23,133/19,280 = 1.20. France therefore has 1.2 times more pharmacies than to be expected from the EU linear regression estimation or EU 'average'.

Acknowledgments: With the support of the Lifelong Learning Program of the European Union programs 142078-LLP-1-2008-BE-ERASMUS-ECDSP and 527194-LLP-1-2012-1-BE-ERASMUS-EMCR.

Abbreviations Used in the PHARMINE Survey

B	Bachelor level (first three years study following secondary school). This may be followed by a number, e.g., B1 = first year of bachelor studies.
M	Master level (fourth and fifth years of study)
D	Doctoral (Ph.D.) level. This will start after five years of study at an HEI (three years B plus two years M)
E&T	Education and training
PET	Pharmacy education and training
HEI	Higher education institution
LLL	Lifelong learning
R&D	Research and development
S	Semester. This may be followed by a number, e.g., S1/B1 = first semester of the first bachelor year

References

1. Kehrer, J.P.; Eberhart, G.; Wing, M.; Horon, K. Pharmacy's role in a modern health continuum. *Can. Pharm. J.* **2013**, *146*, 321–324. Available online: https://www.ncbi.nlm.nih.gov/pmc/articles/PMC3819958/ (accessed on 10 February 2017). [CrossRef] [PubMed]

2. Farrugia, C. Pharmaceutical Industry and the Industrial Pharmacist: A Partnership for the 21st Century. Available online: http://fr.slideshare.net/eipg/the-pharmaceutical-industry-and-the-industrial-pharmacist-a-partnership-for-the-21st-century (accessed on 10 February 2017).

3. The PHAR-QA Project. Quality Assurance in European Pharmacy Education and Training. Available online: www.phar-qa.eu (accessed on 10 February 2017).

4. The PHARMINE (Pharmacy Education in Europe) Consortium. Available online: http://www.pharmine.org/ (accessed on 10 February 2017).

5. European Association of Faculties of Pharmacy (EAFP). Available online: http://www.pharmine.org/ (accessed on 10 February 2017).

6. Pharmacists' Group of the EU (PGEU). Available online: http://www.pgeu.eu/ (accessed on 10 February 2017).

7. European Association of Hospital Pharmacists (EAHP). Available online: http://www.eahp.eu/ (accessed on 10 February 2017).

8. European Industrial Pharmacists' Group (EIPG). Available online: http://www.eipg.eu/ (accessed on 10 February 2017).

9. European Pharmacy Students' Association (EPSA). Available online: http://www.epas.eu/ (accessed on 10 February 2017).

10. EHEA. The European Higher Education Area. Available online: http://www.ehea.info/ (accessed on 10 February 2017).

11. Bologna Declaration 1999. Available online: www.magna-charta.org/.../files/BOLOGNA_DECLARATION.pdf (accessed on 10 February 2017).

12. EC Directive. The EU Directive 2013/55/EU on the Recognition of Professional Qualifications. Available online: http://eur-lex.europa.eu/LexUriServ/LexUriServ.do?uri=OJ:L:2005:255:0022:0142:EN:PDF (accessed on 10 February 2017).

13. Bourlioux, P. Paris, EU TEMPUS Project. Available online: www.phar-qa.eu/wp-content/.../P_Bourlioux_Erasmus-subject-evaluations-1995.pdf (accessed on 10 February 2017).

14. Surveymonkey. The Survey Software—The Survey System. Available online: http://www.surveysystem.com/sscalc.htm (accessed on 10 February 2017).

15. Atkinson, J.; Rombaut, B. The 2011 PHARMINE Report on Pharmacy and Pharmacy Education in the European Union. *Pharm. Pract. (Int.)* **2011**, *9*, 169–187. Available online: https://www.ncbi.nlm.nih.gov/pmc/articles/PMC3818732/ (accessed on 10 February 2017). [CrossRef]

16. Erasmus+. Available online: https://www.erasmusplus.fr/ (accessed on 10 February 2017).

17. European Credit Transfer System (ECTS). Available online: http://www.mastersportal.eu/articles/388/all-you-need-to-know-about-the-european-credit-system-ects.html (accessed on 10 February 2017).

15

Impact of Pharmacist-Conducted Comprehensive Medication Reviews for Older Adult Patients to Reduce Medication Related Problems

Whitney J. Kiel [1],* and Shaun W. Phillips [2]

[1] Bronson Methodist Hospital, 601 John St. Suite M-020, Kalamazoo, MI 49007, USA
[2] Clinical and Pharmacy Services, Bronson Healthcare Group, 300 North Avenue, Battle Creek, MI 49017, USA; phillish@bronsonhg.org
*   Correspondence: kielw@bronsonhg.org

Abstract: Older adults are demanding increased healthcare attention with regards to prescription use due in large part to highly complex medication regimens. As patients age, medications often have a more pronounced effect on older adults, negatively impacting patient safety and increasing healthcare costs. Comprehensive medication reviews (CMRs) optimize medications for elderly patients and help to avoid inappropriate medication use. Previous literature has shown that such CMRs can successfully identify and reduce the number of medication-related problems and improve acute healthcare utilization. The purpose of this pharmacy resident research study is to examine the impact of pharmacist-conducted geriatric medication reviews to reduce medication-related problems within a leading community health system in southwest Michigan. Furthermore, the study examines type of pharmacist interventions made during medication reviews, acute healthcare utilization, and physician assessment of the pharmacist's value. The study was conducted as a retrospective post-hoc analysis on ambulatory patients who received a CMR by a pharmacist at a primary care practice. Inclusion criteria included patients over 65 years of age with concurrent use of at least five medications who were a recent recipient of a CMR. Exclusion criteria included patients with renal failure, or those with multiple providers involved in primary care. The primary outcome was the difference in number of medication-related problems, as defined by the START and STOPP Criteria (Screening Tool to Alert doctors to Right Treatment/Screening Tool of Older Persons' Prescriptions). Secondary outcomes included hospitalizations, emergency department visits, number and type of pharmacist interventions, acceptance rate of pharmacist recommendations, and assessment of the pharmacist's value by clinic providers. There were a total of 26 patients that received a comprehensive medication review from the pharmacist and were compared to a control group, patients that did not receive a CMR. The average patient age for both groups was 76 years old. A total of 11 medication-related problems in the intervention group patients were identified compared with 24 medication-related problems in the control group (p-value 0.002). Pharmacist-led comprehensive medication reviews were associated with a statistically significant different in the number of medication-related problems as defined by the START and STOPP criteria.

Keywords: pharmacist; comprehensive medication review; polypharmacy; medication-related problems; medication therapy management; geriatric; START/STOPP criteria; interdisciplinary team

1. Introduction

Older adults demand increased healthcare attention with regards to prescription medication use due to highly complex regimens and increased vulnerability to poor health outcomes [1,2]. With the advancing age of the Baby Boomer generation, who are now hitting 65 years and older, elderly patient prescriptions now account for over 33% of all prescription medications [3]. As the average life span continues to rise, greater numbers of prescriptions are needed to manage the chronic disease states and conditions commonly encountered in the elderly patient population. Concerns arise due to the fact that medications often have a more pronounced effect on older adults. These effects may include exacerbated confusion, an increased risk of falls, and other adverse drug reactions, further impacting healthcare utilization and increasing costs. The Centers for Medicare and Medicaid Services have provided for medication reviews as part of the Medicare Modernization Act of 2003. These comprehensive medication reviews (CMRs) fall under medication therapy management (MTM) services able to be conducted and billed for by a pharmacist [4].

CMRs optimize medications for elderly patients and avoid inappropriate medication use. Using a pharmacist to conduct these reviews saves the physician time and utilizes a medication expert to identify potential problems with a patient's medication regimen. With the push for healthcare reform, many incentives are being introduced to provide comprehensive health services that improve the quality of health care for patients in non-acute settings. Many have chosen to adopt an interdisciplinary team approach to conquering the advancement in health care services. The American Society of Health-System Pharmacists introduced their Pharmacy Practice Model Initiative in order to guide others in placing pharmacists within these clinical interdisciplinary teams [5]. Previous literature has examined the impact of a pharmacist, conducting such geriatric medication reviews with the goal of improving comprehensive health services for the elderly [2,5].

Various tools have been used to estimate the appropriateness of medications. Arguably the most widely recognized set of criteria is the Beers Criteria for potentially inappropriate medication use in older adults. In 2012, and subsequently in 2015, the American Geriatric Society released the much-anticipated updates to the Beers Criteria [6,7]. While both updates made significant improvements—including updated renal dosing recommendations and a higher level of clinical evidence—other criteria have been proposed to aid in identifying medication related problems. One such criteria is the "Screening Tool to Alert doctors to the Right Treatment and the Screening Tool of Older Persons' potentially inappropriate Prescriptions" (START/STOPP) Criteria. This tool goes a step further from the Beers list in addressing medications possibly indicated for older adults, as well as expanding on those that should be taken away [8,9].

The START/STOPP criteria were used to comprehensively evaluate the appropriateness of medication regimens in older adults in a study by Brahmbhatt et al. [8]. While this study found a significant reduction in the STOPP score between initial and follow up medication reviews, it did not find a significant increase in the START score. The authors commented on the difficulty in initiating medications in the elderly with already complex medication regimens and noted that not all of the criteria are clearly defined. In addition, the study population included home-based veterans, many of whom receive comprehensive healthcare services through other programs. The overarching goal of 'using screening' tools such as the START/STOPP criteria is to help identify potential medications that have an increased risk for falls and adverse effects on the elderly. Through management of their complex, numerous medications, many adverse effects due to multiple medications can be prevented [6,8,9].

Polypharmacy can be defined as taking at least five medications on a regular basis [10]. On average, geriatric patients take eight medications daily, greatly increasing the risk of falls or other adverse events. Falls are a particular concern since they are one of the most common threats to independence for elderly patients. Weber and colleagues found a significant reduction in both total number of medications and number of psychoactive medications in their evaluation of standardized medication reviews in an ambulatory patient population. They further looked at the number of falls among their patients, with the intervention group almost 60% less likely to have one or more fall-related diagnosis. Additional studies have shown reductions in adverse drug reactions, high-risk medications, and falls [3,10–13].

Many studies have sought to improve the appropriateness of medications or decrease medication-related problems. In a study of medication reviews by Vink et al., pharmacists successfully identified medication related problems (MRPs). They showed that 28% of the 232 total MRPs identified in 380 patients were associated with suboptimal therapy, while another 24% consisted of unnecessary medications. Roth and colleagues showed a significant reduction in mean number of medication related problems per patient in their study of 64 elderly patients who were cared for by a pharmacist within a primary care practice. They also noted a significant reduction in acute healthcare utilization of 35%. In a randomized controlled trial by Hanlon and colleagues evaluating medication appropriateness, the inappropriate prescribing scores were reduced significantly in the pharmacist intervention group (24% vs. 6% $p = 0.0006$). They also found a significant acceptance rate from physicians to the pharmacist recommendations in the intervention group ($p < 0.001$) [2,10,14,15].

As indicated in the reports above, a successful comprehensive medication review program would need to impact a wide range of factors in order to address the efficacy and safety of geriatric patients' medications. Studies have shown improvements in clinical outcomes such as blood pressure as well as patient-centered outcomes including adherence and knowledge of medication therapy. As health care costs rise, essential economic outcomes including length of stay and readmission rates are necessary to evaluate among geriatric patients, who are at an especially high risk for readmission. While literature concerning these outcomes is more limited, a study of team-based care [16] including a pharmacist showed a significant reduction in 30-day readmission rates in the intervention group (10% vs. 38.1%, $p = 0.04$); however, these results were not sustained at 60 days post-discharge [10,16,17].

The promising results of current literature have demonstrated that pharmacists have a unique opportunity to help provide comprehensive medication assessments for older adults. With the potential advantages of impacting medication appropriateness, adverse effects, and potentially increased risk of falls, the next step is to identify the best method of delivering these services. Current literature is mixed on which patients to target for this service with the intent of providing the best utilization of resources. Concerns over the cost of providing a medication review service may be balanced by demonstrating a positive impact on readmission rates and acute healthcare utilization while improving patient care. Comprehensive medication reviews for older adults qualify as CMS medication therapy management and can further increase reimbursement for a health system. Additional research on how to implement these services in a cost effective manner is necessary to lead others in advancing patient-centered care [4].

Healthcare reform has created a demand for change in the delivery of healthcare services. Encouraging the introduction of the medication expert in providing patient-centered care is an important element in the advancement of delivering quality clinical services. The purpose of this research study was to examine the impact of pharmacist-conducted geriatric medication reviews on reduction of medication related problems within a leading community health system in southwest Michigan [18].

2. Methods

2.1. Overview of Medication-Review Service

Previously, the hospital worked with the local senior services agency to develop an ambulatory pharmacist geriatric CMR service. This helped to determine a target medical practice with a large volume of geriatric patients. The project was conducted with a licensed pharmacist working in the medical practice approximately one-and-a-half days per week for one month from February to March 2014.

The pharmacist reviewed the scheduled patients for the day to determine those who would benefit from a CMR. After discussing with the patient's provider, the pharmacist offered to review medications with the patient. Patient's had the opportunity to accept or decline the service. If accepted, the pharmacist would meet one-on-one with the patient and/or caregivers and review medications, indications, doses, directions, educate on possible side effects, and answer any questions. The pharmacist completed any missing medication information in the electronic medical record for the patient and identified potential medication-related problems to be addressed with the provider. The patients all received an updated medication list upon visit completion and medication education. Medication education included main counseling points: how to take, major side effects, potential drug interactions, and how to avoid potential medication problems.

2.2. Study Design and Participants

This study was a retrospective post-hoc analysis of ambulatory patients who received a comprehensive medication review by a pharmacist at a primary care office in southwest Michigan between February and March 2014. Patient inclusion criteria were patients 65 years of age and older, taking at least five prescribed medications, and have received a comprehensive medication review from the pharmacist (intervention group). Exclusion criteria are those patients with renal failure (defined as a creatinine clearance less than 30 mL/min), those with multiple primary care providers, and not meeting the above inclusion criteria. The intervention group patients were compared with a control group from the same medical practice. These patients were identified in the same manner as the intervention group through chart review, but never received an actual review due to limitations further outlined in the discussion section below. This study was approved by the Institutional Review Board of Bronson Health Group. The procedures followed were in accord with the ethical standards of the institution's committee on human experimentation or with the Declaration of Helsinki, as revised in 2000 (JAMA. 2000; 284:3043–5).

2.3. Data Collection

Data was collected through retrospective chart review using Medinformatix, the electronic medical record at the family medicine practice. Information collected for review included demographic information, allergy history, major chronic conditions, complete medication profile, and pharmacist interventions made during the medication review. Information regarding hospitalizations and emergency department visits was collected using Cerner Powerchart for Bronson Battle Creek Hospital.

2.4. Primary and Secondary Outcomes

The primary outcome of the study was the difference in medication-related problems, defined according to the START (Screening Tool to Alert doctors to Right Treatment) and STOPP Criteria (Screening Tool of Older Persons' Prescriptions). During review, a number was assigned for each criterion the patient met. The number of medication-related problems was identified and totaled after completion of the medication review and compared to the control group from the same time period.

Secondary outcomes included acceptance of the pharmacists' recommendations, perceived pharmacist's value assessed via a Likert-scale survey administered to medical practice providers, and number and type of pharmacist's interventions. The survey was a paper-based survey with a total of six questions regarding the pharmacist comprehensive medication review service. The survey was distributed and collected by the office administrative staff to each of the 14 primary care providers. Analysis of the survey was completed by the pharmacist, using the mean response to each question. In addition, patients were followed for 90 days after the completion date of comprehensive medication reviews to document hospitalizations and emergency department visits. Pharmacist interventions were categorized according to definition by Cerner PharmNet.

2.5. Statistical Analysis

The primary analysis was conducted on all patients having received a comprehensive medication preview and meeting the above inclusion criteria. Assessment of primary and secondary outcomes was performed using descriptive statistics (frequencies, means, and measures of deviation). For the primary outcome of medication-related problems, inferential statistical testing was performed using the chi-square test, with an a priori alpha of 0.05. Categorical secondary endpoints were also analyzed using the chi-square test and continuous variables were analyzed using the non-paired *t*-test. Data was analyzed using the intent-to-treat principle with last data point carried forward. Statistical testing was performed using Microsoft Excel (2010 Microsoft Corporation, Redmond, WA, USA).

3. Results

3.1. Demographics

There were 26 patients that met study inclusion criteria and received a comprehensive medication review from the pharmacist. The intervention group was compared to a control group of 26 patients for a total of 52 patients included in the study. Demographic and clinical characteristics of the study population are summarized in Table 1. There were no statistically significant differences between the intervention and control groups.

Table 1. Demographic Information.

	CMR (*N* = 26)	Control (*N* = 26)	*p*-Value
Age	76.4 ± 7.7	76.5 ± 8.5	0.49
Male (%)	10 (38%)	9 (35%)	0.68
# Medications	14.2 ± 5.4	12.0 ± 4.4	0.061
SCr	0.93 ± 0.38	0.86 ± 0.29	0.22
BZDs	6	6	-

CMR: Comprehensive Medication Review; SCr: serum creatinine; BZDs: benzodiazepines.

3.2. Primary Outcome

The primary outcome was difference in number of medication-related problems between the intervention group patients that had received a CMR from the pharmacist during the CMR service in February to March 2014 and the control group, patients that did not receive a CMR. The primary outcome is summarized in Table 2. There were a total of 11 medication-related problems defined by the START/STOPP Criteria identified in the intervention group patients, compared with 24 medication-related problems in the control group. This is a statistically significant difference (*p* = 0.002). These medication related problems are further discussed in more detail under secondary outcomes. It is important to note that severity of medication-related problems was not analyzed during our study.

Table 2. Primary Outcome—Number of Medication-related Problems.

	CMR (*N* = 26)	Control (*N* = 26)	*p*-Value
START	4	3	-
STOPP	7	21	-
Total	11	24	0.002

CMR: Comprehensive Medication Review.

3.3. Secondary Outcomes

3.3.1. Pharmacist Interventions

There were a total of 100 pharmacist interventions made during pharmacist-led comprehensive medication reviews during the study period. Figure 1 displays the number and category for these interventions. The most frequent interventions involved thorough chart review from the pharmacist and medication education for all patients. In addition, the patient's medication profile was updated for 21 of the 26 patients (81%), which previously had missing or inaccurate information upon completion of their provider appointment. The remaining five patients already had updated medication records upon completion of their primary care provider appointment, which was confirmed through the comprehensive medication review.

The acceptance rate of pharmacist recommendations for all interventions made was 64% ($N = 100$). The acceptance rate for the primary outcome in regards to recommendations on medication-related problems defined by the START or STOPP Criteria was 35% ($N = 17$). This acceptance rate directly impacts the statistically significant difference identified in our primary outcome.

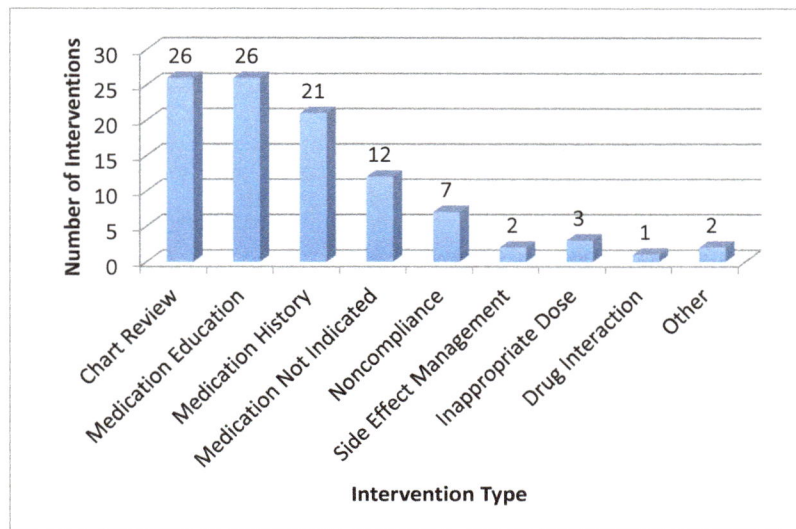

Figure 1. Frequency and Type of Pharmacist Interventions during Pharmacist CMRs.

3.3.2. Acute Healthcare Utilization

There were a total of seven emergency department visits in the intervention group. Of these seven ED visits, three were fall-related with no resulting admissions for falls. One of the seven ED visits was considered to be medication-related due to noncompliance with blood pressure medications and a resulting admission for uncontrolled hypertension. In the control group, there was a total of six ED visits, one of which may have been medication-related as the patient went to the ED with a chief complaint of difficulty breathing. The patient was recently taken off a diuretic and had a history of congestive heart failure. There were no statistically significant differences in emergency department visits between the two groups.

A total of three patients were hospitalized during the follow-up period in the intervention group. No admissions could be directly attributed to falls or medications. In the control group, there were four hospitalizations identified during chart review. There were no statistically significant differences in hospitalizations between the two groups. See Table 3 for a summary of acute healthcare utilization.

Table 3. Acute Healthcare Utilization.

	CMR	Control	p-Value
ED Visits (total)	7	6	0.413
Fall-related	3	0	0.100
Medication-related	1	1	-
Hospitalizations (total)	3	4	0.379
Fall-related admissions	0	0	-
Medication Related	1	1	-
Mean Length of Stay (days)	4.33	3	

CMR = comprehensive medication review group.

Finally, a survey was administered to 14 members of the medical staff of the hosting primary care clinic. A response was received from 12 participants, giving a response rate of 86%. The results of the survey are summarized in Table 4 and Figure 2. Additional feedback comments on the survey included, "I loved having access to a pharmacist for questions on difficult patients with polypharmacy", and "nice interacting with a medication expert".

Table 4. Provider Survey.

Question
1. Our providers/I benefited from utilizing the pharmacist within our medical practice
2. Our patients benefited from a comprehensive medication review by the pharmacist
3. The pharmacist was a positive attribute to our medical practice
4. Utilizing an interdisciplinary approach provides for patient-centered healthcare
5. I would consult with a pharmacist (if available) to assess medication therapy for my/our patients
6. Medication management is a difficult task for our elderly patients

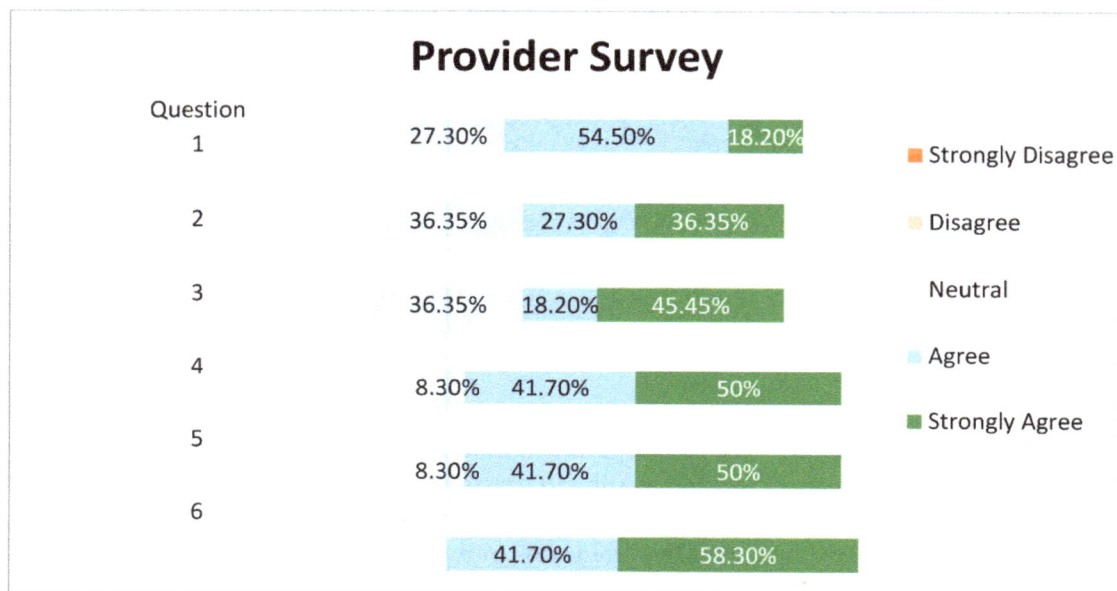

Figure 2. Results of provider survey for pharmacist CMR service.

4. Discussion

This study found a significant difference in number of medication-related problems for geriatric patients after receiving a comprehensive medication review with a pharmacist compared to patients that did not receive a CMR. This research further acknowledges the pharmacist's role in medication therapy management services and confirms findings from previous studies [1–3,8,10–17]. As CMRs can be billed to Medicare, providing these clinical services will pave the way for future ambulatory pharmacy practice.

The pharmacist was able to provide a variety of interventions, indicating that with the complexity of geriatric patients, this population is an optimal target to improve medication management. The fact that over 80% of patients had missing or inaccurate medication profiles after the completion of their primary care provider appointment shows the gap that remains in the medication reconciliation process, which the pharmacist was able to fulfill when providing CMRs. While the acceptance rate for the START and STOPP Criteria interventions was lower than anticipated, the overall acceptance rate was typical to rates observed at Bronson Battle Creek inpatient settings for smaller intervention types. This lower rate is most likely attributed to the lack of discontinuation of benzodiazepines, a problematic class of medications, which require tapering to prevent withdrawal effects. More education and frequent discussions on the use of benzodiazepines may be warranted for this non-acute, clinical setting.

There were no statistically significant differences in emergency department visits or hospitalizations between the two groups. There was a trend observed in that more fall-related emergency department visits occurred in the intervention group. It should be noted that two of the three falls were for the same patient and no falls could directly be attributed to high-risk medications. Healthcare utilization remains a point of interest for further research in hopes of identifying whether CMRs have an impact on acute healthcare utilization and associated costs.

Finally, ambulatory pharmacy services are greatly limited by the lack of billing opportunities and adoption by physicians as a necessity to their practices. Using a provider survey, we were able to identify that the pharmacist was a positive addition to a family medicine office practice to improve medication regimens, drug-information consults, and provide patient-centered, interdisciplinary care.

Strengths of this study include the direct integration of a pharmacist into a primary care practice and the positive outcomes resulting from the addition of medication therapy management services. However, it is important to also take note of the limitations of this study. A relatively small population size limited our results with only 26 patients in each group, and a sample size calculation was not performed. Next, the follow-up period was short (90 days) due to the scope of this research project. Further evaluations in the future can expand this time period and follow-up with any potential differences in results. Finally, a lack of scheduling appointments for a comprehensive medication review with the pharmacist presented numerous barriers to the study. Many patients were missed, simply by providers or medical assistants forgetting to have the patient meet with the pharmacist at the end of their appointment. This lack of participation from physicians and mid-level providers remained, despite our education for providers on the purpose and scope of the project.

5. Conclusions

In conclusion, a comprehensive medication review performed by a pharmacist was associated with a statistically significant decrease in the number of medication-related problems defined according to the START and STOPP Criteria, compared with those patients that did not receive a CMR. Pharmacist interventions improved medication use in primary care, however physicians did not necessarily adopt even well-established recommendations. Despite these shortfalls, the presence of a pharmacist to assist in medication management was well supported by the primary care practice. Our hope is that this project provides direction and guidance for one method to establish an ambulatory pharmacist CMR service.

Acknowledgments: The authors would like to thank Robert Coffey; Todd Super; Amanda Ackerman and Day One Family Healthcare for their contributions and support of this research project.

Author Contributions: The co-author Whitney Kiel contributed to this research project by conceiving and designing the research, performing the research, analyzing the data, and writing and editing the manuscript. The co-author Shaun Phillips contributed to this research project by conceiving and designing the research, analyzing the data, and editing the manuscript.

References

1.   Touchette, D.R.; Masica, A.L.; Dolor, R.J.; Schumock, G.T.; Choi, Y.K.; Kim, Y.; Smith, S.R. Safety-focused medication therapy management: A randomized controlled trial. *J. Am. Pharm. Assoc.* **2012**, *52*, 603–612. [CrossRef] [PubMed]

2.   Roth, M.T.; Ivey, J.L.; Esserman, D.A.; Crisp, G.; Kurz, J.; Weinberger, M. Individualized medication assessment and planning: Optimizing medication use in older adults in the primary care setting. *Pharmacotherapy* **2013**, *33*, 787–797. [CrossRef] [PubMed]

3.   Lee, J.K.; Slack, M.K.; Martin, J.; Ehrman, C.; Chisholm-Burns, M. Geriatric patient care by U.S. Pharmacists in healthcare teams: Systematic review and meta-analyses. *J. Am. Geriatr. Soc.* **2013**, *61*, 1119–1127. [CrossRef] [PubMed]

4.   Medication Therapy Management. Centers for Medicare & Medicaid Services. Available online: http://www. cms.gov/Medicare/Prescription-Drug-Coverage/PrescriptionDrugCovContra/MTM.html (accessed on 1 October 2013).

5.   Anonymous. The consensus of the Pharmacy Practice Model Summit. *Am. J. Health Syst. Pharm.* **2011**, *68*, 1148–1152.

6.   American Geriatrics Society 2012 Beers Criteria Update Expert Panel. American Geriatrics Society updated Beers Criteria for potentially inappropriate medication use in older adults. *J. Am. Geriatr. Soc.* **2012**, *60*, 616–631.

7.   American Geriatrics Society 2015 Beers Criteria Update Expert Panel. American Geriatrics Society 2015 Updated Beers Criteria for potentially inappropriate medication use in older adults. *J. Am. Geriatr. Soc.* **2015**, *63*, 2227–2246.

8.   Brahmbhatt, M.; Palla, K.; Kossifologos, A.; Mitchell, D.; Lee, T. Appropriateness of medication prescribing using the STOPP/START criteria in veterans receiving home-based primary care. *Consult. Pharm.* **2013**, *28*, 361–369. [CrossRef] [PubMed]

9.   PL Detail-Document, STARTing and STOPPing Medications in the Elderly. Pharmacist's Letter/Prescriber's Letter, 2011. Available online: http://hospitalpharmacistsletter.therapeuticresearch.com/pl/ArticleDD. aspx?nidchk=1&cs=ROSTER&s=PLH&pt=2&fpt=31&dd=270906&pb=PLH&searchid=62872708& segment=3580 (accessed on 1 October 2017).

10.   Hanlon, J.T.; Weinberger, M.; Samsa, G.P.; Schmader, K.E.; Uttech, K.M.; Lewis, I.K.; Cowper, P.A.; Landsman, P.B.; Cohen, H.J.; Feussner, J.R. A randomized, controlled trial of a clinical pharmacist intervention to improve inappropriate prescribing in elderly outpatients with polypharmacy. *Am. J. Med.* **1996**, *100*, 428–437. [CrossRef]

11.   Weber, V.; White, A.; McIlvried, R. An electronic medical record (EMR)-based intervention to reduce polypharmacy and falls in an ambulatory rural elderly population. *J. Gen. Intern. Med.* **2008**, *23*, 399–404. [CrossRef] [PubMed]

12.   Blalock, S.J.; Casteel, C.; Roth, M.T.; Ferreri, S.; Demby, K.B.; Shankar, V. Impact of enhanced pharmacologic care on the prevention of falls: A randomized controlled trial. *Am. J. Geriatr. Pharmacother.* **2010**, *8*, 428–440. [CrossRef] [PubMed]

13.   Schmader, K.E.; Hanlon, J.T.; Pieper, C.F.; Sloane, R.; Ruby, C.M.; Twersky, J.; Francis, S.D.; Branch, L.G.; Lindblad, C.I.; Artz, M.; et al. Effects of geriatric evaluation and management on adverse drug reactions and suboptimal prescribing in the frail elderly. *Am. J. Med.* **2004**, *116*, 394–401. [CrossRef] [PubMed]

14.   Bao, Y.; Shao, H.; Bishop, T.F.; Schackman, B.R.; Bruce, M.L. Inappropriate medication in a national sample of US elderly patients receiving home health care. *J. Gen. Intern. Med.* **2012**, *27*, 304–310. [CrossRef] [PubMed]

15.   Vink, J.; Morton, D.; Ferreri, S. Pharmacist identification of medication-related problems in the home care setting. *Consult. Pharm.* **2011**, *26*, 477–484. [CrossRef] [PubMed]

16.   Koehler, B.E.; Richter, K.M.; Youngblood, L.; Cohen, B.A.; Prengler, I.D.; Cheng, D.; Masica, A.L. Reduction of 30-day post discharge hospital readmission or emergency department (ED) visit rates in high-risk elderly medical patients through delivery of a targeted care bundle. *J. Hosp. Med.* **2009**, *4*, 211–218. [CrossRef] [PubMed]

17.   Lee, J.K.; Grace, K.A.; Taylor, A.J. Effect of a pharmacy care program on medication adherence and persistence, blood pressure, and low-density lipoprotein cholesterol: A randomized controlled trial. *JAMA* **2006**, *296*, 2563–2571. [CrossRef] [PubMed]

18.   Bronson Battle Creek Hospital. Bronson Health Group [Internet]. Available online: http://www. bronsonhealth.com/locations/bronson-battle-creek-hospital (accessed on 1 October 2013).

16

Pharmacy Practice and Education

Valentina Petkova [1] **and Jeffrey Atkinson** [2,*]

[1] Faculty of Pharmacy, Medical University-Sofia, 2-Dunav Street, 1000 Sofia, Bulgaria;
    petkovav1972@yahoo.com
[2] Pharmacolor Consultants Nancy, 12 rue de Versigny, 54600 Villers, France
*   Correspondence: jeffrey.atkinson@univ-lorraine.fr

Academic Editor: Antonio Sanchez-Pozo

Abstract: Pharmacies in Bulgaria have a monopoly on the dispensing of medicinal products that are authorized in the Republic of Bulgaria, as well as medical devices, food additives, cosmetics, and sanitary/hygienic articles. *Aptekari* (pharmacists) act as responsible pharmacists, pharmacy owners, and managers. They follow a five year Masters of Science in Pharmacy (M.Sc. Pharm.) degree course with a six month traineeship. *Pomoshnik-farmacevti* (assistant pharmacists) follow a three year degree with a six month traineeship. They can prepare medicines and dispense OTC medicines under the supervision of a pharmacist. The first and second year of the M.Sc. Pharm. degree are devoted to chemical sciences, mathematics, botany and medical sciences. Years three and four center on pharmaceutical technology, pharmacology, pharmacognosy, pharmaco-economics, and social pharmacy, while year five focuses on pharmaceutical care, patient counselling, pharmacotherapy, and medical sciences. A six month traineeship finishes the fifth year together with redaction of a master thesis, and the four state examinations with which university studies end. Industrial pharmacy and clinical (hospital) pharmacy practice are integrated disciplines in some Bulgarian higher education institutions such as the Faculty of Pharmacy of the Medical University of Sofia. Pharmacy practice and education in Bulgaria are organized in a fashion very similar to that in most member states of the European Union.

Keywords: pharmacy; education; practice; Bulgaria

1. Introduction

Concerning general health in Bulgaria, the World Health Organization (WHO) estimated that a person born in Bulgaria in 2016 can expect to live 74.6 years on average: 78 years if female and 71.2 years if male (Table 1). WHO also estimated that life expectancy at birth for both sexes increased by 3 years over the period of 2000–2012; the WHO regional average increased by 4 years in the same period. In 2012, healthy life expectancy, in both sexes, was 9 years lower than the European average. This lost healthy life expectancy represents 9 equivalent years of full health lost through years lived with morbidity and disability.

Table 1. Health statistics for Bulgaria [1].

Total Population	7,067,024
Life expectancy at birth m/f (years)	71.2/78 (2016)
Healthy life expectancy at birth m/f (years)	63/67 (2015)
Total expenditure on health per capita	1399$ (2014)
Total expenditure on health as % of GDP	8.4 (2014)

Statistics 30 January 2017 unless indicated.

Despite these somewhat disappointing figures, progress has been made in the past 30 years. Since the disruption of the established order of the Soviet Union in 1989, the on-going economic, political, and social changes in Bulgaria have had an important impact on all aspects of social life in the country, including pharmaceutical activities. Until 1989, the pharmaceutical system was centralized—community pharmacies, hospital pharmacies, wholesalers, pharmaceutical factories, and institutes were owned by the state. The importation and exportation of drugs were controlled by the state.

Following the changes in 1989, the Bulgarian pharmaceutical system is oriented towards the private sector. Community pharmacies, wholesalers, and many drug manufacturers are now private entities. The first Bulgarian Law on drugs and pharmacies in human medicine was introduced in 1995 [2]. It lays out the structure for harmonization of Bulgarian drug regulatory affairs with those of the European Union.

All these specific circumstances, together with a more global perspective on new drug discoveries and pharmaceutical technologies and methodologies, are a constant challenge leading to re-evaluation of the role of pharmacists in the Bulgarian health care system. Before these changes, a majority of Bulgarian pharmacists' time was spent manufacturing drugs in the pharmacy. Nowadays, pharmacists apply different skills that require a detailed knowledge of communications and human behavior to scientifically dispense medications, and to counsel patients about their health and the correct use of their prescribed and OTC drugs. They are also responsible for monitoring patients to avoid adverse drug reactions and to achieve maximum benefit from the treatment. A very recent development is the implementation of the concept of "pharmaceutical care" as a central element of pharmacy practice.

The Medical University in Sofia will be taken as an example for Bulgaria. The university has four faculties: medicine, dentistry, pharmacy, and social health. The pharmacy faculty is the oldest in Bulgaria in educating pharmaceutical specialists. The duration of the education is five years for community, hospital, and industrial pharmacists. All the graduates receive a M.Sc. Pharm. degree. One hundred to 120 Bulgarian and 80–100 foreign students are accepted for pharmacy education and training every year.

There are six departments in the Faculty of Pharmacy in the Medical University in Sofia:

1. Pharmaceutical Technology and Bio-Pharmacy
2. Pharmacognosy and Pharmaceutical Botany
3. Pharmaceutical Chemistry
4. Chemistry
5. Pharmacology and Toxicology
6. Social Pharmacy

Following graduation, students have the opportunity to specialize for a further 3 years. Whilst working in a hospital or industrial environment, they follow a study program with courses at the faculty of pharmacy two weeks per year. After the third year of such specialization they pass a state examination in a given specialty. This possibility is granted by the Ministry of Education to all pharmaceutical students and graduates.

Since 1989, there have been many changes in the curriculum to harmonize courses and diplomas with those of the other schools in the European Union (EU). Many new study areas have been introduced such as: bio-pharmacy, clinical laboratory testing and analysis, and biology. The Department of Social Pharmacy has introduced new study areas such as: history of pharmacy, pharmaco-epidemiology, pharmaco-economics, pharmaceutical law, pharmaceutical marketing, and pharmaceutical management.

In 2000, a new course in pharmaceutical care was introduced. The lectures and seminars on this subject are given during the first semester of the fifth year. The lectures synthesize the knowledge gained during the five-year pharmacy course and blend this with communication skills and the development of the logic of pharmaceutical care. University lecturers together with pharmacy practitioners, provide the training.

2. Design

Given the changes in pharmacy practice and education in Bulgaria outlined above, the PHARMINE (*Pharmacy Education in Europe*) European consortium surveyed the state of pharmacy education and practice in Bulgaria in 2012, with an update in 2017. The PHARMINE consortium was interested in general practice and education and in specialization in pharmacy education for hospital and industrial pharmacy practice. The survey also looked at the impact of the Bologna agreement on harmonization of the various European degree courses [3], and on the directive of the European Commission on education and training for the sectoral profession of pharmacy [4]. These two documents are somewhat contradictory in that the Bologna agreement proposes a bachelor plus master degree structure for all degrees including pharmacy, whereas as the European directive lays down a five-year "tunnel" degree structure for pharmacy, i.e., a degree course that has no possibility for intermediate entry or exit for example after a three-year bachelor period. The methodology used in the PHARMINE survey [5] and the principal results obtained in the EU [6] have already been published.

3. Evaluation and Assessment

3.1. Organisation of the Activities of Pharmacists, Professional Bodies

Table 2 provides details of the numbers and activities of community pharmacists and pharmacies in Bulgaria.

Table 2. Numbers and activities of community pharmacists and pharmacies.

Item	Numbers	Comments
Pharmacists	5500–6000	1284 Inhabitants/Pharmacist
Pharmacies	4208	1.2–1.3 pharmacists per pharmacy 1679 inhabitants/pharmacy
Competences and roles of community pharmacists		After graduation from university, pharmacists can work in a pharmacy and can perform drug preparation, dispensing of drugs and consulting of patients on the proper drug treatment and prepare a pharmaceutical care plan (identifying drug-related problems, making a plan for proper drug treatment, monitoring of the treatment, etc.)
Is ownership of a community pharmacy limited to pharmacists?	No	The following are entitled to carry out retail trade in medicinal products: A natural or legal person. One who is registered as a pharmacy trader under the Bulgarian legislation or under the legislation of an EU member state. One who has signed a labour contract or a contract for management of a pharmacy with a pharmacist (in possession of an M.Sc. Pharm. degree. Or one who, in the cases provided under the law (no pharmacist available and until the arrival of master of a pharmacist), has signed a contract with an assistant pharmacist (for dispensation of OTC drugs only) One person may open no more than 4 pharmacies in Bulgaria [7].
Rules on geographical distribution of pharmacies?	No	There are no governmental restrictions on the geographical distribution of community pharmacies as a function of population density for instance.
Are drugs and healthcare products available to the general public by channels other than pharmacies?	No	Medicinal products, medical devices authorised in the Republic of Bulgaria, with or without medical prescription, as well as food additives, cosmetic, and sanitary-hygienic articles, are sold only in pharmacies. There are no mail-order pharmacies in Bulgaria. Any attempt to sell drug products at a lower price than originally planned is prohibited. Medicinal products not subject to a medical prescription may be sold on the internet only by a pharmacy or drugstore that has been granted authorisation under the terms and conditions of Medicinal Products in the Bulgarian Human Medicine Act [7].

The data in Table 2 shows that compared to the EU linear regression estimation (for definition and calculation see reference 5) the ratio of the actual number of community pharmacists in Bulgaria (/population) compared to the linear regression estimation for Bulgaria = 1.16. Thus number of pharmacists per population is very close to the EU norm. The same comparison for community pharmacies produces a ratio of 1.99. Thus the number of community pharmacies in Bulgaria is double the EU average.

The activities and occupations of pharmacists in Bulgaria are similar to those of community pharmacists in other member states [5]. The organization of community pharmacists regarding ownership, etc. is similar to that elsewhere in the EU; it should be noted that there are no government-imposed rules on the geographical distribution of community pharmacies in Bulgaria. The sale of medicinal products on the internet is limited to authorized pharmacies.

Table 3 provides details of the numbers and activities of assistant pharmacists in Bulgaria.

Table 3. Numbers and activities of assistant pharmacists.

Are persons other than pharmacists involved in community practice?	Yes	In addition to pharmacists, assistant pharmacists are also considered to be professional pharmacy staff. Article 220/3 of the "Medicinal Products in Human Medicine Act" states that "An assistant pharmacist may carry out all operations under the control of a Master of Pharmacy, with the exception of: dispensation of a medicinal product under medical prescription, control, and consultations connected with medicinal products..." [7]. The assistant pharmacist´s code 5.7 states: "The students graduated from that speciality can work at the clinical pharmacy, at herbal stores, sanitary and drug stores, pharmacy stores, pharmacy laboratories, science institutes, and pharmaceutical factories." [8].
Their titles and number(s)		There is no official data. There is no upper limit on the number; some pharmacies work without assistant pharmacists. There is a register of the pharmacists on the site of the Bulgarian Pharmaceutical Union [9]—but not of the assistant pharmacists.
Organizations providing and validating education and training of assistant pharmacists		Five pharmaceutical colleges provide education for assistant pharmacists: Medical College-Sofia: http://mu-sofia.bg/node/32 Medical College-Varna: http://www.mu-varna.bg/muVarna/index.php?option= com_content&task=view&id=193&Itemid=122 Medical College-Plovdiv: http://www.medcollege-plovdiv.org/ Medical College-Bourgas: http://www.btu.bg/bg/homebg.htm Pleven: http://www.mu-pleven.bg/index.php?lang=en&Itemid=254:
Duration of studies (years)	3	The studies of assistant pharmacists cannot be compared to bachelor studies at a university. There is no bachelor degree of "pharmaceutical education" in Bulgaria. There are uniform requirements for achievement of higher education as assistant pharmacist.
Conditions of entry		The entrance examination is in biology (that for pharmacy is in biology and chemistry). In some colleges there is also an interview.
Subject areas		Basic pharmaceutical sciences such as pharmaceutical chemistry, pharmaceutical technology, drug legislation, etc. The course lasts a minimum of 1200 h.
Competences and roles		Assist a pharmacist in the dispensation of OTC medicines only while under the supervision of a pharmacist.

Bulgarian legislation recognizes that assistant pharmacists are health care professionals and defines their role in the health care system. Five pharmaceutical colleges provide education and training for assistant pharmacists. Although this is in the form of a three-year course, it cannot be compared to a "B. Pharm." as defined by the Bologna declaration (see above).

Table 4 provides details of the numbers and activities of hospital pharmacists in Bulgaria.

Bulgarian legislation recognizes the existence of a hospital pharmacy, although the number of hospital pharmacists is low compared to the EU average. The ratio of the actual number of hospital pharmacists in Bulgaria (/population) compared to the linear regression estimation for Bulgaria = 0.29, (for definition and calculation see reference 5). The estimated number of hospital pharmacies is higher than that of hospital pharmacists. It appears therefore that the function of "hospital pharmacist" in Bulgaria is defined by competences and roles and/or by place of work. In the latter case, health care personnel other than pharmacists are involved.

Table 4. Numbers and activities of hospital pharmacists.

Does such a function exist?	Yes	The Bulgarian branch of the European Association of Hospital Pharmacists is the professional organization of the Bulgarian hospital pharmacies [10].
Number of hospital pharmacists	197	This is the number of pharmacists registered with the Bulgarian Association of Hospital Pharmacists [11]
Number of hospital pharmacies		There are 344 (2011) hospitals in Bulgaria—most have a hospital pharmacy.
Competences and roles of hospital pharmacists		Preparation and dispensing of drugs on hospital wards and also: Part of multidisciplinary patient-care team. Purchasing of drugs and medical material. Monitoring of drug use. Production of patient-specific medicines. Participation in clinical studies.

Table 5 provides details of the numbers and activities of industrial pharmacists and pharmacists in other sectors, in Bulgaria.

Table 5. Numbers and activities of industrial pharmacists and pharmacists in other sectors.

Industrial Pharmacy and Pharmacists		
Number of pharmaceutical companies with production, R&D and distribution	22	The European Federation of Pharmaceutical Industries and Associations (EFPIA) has 22 members in Bulgaria [12]. The Bulgarian representative is the Association of the Research-based Pharmaceutical Manufacturers in Bulgaria [13].
Number of companies producing generic drugs only	9	Examples: Actavis http://www.actavis.bg/bg/default.htm Sopharma http://www.sopharma.bg/
Number of pharmacists working in industry	About 1000	The number is estimated from the number of students graduating with the industrial pharmacy degree option; students taking the industrial pharmacy option account for <10% of the class size. EFPIA has estimated that the total number of people employed in the pharmaceutical industry equals 9900 [14].
Competences and roles		Drug manufacturing, control, analysis, registration, etc.
Pharmacists Working in Other Sectors		
Sectors in which pharmacists are employed		Academia (faculties of pharmacy) Wholesale Medical and pharmaceutical information Bulgarian Drug Agency Ministry of health Representative offices of Bulgarian and foreign drug companies Drug manufacturing in the Bulgarian drug companies.
Competences and roles in other sectors		Teaching, tutoring, drug accounting, communication, advertising, etc. The exact number of pharmacists working in other sectors in Bulgaria is impossible to determine.

Industrial pharmacists in Bulgaria have similar practices and duties to those in other EU countries [5]. As numbers of industrial pharmacists were not available for most European countries a comparison with the EU average is not possible.

Table 6 provides information on professional associations for pharmacists in Bulgaria.

Table 6. Professional associations for pharmacists in Bulgaria.

Registration of pharmacists	Yes	The Bulgarian Pharmaceutical Union [15] provides a certificate of entry onto the register of the corresponding Regional College of the Bulgarian Pharmaceutical Union, to every Master of Pharmacy who is at the head of a pharmacy. In order to be registered as a professional pharmacist one has to submit to the Bulgarian Pharmaceutical Union: Diploma of a higher educational pharmaceutical department. Diploma(s) for specialization (hospital, industrial) or Ph.D./DSc/Associate professor/Professor. Certificate from the working place attesting that he/she is working as a pharmacist. A certificate showing no previous criminal conviction. After approval, the pharmacist becomes a member of the Bulgarian Pharmaceutical Union and gains his/her unique identification number as a pharmacist.
Creation of pharmacies and control of territorial distribution	Yes	The Bulgarian Drug Agency issues an authorisation for retail trade in medicinal products in a pharmacy and controls the implementation of requirements for the retail trade of medicines.
Ethical and other aspects of professional conduct	Yes	The Bulgarian Pharmaceutical Union has an ethical code for pharmacy practice.
Quality assurance and validation of university courses	Yes	University courses are controlled by the quality commission of the Bulgarian Pharmaceutical Union [16]. http://bphu.eu/

The Bulgarian pharmaceutical union, which is the representative organisation of pharmacists in the country, oversees pharmacy education and training (PET), pharmacy practice, and ethics in a fashion similar to that in other member states of the EU [5].

3.2. Pharmacy Faculties, Students, and Courses

Table 7 provides details of pharmacy higher education institutions (HEIs), staff and students in Bulgaria.

Table 7. Pharmacy higher education institutions (HEIs), staff, and students in Bulgaria.

Item	Number	Comments
Number of pharmacy HEIs in Bulgaria	5	Pharmacy HEIs: Medical University of Sofia : www.pharmfac.net University of Plovdiv: http://meduniversity-plovdiv.bg/index.php?lang_id=2&prm=fac&subprm=farf University of Varna: http://www.mu-varna.bg/ (started accepting students in 2009) Sofia University: http://www.uni-sofia.bg/index.php/eng/faculties/faculty_of_chemistry_and_pharmacy Medical University of Pleven: http://www.mu-pleven.bg/index.php/structure/faculty-of-pharmacy?lang=en
Public pharmacy HEIs	5	There are no private pharmacy HEIs in Bulgaria.
Faculty attachment		The faculties of pharmacy in Sofia (Medical University of Sofia), Plovdiv, Pleven and Varna are faculties of the corresponding medical universities. The faculty of Chemistry and Pharmacy (number 4 above) is part of Sofia University.
Do HEIs offer B and M degrees?	No	Only an M.Sc. Pharm. Degree is offered; there is no Bulgarian B. Pharm degree (see later).

Table 7. *Cont.*

Item	Number	Comments
		Teaching staff
Staff (nationals)	250	
Professionals from outside the HEIs	20	They are from the pharmacies (supervision of student traineeships), pharmaceutical companies, wholesalers, etc.
		Students
Graduates that become registered pharmacists.	More than 400 per year	The number of graduates during the past five years was increased due to the increase in the number of the faculties and the introduction of a pharmacy course in English in most of the faculties—especially Sofia and Plovdiv.
Number of places on entry following secondary school	260+ per year	For 2012 [17]: Medical university of Sofia: 120 Plovdiv: 60 Varna: 30 Sofia University: 50 Pleven: not available
Number of applicants for each entry place		Medical University of Sofia: 3.4 Plovdiv: 1.8 Figures from reference 18.
Number of non EU international students	≥ 50 per year	Mainly from Macedonia, Turkey, Morocco, Tunisia and Serbia.
		Entry requirements following secondary school
Specific national entrance examination for pharmacy	Yes	National entrance examination in biology and chemistry.
Is there a national *numerus clausus*?	No	
		Fees per year
For home students		375€
For EU MS students		375€
For non EU students		7000€

The ratios of the actual number of HEIs, staff, and students in Bulgaria (/population) compared to the linear regression estimations for Bulgaria are 1.07, 1.01, and 0.76, respectively (for definition and calculation see reference [5]). Thus, figures for Bulgarian PET reflect those of the EU average for the country with a population the size of that of Bulgaria. Student numbers show a substantial international intake. It should be noted that the Erasmus Programme (European Region Action Scheme for the Mobility of University Students) is an EU student exchange program. Table 8 provides details of specialization electives in pharmacy HEIs.

Both pre- and post-graduate specialization are possible in Bulgaria. The last wave of pharmacists in post-graduate specialization in the medical university of Sofia was composed as follows—social pharmacy: 25; pharmacognosy: one; pharmaceutical analysis: one; pharmaceutical technology: one; industrial pharmacy: three. In this context, social pharmacy can be considered to consist of all the social factors that influence medicine use.

Table 9 provides details of past and present changes in education and training in Bulgarian pharmacy HEIs.

Table 8. Specialization electives in pharmacy HEIs.

Do HEIs Provide Specialized Courses?	Yes	Comments
In which years?	third, fourth and fifth; also post-graduate	
In which specialisation (industry, hospital …)?		Industry and clinical pharmacy after the third year.
What are the student numbers in each specialization?	15 (industry) and 12 (clinical pharmacy)/year for pre-graduate	Following graduation there is a possibility to start post-graduate specialization (three year course) in one of five different areas: industrial pharmacy; social pharmacy; pharmacognosy; pharmaceutical analysis; and pharmaceutical technology.

Table 9. Past and present changes in education and training in Bulgarian pharmacy HEIs.

Have there been any major changes since 1999?	Yes	The main changes were towards harmonising with the EU requirements—more practical than theoretical subjects. Teaching of "new" subjects such as, pharmaceutical care, pharmaco-economics, bromatology/food science, history of pharmacy, etc. Changes were made in the state exam in order to harmonize the final examinations to those of EU HEIs.
Are any major changes envisaged before 2019?	Yes	Changes in the relative number of hours of some subject areas. Chemical subjects will decrease while the special subjects like pharmaceutical technology will increase their number of hours.

3.3. Teaching and Learning Methods

Table 10 provides details of student hours [18] by learning method. The data from Sofia is taken as an example in this table and Table 11.

Table 10. Student hours by learning method.

Method	Year 1	Year 2	Year 3	Year 4	Year 5	Total
Lecture	210	315	330	435	210	1500
Practical	540	525	585	825	345	2820
Hospital/community traineeship					800	800
Electives			90	120		
Total	750	840	915	1260	1355	5120

Regarding the validation of traineeship, the pharmacist responsible for the trainee fills in a monthly and a final report at the end of the six months and these are validated (or not) by the HEI. It is to be noted that "practical" work is carried out by students at the university in the form of personnel projects, etc., whereas "traineeship" refers to work in a pharmacy setting.

3.4. Subject Areas.

Table 11 provides details of student hours by subject area.

Table 11. Student hours by subject area (for definition of subject areas see [4]). The numbers are calculated according to the schema of the Uniform State Requirements of Bulgaria [14].

Subject Area	Year 1	Year 2	Year 3	Year 4	Year 5	Total
CHEMSCI	165	510	225	225	150	1275
PHYSMATH	300					300
BIOLSCI	60	165	75	150		450
PHARMTECH			210	315		525
MEDISCI	45	120		690	120	975
LAWSOC	30		90	45	120	285
GENERIC	300					300
GENERIC + TRAINEESHIP	300				800	800
Total	900	795	600	1425	1190	4910

CHEMSOC: chemical sciences; PHYSMATH: physical and mathematical sciences; BIOLSCI: biological sciences; PHARMTECH: pharmaceutical technology; MEDISCI: medicinal sciences; LAWSOC: law and social sciences; GENERIC: generic competences. Taking the MEDISCI/CHEMSCI ratio as an indicator [19] of the nature of the M. Pharm. degree course (ratio = 975/1,275 = 0.8) it appears that the Bulgarian course is more a "chemical science" course similar to that in Germany (ratio = 0.7), but different from "medicinal science" course given in Ireland (ratio = 2.6) [18].

3.5. Impact of the Bologna Principles [3]

Table 12 provides details the various ways in which the Bologna declaration impacts on Bulgarian pharmacy HEIs.

Table 12. Ways in which the Bologna declaration impacts on Bulgarian pharmacy HEIs.

"Comparable degrees with diploma supplement"	Yes	The comparability of degrees is achieved through calculation of the hours and comparison with other EU countries. The Diploma Supplement provided is in English. The Diploma Supplement describes the nature, level, context, content, and status of the studies that were pursued. With the texts of the Law on Higher Education adopted by the Bulgarian Parliament on 4 June 2004 both the system for collection and transfer of credits and the Diploma Supplement were legally introduced.
"Two main cycles (B and M) with entry and exit at B level"	No	There is a five-year "tunnel" degree structure.
"European Credit Transfer System (ECTS) system of credits with links to life-long learning (LLL)"	Yes	The ECTS system of credits is applied during the fiv year period of learning and after graduation in the different courses of LLL.
"Addressing obstacles to mobility"	Partial	As the English language is not used extensively in Bulgaria there are language barriers for the proper application of mobility. Financial problems also exist.
"Application of European QA"	Partial	PET is regulated at a national level by the ministry of education, but it is harmonized to EU requirements
ERASMUS staff exchange to Sofia from elsewhere		Staff months: zero
ERASMUS staff exchange from Sofia to other HEIs		Staff months: one
ERASMUS student exchange to Sofia from elsewhere		Student months: 28
ERASMUS student exchange from Sofia to other HEIs		Student months: 72

Data in the above table are in exchange months per year. The faculty of pharmacy in Sofia has ERASMUS exchange programs with:

○ Belgium, University of Antwerp and Vrije Universiteit Brussels
○ France, Université de Lorraine, Nancy and Université de Limoges
○ Germany, Ruprecht-Karls-Universität Heidelberg, Anhalt University of Applied Sciences Kothen and Freie Universität Berlin
○ Czech Republic—University of Veterinary and Pharmaceutical Sciences, Brno
○ Italy—Universita' degli studi di Siena and Sapienza, University of Rome
○ Spain—University of Navarra and Universitat autonoma de Barcelona

There is also an exchange program with Turkey—Mersin University.

3.6. Impact of EU Directive 2013/55/EC

Table 13 provides details the various ways in which the EC directive impacts on Bulgarian pharmacy HEIs [3].

Table 13. Ways (right column) in which the elements of the EC directive (left column) impact on Bulgarian pharmacy HEIs.

"Evidence of formal qualifications as a pharmacist shall attest to training of at least five years' duration, … "	The training of pharmacists M.Sc. in Bulgaria is five years induration. The curriculum covers the EU requirements.
" … four years of full-time theoretical and practical training at a university or at a higher institute of a level recognised as equivalent, or under the supervision of a university;"	Bulgaria complies.
" … six-month traineeship in a pharmacy which is open to the public or in a hospital, under the supervision of that hospital's pharmaceutical department."	Bulgaria complies.

Bulgarian PET mainly conforms to the different aspects of the EC directive with notably a five-year tunnel degree. Aspects of the Bologna agreement such as European Credit Transfer System (ECTS) and the Diploma Supplement are included.

Figure 1 shows the scheme of PET in Bulgaria.

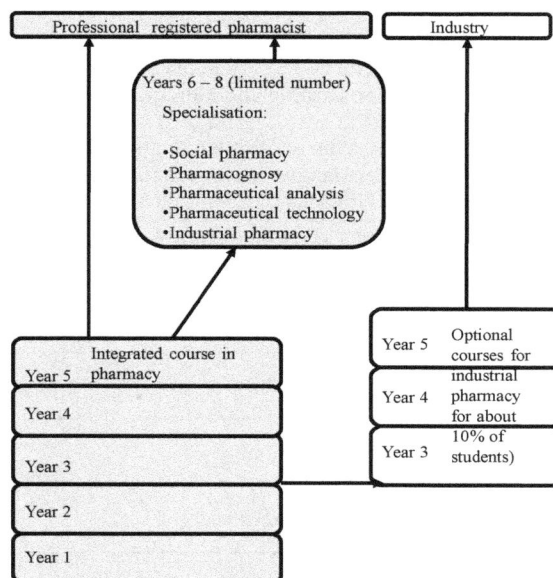

Figure 1. The scheme of pharmacy education and training (PET), in Bulgaria.

4. Discussion and Conclusions

Pharmacies in Bulgaria have a monopoly on the dispensing of medicinal products in Bulgaria. Pharmacists follow a five-year (M.Sc. Pharm.) degree course with a six months traineeship. The first and second year of the M.Sc. Pharm. degree are devoted to chemical sciences, mathematics, botany, and medical sciences. Years three and four center on pharmaceutical technology, pharmacology, pharmacognosy, pharmaco-economics, and social pharmacy, and year five on pharmaceutical care, patient counselling, pharmacotherapy, and medical sciences. A six month traineeship finishes the fifth year together with redaction of a master thesis, and the four state examinations with which university studies end. Industrial pharmacy and clinical (hospital) pharmacy practice are integrated disciplines in some Bulgarian HEIs, such as the Faculty of Pharmacy of the Medical University of Sofia.

Following the changes in Bulgaria in 1989, pharmacy practice and education are organized in a fashion very similar to that in (most member states of) the European Union. Whilst new developments in pharmaceutical care with elements such as immunization, advice on tobacco use cessation, management of medication adherence, and provision of health screening to detect hypertension do not at the present time receive financial backing from the government, the fact that these elements are supported at the academic level, should reinforce the future role of the pharmacist in the promotion of patient well-being in Bulgaria.

Acknowledgments: Valentina BELCHEVA, Sanofi-Aventis, 103, Al. Stamboliiski Blvd.-level 8, Sofia Tower building, 1303 Sofia, Bulgaria (valentina.belcheva@sanofi-aventis.com) participated in the production of the 2012 version of this country profile. With the support of the Lifelong Learning Program of the European Union (142078-LLP-1-2008-BE-ERASMUS-ECDSP).

Author Contributions: Valentina Petkova provided all the data and information and helped in the revisions of the manuscript; Jeffrey Atkinson wrote the first manuscript and dealt with revisions.

References

1. The WHO Statistical Profile of Bulgaria. Available online: http://www.who.int/gho/countries/bgr.pdf?ua=1 (accessed on 10 February 2017).
2. Bulgarian Law on Drugs and Pharmacies in Human Medicine. Available online: http://www.zdrave.net/document/institute/e-library/BG_Health_Acts/Drugs_Act.htm (accessed on 10 February 2017).
3. Bologna Agreement of Harmonisation of European University Degree Courses. Available online: http://www.ehea.info/ (accessed on 10 February 2017).
4. The European Commission Directive on Education and Training for Sectoral Practice Such as That of Pharmacy. Available online: http://eur-lex.europa.eu/legal-content/FR/TXT/?uri=celex:32013L0055 (accessed on 10 February 2017).
5. Atkinson, J. The PHARMINE Survey Methodology. Submitted.
6. Atkinson, J.; Rombaut, B. The 2011 PHARMINE report on pharmacy and pharmacy education in the European Union. *Pharm. Pract.* **2011**, *9*, 169–187. [CrossRef]
7. Bulgarian Drug Agency. Available online: http://bda.bg/bg/?lang=enimages/stories/documents/legal_acts/ZLPHM_en.pdf (accessed on 10 February 2017).
8. Bulgarian Assistant Pharmacists' Code. Available online: http://old.mu-sofia.bg/index.php?p=166&l=1 (accessed on 10 February 2017).
9. Register of the Pharmacists of the Bulgarian Pharmaceutical Union. Available online: https://bphu.bg/19_Register.htm (accessed on 10 February 2017).
10. Bulgarian Branch of the European Association of Hospital Pharmacists (EAHP). Available online: http://www.eahp.eu/about-us/members/bulgaria (accessed on 10 February 2017).
11. Bulgarian Association of Hospital Pharmacists. Available online: http://www.ohpb.org/styled/page5/index.php (accessed on 10 February 2017).
12. European Federation of Pharmaceutical Industries and Associations (EFPIA) Bulgaria. Available online: http://www.arpharm.org/en (accessed on 10 February 2017).

13. Association of the Research-Based Pharmaceutical Manufacturers in Bulgaria (ARPharM). Available online: www.arpharm.org/en (accessed on 10 February 2017).

14. European Federation of Pharmaceutical Industries and Associations (EFPIA): The Pharmaceutical Industry in Figures 2016. Available online: http://www.efpia.eu/publications/data-center/ (accessed on 10 February 2017).

15. The Bulgarian Pharmaceutical Union Certification. Available online: http://bphu.eu/about_us.php?id_page=1 (accessed on 10 February 2017).

16. Quality Commission of the Bulgarian Pharmaceutical Union. Available online: https://bphu.bg/bg.htm (accessed on 10 February 2017).

17. Student Numbers in Bulgarian pharmacy HEIs. Available online: http://www.medfaculty. ECDirectiveonSectoralProfessionsorg/forum/index.php?action=printpage;topic=6177.0 (accessed on 10 February 2017).

18. Details of Courses in Sofia. Available online: http://www.pharmfac.net/course.htm (accessed on 10 February 2017).

19. Atkinson, J.; De Paepe, K.; Sánchez Pozo, A.; Rekkas, D.; Volmer, D.; Hirvonen, J.; Bozic, B.; Skowron, A.; Mircioiu, C.; Marcincal, A.; et al. Does the Subject Content of the Pharmacy Degree Course Influence the Community Pharmacist's Views on Competencies for Practice? *Pharmacy* **2015**, *3*, 137–153. [CrossRef]

17

A 15 Year Ecological Comparison for the Market Dynamics of Minnesota Community Pharmacies from 2002 to 2017

Anthony W. Olson * [ID], Jon C. Schommer and Ronald S. Hadsall

College of Pharmacy, University of Minnesota, 308 Harvard Street, S.E., Minneapolis, MN 55455, USA; schom010@umn.edu (J.C.S.); hadsa001@umn.edu (R.S.H.)
* Correspondence: olso2001@umn.edu

Abstract: Background: Understanding the factors that influence the market entry, exit, and stability of community pharmacies (i.e., market dynamics) is important for stakeholders ranging from patients to health policymakers and small business owners to large corporate institutions. **Objective:** The study's first objective was to describe the market dynamics of community pharmacies for Minnesota counties in 2002, 2007, 2012, and 2017 by associating county (a) population density and (b) metropolitan designation with the change in the number of 'All community pharmacies', 'Chain community pharmacies', and 'Independent community pharmacies' . The study's second objective was to describe the number and proportion of community pharmacies for Minnesota counties in 2002, 2007, 2012, and 2017 by (1) 'Business Organization Structure' and (2) 'Pharmacy Type'. **Methods:** County-level data were obtained from the Minnesota Board of Pharmacy, US Census Bureau, and Minnesota State Demographic Center for 2002, 2007, 2012, and 2017. Findings were summarized and the associations between study variables described using descriptive statistics. **Results:** The ratio of 'Independent community pharmacies' to 'Chain community pharmacies' was about 1:1 (466:530) in 2002, 1:2 (352:718) in 2007, 1:2 (387:707) in 2012, and 1:3 (256:807) in 2017. There was not a consistent relationship that carried through the 15 year analysis between county population density and metropolitan designation and the market dynamic patterns of community pharmacies. The types of pharmacy in Minnesota changed significantly over the study with increases in state, regional, and national chains and declines in single entity and small chain independents. There were also notable declines in mass merchandiser community pharmacies and increases in clinic and medical center community pharmacies. **Discussion:** The findings suggest that different or additional factors beyond traditional market dynamic predictors of population density and metropolitan designation were at play in each five year interval of this study. We propose that the traditional dichotomy of independent and chain community pharmacy groupings no longer provide an optimal characterization for the market dynamics of pharmacies today. Instead, community pharmacies may be better organized by their capacity to operate as healthcare access points that provide and are reimbursed for patient care and public health services like medication therapy management, immunizations, and more. **Conclusions:** The findings showed that community pharmacy distribution in Minnesota's 87 counties has shifted between 2002 and 2017 from traditional retail models to emerging healthcare models based on population health needs. This signals the need for not only a new approach for tracking community pharmacy market dynamics but also adjustments by community pharmacies to remain relevant in a new environment of patient care services.

Keywords: community pharmacy; market dynamics; independent community pharmacy; chain community pharmacy; Minnesota

1. Introduction

1.1. Background

Over half of actively practicing pharmacists work in a community pharmacy, making the market dynamics of this practice setting very impactful on the pharmacist labor market [1,2]. Community pharmacies in the United States are an important access point for healthcare products and services involving medication, disease management, and public health [3–6]. An understanding of the factors that influence the market entry, exit, and stability of community pharmacies (i.e., market dynamics) of all types (e.g., mass merchandiser, clinic, etc.) is important for stakeholders ranging from patients to health policymakers and small business owners to large corporate institutions [7].

Previous research by Schommer et al. has demonstrated that market entry, exit, and geographical distribution of community pharmacies (i.e., market dynamics) on the county level in Minnesota between 1992 and 2012 could be explained using environmental attributes drawn from organizational behavior theory [8,9]. This approach suggests that environmental factors like population density and a county's designation as a rural or metropolitan area affect the business decisions made by community pharmacies, which influences access to community pharmacy services. The results of this research found that county characteristics like a metropolitan designation and growth in population density were significantly associated with gains in the overall number of community pharmacies, but relative declines in the number of independent community pharmacies. The increases in chain community pharmacies and all community pharmacies overall was attributed to metropolitan counties possessing the infrastructure (e.g., transportation, communication, health systems), workforce pool (i.e., source of pharmacists to fulfill staffing requirements), and market demands for items other than medications. Meanwhile, independent community pharmacies declined while chain community pharmacies grew in these counties potentially because the former were unable to capitalize on these resources to the same extent as the latter. In counties with low or negative population density growth, the number independent community pharmacies declined likely due to insufficient demands in the marketplace for sustainably operating a pharmacy as generally there was no chain community pharmacy growth in these areas. Schommer et al'.s research also documented changes in the face of community pharmacies in Minnesota, with the gradual rise of community pharmacies in mass merchandiser stores, regional supermarkets, and health care clinics/medical centers amongst declines in traditional retail pharmacy.

Since the publication of this research, the role, and importance of community pharmacies has changed and grown in terms of providing public health (e.g., immunizations, opioid rescue drugs, drug disposal) and population health services (medication management, health screening, specialty pharmacy) [3,10–17]. Other changes like the recovery from the economic downturn of 2008, healthcare legislation (e.g., Patient Protection and Affordable Care Act, Health Care and Education Reconciliation Act), the growth of continuity of care models, and the rise of outcome-based reimbursement systems warrant continued investigation of the market dynamics of community pharmacies in Minnesota [18–20].

1.2. Objectives

The first objective of this study was to describe the market dynamics of community pharmacies for each county in the state of Minnesota every five years over a 15 year period (i.e., 2002–2017). The development of methods for fulfilling this objective was guided by previous work done by Schommer et al. which associated county (a) population density and (b) metropolitan designation with the change in the number of 'All community pharmacies', 'Chain community pharmacies', and 'Independent community pharmacies [9]'.

The second objective was to describe the number and proportion of community pharmacies for each county in the state of Minnesota every five years over a 15 year period (i.e., 2002–2017) by (1) 'Business Organization Structure' and (2) 'Pharmacy Type'. These two variables reflect varying approaches to generating revenue and providing health services by community pharmacies in response to environmental factors (i.e., market dynamics).

2. Methods

2.1. Data Sources

County-level data for the number, names, and locations of community pharmacies in Minnesota was obtained from the Minnesota Board of Pharmacy for 2002, 2007, 2012, and 2017 [21]. Population density and metropolitan designation information for each county were obtained from the US Census Bureau and Minnesota State Demographic Center [22,23].

2.2. Data Analysis

Each pharmacy in Minnesota was categorized from state licensing board records by their location (i.e., county), 'Business Organization Structure', and 'Pharmacy Type'. Descriptive statistics were used for tabulating and summarizing the findings for the years 2002, 2007, 2012, and 2017. Temporal associations between independent and dependent variables were described using Pearson Chi-square analysis given there were only 87 cases (i.e., counties). A p-value of less than 0.05 was the significance threshold used for each test and was computed using IBM SPSS version 24.0 at the University of Minnesota, College of Pharmacy. Additional statistical computations for likelihood-ratio and fisher's exact tests were also run for each association to detect any findings unstable and affected by cell size. p-values for all study comparisons were found to be stable, nearly identical, and therefore none altering the interpretation of significance.

2.3. Study Objective 1

2.3.1. Dependent Variables

Changes in frequency for three dependent variables were used to fulfill study objective 1: 'All Community Pharmacies', 'Independent community pharmacies', and 'Chain community pharmacies'. There were operationally defined as:

- All community pharmacies: Per the state of Minnesota, an "established place(s) in which prescriptions, drugs, medicines, chemicals, and poisons are prepared, compounded, dispensed, vended, distributed, or sold to or for the use of non-hospitalized patients and from which related pharmaceutical care services are provided [24]".
- Independent community pharmacies: A community pharmacy owned as a single entity or as part of an organization comprising of 10 or fewer community pharmacies.
- Chain community pharmacies: Any community pharmacy owned as part of an organization comprising of more than 10 community pharmacies.

Frequency changes for each dependent variable were totaled and tracked for each Minnesota county in 2002, 2007, 2012, and 2017. Each of these variables was coded as: −1 if the county lost pharmacies, 0 if the number of pharmacies in county stayed the same, and 1 if the county gained pharmacies.

2.3.2. Independent Variables

'Change in Population Density' was defined as the change in person per square mile in each county for every five years from 2002–2017. This variable was coded as: −1 = negative change, 0 = change was from 0 to 5 people per square mile, and 1 = change was greater than 5 people per square mile. This variable represented the change in population for each county in a standardized unit of measurement. Metropolitan designation was defined by the US Census Bureau (core urban area of 50,000 or more population) wherein counties were coded as 0 = non-metro area and 1 = metro area.

2.4. Study Objective 2

Variables

Two variables were used to study the second objective: (1) 'Business Organization Structure' and (2) 'Pharmacy Type'. 'Business Organization Structure' related to the number of pharmacies under common ownership and the size of the organization's geographic markets. It was operationally defined as:

- Single entity: A business organization comprised of one pharmacy in a local market that would be classified under 'Independent community pharmacies' for objective 1.
- Small chain: A business organization comprised of 2–10 community pharmacies under common ownership (typically located in a local market) that would be classified under 'Independent community pharmacies' for objective 1.
- State/regional chain: A business organization comprised of greater than 10 community pharmacies under common ownership; distributed throughout Minnesota or the Midwest Region (Iowa, Illinois, Indiana, Kansas, Michigan, Minnesota, Missouri, North Dakota, Nebraska, Ohio, South Dakota, Wisconsin) and that would be classified under 'Chain community pharmacies' for objective 1.
- National chain: greater than 10 community pharmacies under common ownership; typically comprised of more than 1000 community pharmacies nationwide, located in most of the 50 states, and that would be classified under 'Chain community pharmacies' for objective 1.

The variable of 'Pharmacy Type' relates to the square footage devoted to the pharmacy department, the proportion of the business' revenue coming from the pharmacy department, and the typical reason for patronizing the business [1,2]. It was operationally defined as:

- Health & Personal Care: establishment is considered a pharmacy that also has a "front end". A relatively large amount of square footage is devoted to the pharmacy and over-the-counter products. Revenue from the pharmacy and over-the-counter product sales is relatively large. The typical reason for patronizing the business is to "go to the pharmacy". Locational convenience is a primary patronage motive. This type of pharmacy has also been known as a retail pharmacy.
- Mass merchandiser: establishment is considered a big box retail store that also has a "pharmacy". A relatively small amount of square footage is devoted to the pharmacy and over-the-counter products. Revenue from the pharmacy and over-the-counter product sales is relatively small. The typical reason for patrons to visit the business is to "go to the big box retailer". Retail shopping convenience is a primary patronage motive.
- Supermarket: establishment is considered a grocery store that also has a "pharmacy". A relatively small amount of square footage is devoted to the pharmacy and over-the-counter products. Revenue from the pharmacy and over-the-counter product sales is relatively small. The typical reason for patronizing the business is to "go to the grocery store". Grocery shopping convenience is a primary patronage motive.
- Clinic/medical center: establishment is considered a clinic that also has a "pharmacy". A relatively small amount of square footage is devoted to the pharmacy and over-the-counter products. Revenue from the pharmacy and over-the-counter product sales is relatively small. The typical reason for patronizing the business is to "go to the clinic". In some cases, the pharmacy is a stand-alone business but is still considered to be closely associated with the clinic or medical center that is nearby. In many cases, the pharmacy name is the same as the clinic name (XYZ Clinic, XYZ Medical Center, XYZ Pharmacy). Health care visit convenience is a primary patronage motive.
- Specialty: establishment is considered a specialty business. Typically, all of the square footage is devoted to the pharmacy. Revenue for this business typically comes completely from the specialty services offered by the pharmacy. The typical reason for patronizing the business is to "receive

unique pharmaceutical services" to meet patient care needs. Examples of specialty pharmacies include those focused upon renal services, compounding, veterinary pharmacy, long-term care, oncology, infusion, nuclear, outpatient treatment centers, HIV medication services, specialty pharmaceuticals. Need for specialty services is a primary patronage motive.

3. Results

The first objective of this study was to describe the market dynamics of community pharmacies for each county in the state of Minnesota every five years over a 15 year period (i.e., 2002–2017). Figures A1–A4 in the Appendix A depict the county totals of 'All community pharmacies', 'Independent community pharmacies', and 'Chain community pharmacies' in Minnesota for 2002, 2007, 2012, and 2017. The results show that every county in Minnesota had at least one community pharmacy for all years which data were collected, but only four counties had only one community pharmacy throughout the study. The total number of community pharmacies in Minnesota grew by 7 percentage points between 2002 and 2007, grew by 2 percentage points between 2007 and 2012, and fell by 3 percentage points between 2012 and 2017. The number of 'Independent community pharmacies' in Minnesota fell by 25 percentage points between 2002 and 2007, grew by 10 percentage points between 2007 and 2012, and fell by 33 percentage points between 2012 and 2017. The ratio of 'Independent community pharmacies' to 'Chain community pharmacies' registered roughly 1:1 (466:530) in 2002, 1:2 (352:718) in 2007, 1:2 (387:707) in 2012, and 1:3 (256:807) in 2017.

The market dynamics for Minnesota's 87 counties for each five year interval between 2002 and 2017 are shown in Table 1. The proportion of Minnesota's counties that gained community pharmacies in each five year interval declined over time (46% for 2002–2007, 29% for 2007–2012, and 22% for 2012–2017). The proportion of Minnesota's counties that lost community pharmacies in each five year interval increased over time (18% for 2002–2007, 29% for 2007–2012, and 38% for 2012–2017). The proportion of Minnesota's counties that maintained the same number of community pharmacies in each five year interval remained fairly stable over time (36% for 2002–2007, 43% for 2007–2012, and 40% for 2012–2017). The five year interval for 2007–2012 stood in contrast to the time periods before and after it, with opposing effects on 'Independent community pharmacies' and 'Chain community pharmacies'. During this time period, 'Independent community pharmacies' in Minnesota counties showed greater gains (38% in 2007–2012 vs. 20% in 2002–2007 & 16% in 2012–2017) and fewer losses (33% in 2007–2012 vs. 55% in 2002–2007 & 54% in 2012–2017). Meanwhile, 'Chain community pharmacies' in Minnesota counties showed greater losses (31% in 2007–2012 vs. 8% in 2002–2007 & 16% in 2012–2017) and fewer gains (31% in 2007–2012 vs. 56% in 2002–2007 & 39% in 2012–2017).

Figures 1–3 present findings that relate the change in population density and market dynamics for each five year interval between 2002 and 2017 for the 87 counties of Minnesota. Overall, counties with greater growth in population density lost fewer and gained more community pharmacies than counties with less growth in population density. This association between population density and the change in the total number of community pharmacies can be found in Figure 1 and was statistically significant for 2002–2007 ($p = 0.002$; See Appendix A Table A1), but not 2007–2012 ($p = 0.052$; See Appendix A Table A2) and 2012–2017 ($p = 0.349$; See Appendix A Table A3).

Table 1. Market dynamics for community pharmacies in Minnesota counties every five years between 2002 and 2017 (N = 87).

Pharmacy Category Market Dynamic	2002–2007	2007–2012	2012–2017
All community pharmacies			
Lost pharmacies	18%	29%	38%
Stayed the same	36%	43%	40%
Gained pharmacies	46%	29%	22%

Table 1. *Cont.*

Pharmacy Category Market Dynamic	2002–2007	2007–2012	2012–2017
Independent pharmacies			
Lost pharmacies	55%	33%	54%
Stayed the same	25%	29%	30%
Gained pharmacies	20%	38%	16%
Chain pharmacies			
Lost pharmacies	8%	31%	16%
Stayed the same	36%	38%	45%
Gained pharmacies	56%	31%	39%

Notes: percentages may not total 100% due to rounding.

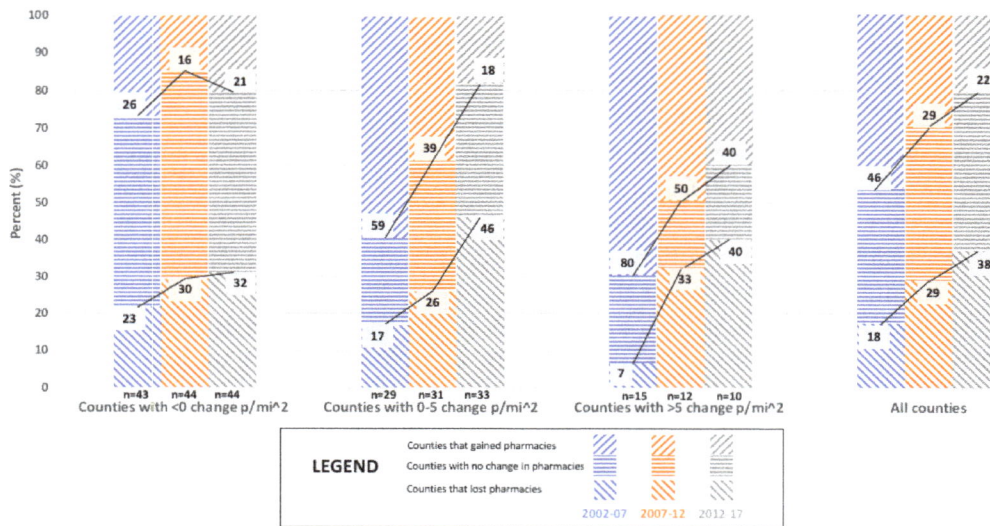

Figure 1. The relationship between change in population density (p/mi^2) and market dynamics for 'All community pharmacies' in Minnesota counties for 2002, 2007, 2012, and 2017 (N = 87).

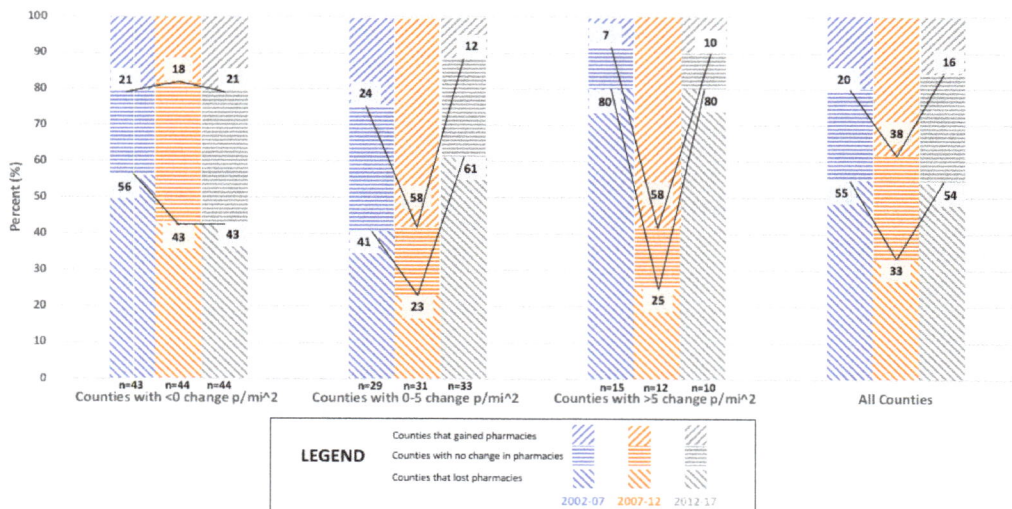

Figure 2. The relationship between change in population density (p/mi^2) and market dynamics for 'Independent community pharmacies' in Minnesota counties for 2002, 2007, 2012, and 2017 (N = 87).

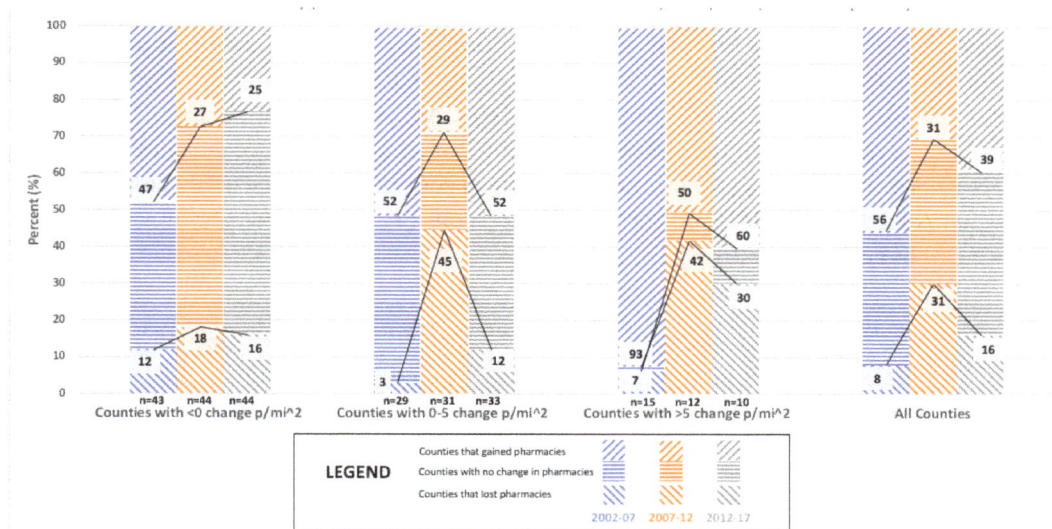

Figure 3. The relationship between change in population density (p/mi^2) and market dynamics for 'Chain community pharmacies' in Minnesota counties for 2002, 2007, 2012, and 2017 (N = 87).

The relationship between population density with the number of 'Independent community pharmacies' is shown in Figure 2, which varied in direction and significance between the five year intervals. For 2002–2007, more than half of counties lost 'Independent community pharmacies'. For 2007–2012, the greatest proportional increases for 'Independent community pharmacies' occurred in counties that grew in population density. For 2012–2017, more than half of Minnesota counties lost pharmacies with the proportional losses positively relating to greater levels of population density. The association between population density and change in the number of 'Independent community pharmacies' was statistically significant for 2007–2012 ($p = 0.005$; See Appendix A Table A2), but not for 2002–2007 ($p = 0.185$; See Appendix A Table A1) and 2012–2017 ($p = 0.234$; See Appendix A Table A3).

Figure 3 shows the relationship between population density with the number of 'Chain community pharmacies' varied in direction and significance between the five year intervals. For 2002–2007, almost 50% of counties in each population density category gained 'Chain community pharmacies', with no more than 12% losing 'Chain community pharmacies'. For 2007–2012, almost a third of all Minnesota counties lost 'Chain community pharmacies' with the greatest proportional declines occurring in counties that grew in population density. However, counties with population density growth greater than 5 persons per square mile gained more 'Chain community pharmacies' than counties with less growth or decline in population density. The proportion of counties with large increases in population density lost as many pharmacies as were gained (31% lost vs. 31% gained). For 2012–2017, a little over 20% of all Minnesota counties gained pharmacies with most of the proportional increases occurring in counties that grew in population density. A similar proportion of counties lost pharmacies across the three population density groupings (<0 p/mi^2: 32%, 0–5 p/mi^2: 46%, >5 p/mi^2: 40%). The association between population density and the change in the number of 'Chain community pharmacies' was statistically significant for 2002–2007 ($p = 0.014$; See Appendix A Table A1), 2007–2012 ($p = 0.009$; See Appendix A Table A2) and 2012–2017 ($p = 0.022$; See Appendix A Table A3).

Figures 4–6 present findings that relate metropolitan designation and market dynamics for each five year interval between 2002 and 2017 for the 87 counties of Minnesota. Metropolitan designation of Minnesota counties was not shown to significantly associate with the change in the total number of community pharmacies for any of the time periods analyzed, which are depicted in Figure 4. However, metropolitan designation of Minnesota counties was shown to significantly associate with the change in the number of 'Chain community pharmacies' for 2012–2017 ($p = 0.013$; See Appendix A Table A6), but not for 2002–2007 ($p = 0.108$; See Appendix A Table A4) and 2007–2012 ($p = 0.138$; See Appendix A

Table A5) as displayed in Figure 5. Additionally, metropolitan designation of Minnesota counties was shown to significantly associate with the change in the number of 'Independent community pharmacies' for 2002–2007 ($p = 0.021$; See Appendix A Table A4), but not for 2007–2012 ($p = 0.171$; See Appendix A Table A5) and 2012–2017 ($p = 0.282$; See Appendix A Table A6) as shown in Figure 6. Results from the 2012–2017 time interval show that almost one third (30%) of counties with a metropolitan designation gained pharmacies compared to less than one fifth (18%) of counties without a metropolitan designation doing the same. A fairly equivalent proportion of both types of counties lost pharmacies (Metro: 41%, Non-Metro: 37%) over the same time period.

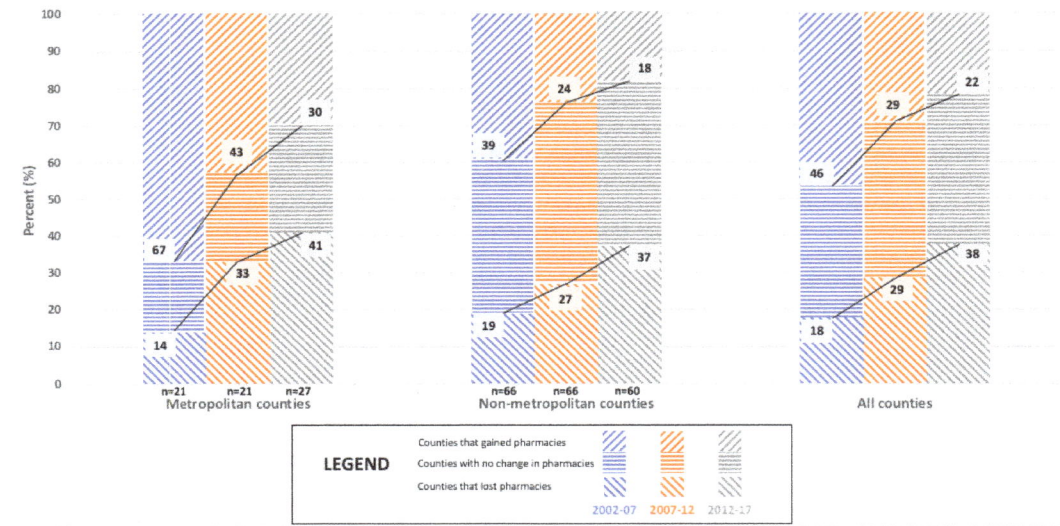

Figure 4. The relationship between Metropolitan Designation and market dynamics for 'All community pharmacies' in Minnesota counties for 2002, 2007, 2012, and 2017 (N = 87).

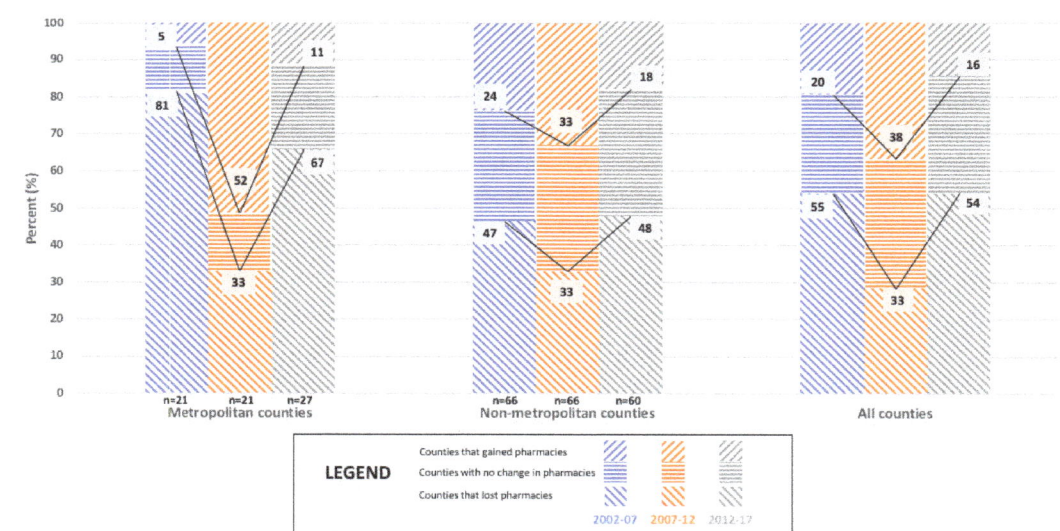

Figure 5. The relationship between Metropolitan Designation and market dynamics for 'Independent community pharmacies' in Minnesota counties for 2002, 2007, 2012, and 2017 (N = 87).

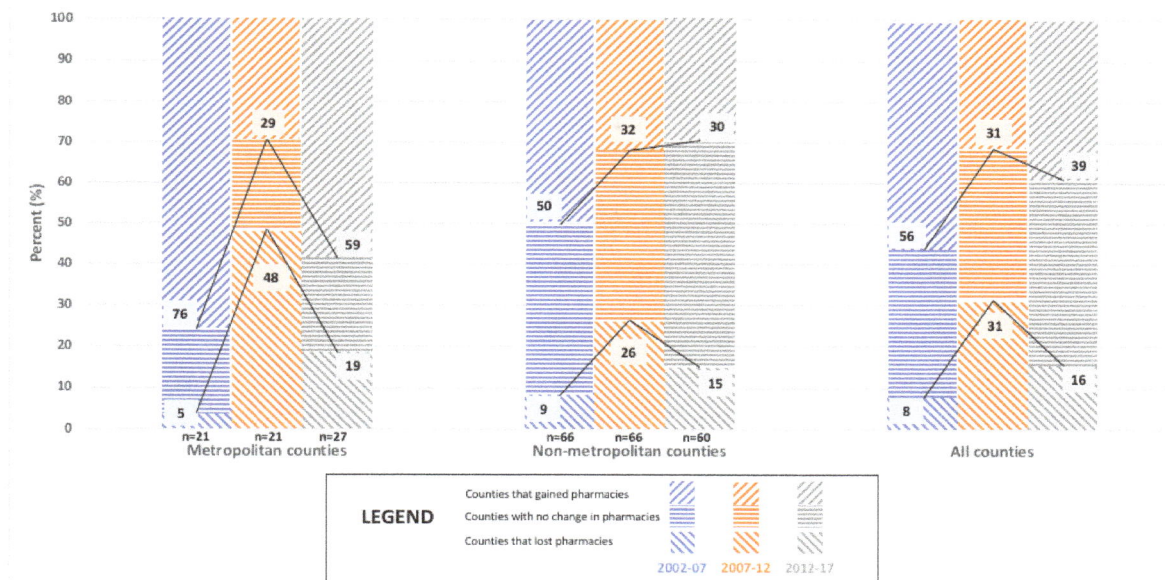

Figure 6. The relationship between Metropolitan Designation and market dynamics for 'Chain community pharmacies' in Minnesota counties for 2002, 2007, 2012, and 2017 (N = 87).

The second objective was to describe the number and proportion of community pharmacies for each county in the state of Minnesota every five years over a 15 year period from 2002 through 2017 by (1) 'Business Organization Structure' and (2) 'Pharmacy Type'.

Table 2 shows a summary of Minnesota's pharmacies by 'Business Organization Structures' and 'Pharmacy Type' for 2002, 2007, 2012, and 2017. The number of community pharmacies in Minnesota was 996 in 2002, 1070 in 2007, 1094 in 2012, and 1063 in 2017. 'Independent community pharmacies' (i.e., Single entity + Small chain) made up 47% (N = 466) of 'All community pharmacies' in 2002, with the remaining 53% (N = 530) classified as 'Chain community pharmacies' (i.e., State/regional chain + National chain). In 2007, 'Independent community pharmacies' made up 33% (N = 352) of 'All community pharmacies', with the remaining 67% (N = 718) classified as 'Chain community pharmacies'. In 2012, 'Independent community pharmacies' made up 35% (N = 387) of 'All community pharmacies', with the remaining 65% (707) classified as 'Chain community pharmacies'. By 2017, 'Independent community pharmacies' made up only 24% (N = 256) of 'All community pharmacies', with the remaining 76% (N = 807) classified as 'Chain community pharmacies' (see Figure 7).

Figure 8 depicts the proportional makeup of community pharmacies in Minnesota by business organization structures for 2002, 2007, 2012, and 2017. 'Single entity' pharmacies decreased from 35% in 2002 to 21% in 2007, rose to 24% in 2012 and then fell to 14% in 2017. 'Small chain' pharmacies remained stable at 12% from 2002 through 2007 and 2012 but decreased to 10% in 2017. 'State/regional chain' pharmacies rose from 31% in 2002 to 33% in 2007, fell to 30% in 2012 and then rose 36% in 2017. 'National chain' community pharmacies rose from 23% in 2002 to 34% in 2007, remained stable at 34% in 2012 and then rose to 40% in 2017.

Table 2. Community pharmacy business organization structures and pharmacy types in Minnesota for 2002, 2007, 2012, 2017 (Number, column %).

Business Organization Structure	Pharmacy Type	2002 N = 996	2007 N = 1070	2012 N = 1094	2017 N = 1063
Single entity	Health & Personal Care	281 (28%)	185 (17%)	199 (18%)	127 (12%)
	Mass merchandiser	0 (0%)	0 (0%)	0 (0%)	0 (0%)
	Supermarket	0 (0%)	0 (0%)	0 (0%)	0 (0%)
	Clinic/medical center	36 (4%)	32 (3%)	28 (3%)	19 (2%)
	Specialty	29 (3%)	10 (1%)	33 (3%)	5 (1%)
Total		346 (35%)	227 (21%)	260 (24%)	151 (14%)
Small chain	Health & Personal Care	98 (10%)	97 (9%)	91 (8%)	83 (8%)
	Mass merchandiser	0 (0%)	0 (0%)	0 (0%)	0 (0%)
	Supermarket	0 (0%)	0 (0%)	0 (0%)	0 (0%)
	Clinic/medical center	20 (2%)	26 (2%)	30 (3%)	17 (2%)
	Specialty	2 (<1%)	2 (<1%)	6 (1%)	5 (1%)
Total		120 (12%)	125 (12%)	127 (12%)	105 (10%)
ALL INDEPENDENTS (=Single entity +Small chain)		466 (47%)	352 (33%)	387 (35%)	256 (24%)
State/regional chain	Health & Personal Care	99 (10%)	120 (11%)	63 (6%)	66 (6%)
	Mass merchandiser	13 (1%)	0 (0%)	17 (2%)	0 (0%)
	Supermarket	127 (13%)	139 (13%)	155 (14%)	150 (14%)
	Clinic/medical center	61 (6%)	96 (9%)	83 (8%)	162 (15%)
	Specialty	5 (1%)	0 (0%)	12 (1%)	5 (1%)
Total		305 (31%)	355 (33%)	330 (30%)	383 (36%)
National chain	Health & Personal Care	81 (8%)	152 (14%)	201 (18%)	294 (28%)
	Mass merchandiser	144 (14%)	209 (20%)	173 (16%)	127 (12%)
	Supermarket	0 (0%)	0 (0%)	0 (0%)	0 (0%)
	Clinic/medical center	0 (0%)	0 (0%)	0 (0%)	0 (0%)
	Specialty	0 (0%)	2 (<1%)	3 (<1%)	2 (<1%)
Total		225 (23%)	363 (34%)	377 (34%)	423 (40%)
ALL CHAIN (=State/regional chain + National chain)		530 (53%)	718 (67%)	707 (65%)	807 (76%)

Notes: percentages may not total 100% due to rounding.

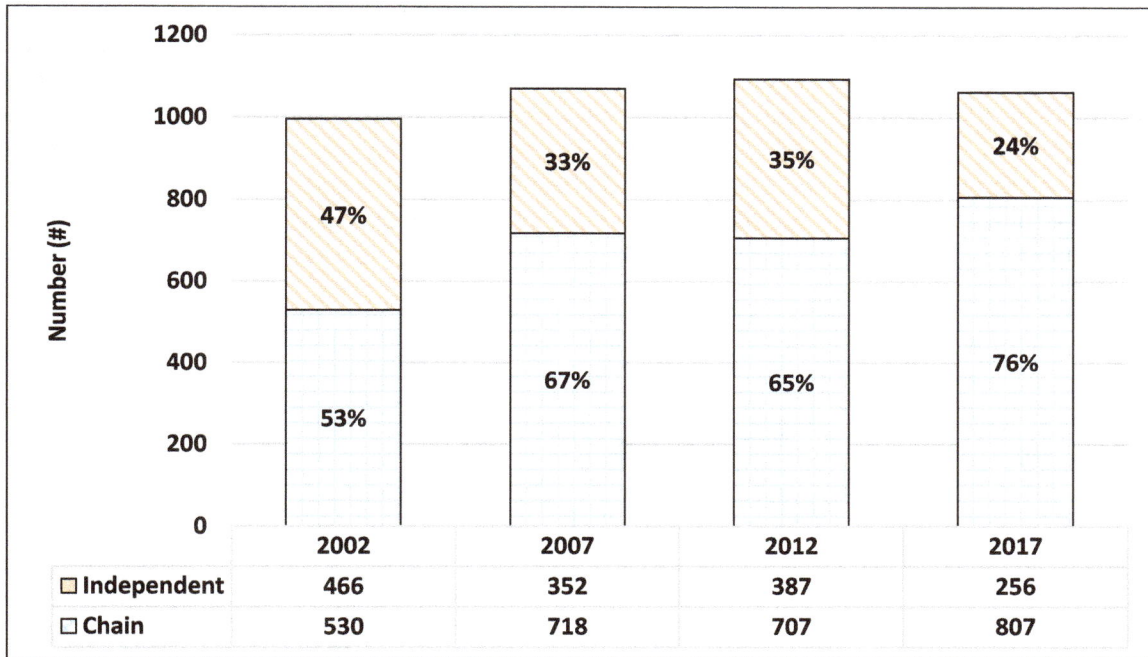

Figure 7. The number of 'Independent community pharmacies' and 'Chain community pharmacies' in Minnesota for 2002, 2007, 2012, and 2017.

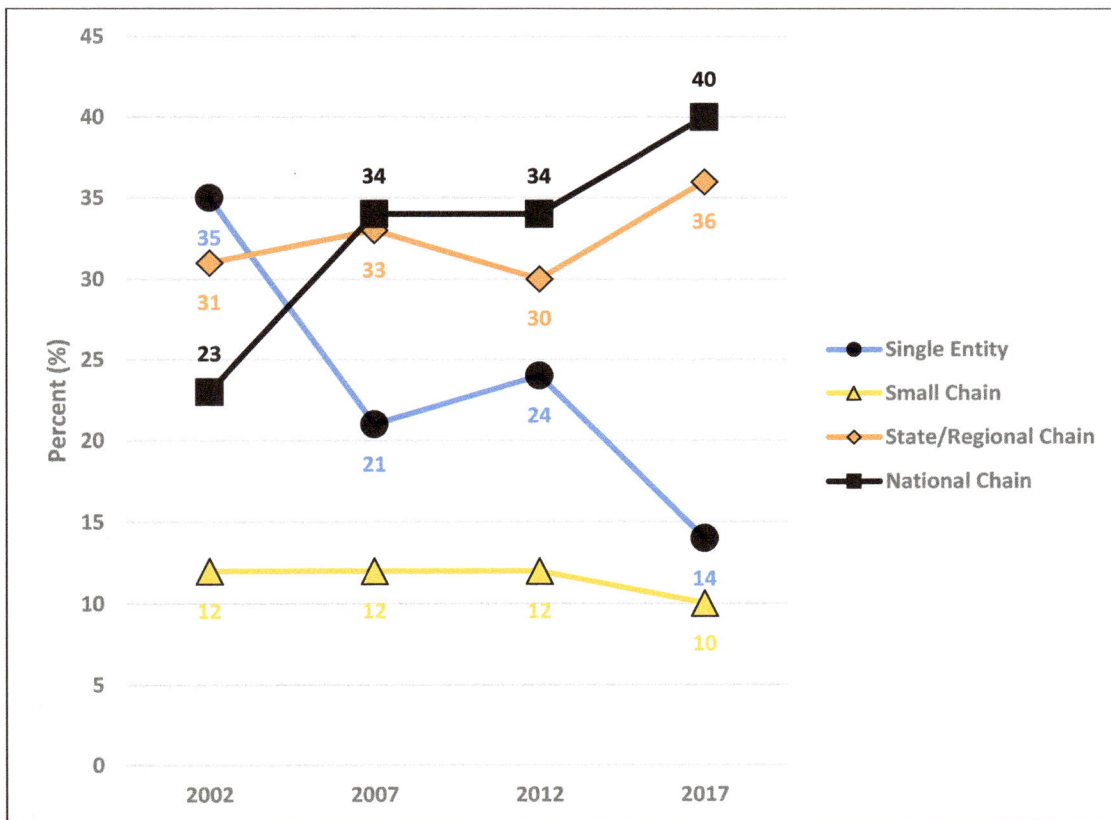

Figure 8. The proportion of business organization structures for community pharmacies in Minnesota for 2002, 2007, 2012, and 2017.

Figure 9 depicts the proportional makeup of community pharmacies in Minnesota by health and personal care pharmacy types for 2002, 2007, 2012, and 2017. Health and personal care pharmacy types decreased from 56% of 'All community pharmacies' in 2002 to 52% in 2007 and 50% in 2012, but then rose to 54% in 2017. 'Mass Merchandiser' pharmacies grew from 15% in 2002 to 19% in 2007, but fell to 18% in 2012 and then 12% in 2017. 'Supermarket' pharmacies stayed stable at 13% from 2002 to 2007 and the rose to 14% in 2012 and 2017. 'Clinic/Medical Center' pharmacies rose from 12% in 2002 to 14% in 2007 and 2012 and then increased again to 19% in 2017. Finally, 'Specialty' pharmacies fell from 4% in 2002 to 1% in 2007, before rising up to 5% in 2012 and falling again to 2% in 2017.

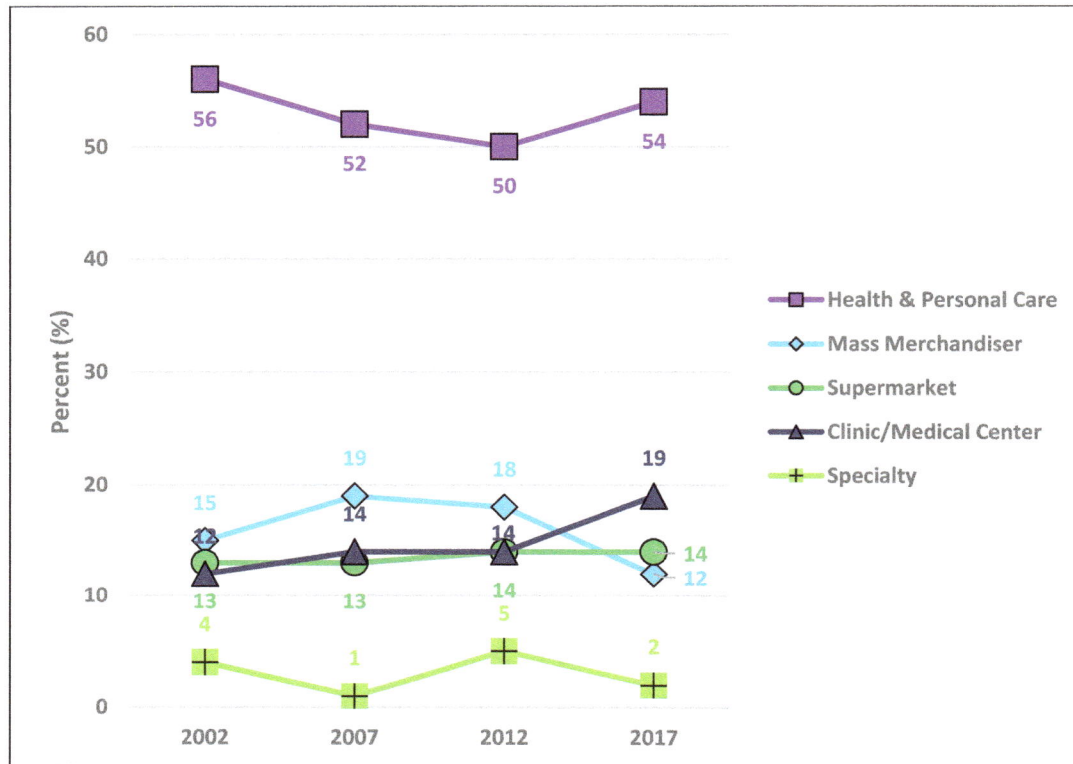

Figure 9. The proportion of community pharmacy types in Minnesota for 2002, 2007, 2012, and 2017.

4. Discussion

The first objective of this study was to describe the market dynamics of community pharmacies for each county in the state of Minnesota every five years over a 15 year period (i.e., 2002–2017).

The results show that the total number of community pharmacies grew from 2002–2007 (966 to 1070) and 2007–2012 (1070 to 1094) but declined from 2012–2017 (1094 to 1063) resulting in an overall net increase of 97 community pharmacies over 15 years (see Table 2). The bulk of this overall increase took place in only a handful of Minnesota counties as each sequential five year period saw smaller proportions of counties gaining pharmacies and larger proportions of counties losing pharmacies. Each successive 5 year interval analyzed saw a weakening in the explanatory power of the independent variables of population density (p-values: $0.002 < 0.052 < 0.349$; see Appendix A Tables A1–A3) and metropolitan designation (p-values: $0.083 < 0.111 < 0.323$; see Appendix A Tables A4–A6) for the market dynamics of 'All community pharmacies'. This result deviates from previous research on the topic and indicates the need for additional investigation into the potential causes.

The total number of 'Independent community pharmacies' fell between 2002–2007 (466 to 352), then rose between 2007–2012 (352 to 387), before falling again in 2012–2017 (387 to 256) resulting in a net decrease of 210 'Independent community pharmacies' over 15 years (see Table 2). The only statistically significant relationships with the market dynamics of 'Independent community pharmacies' were population density for 2007–2012 ($p = 0.005$; see Appendix A Table A2) and metropolitan designation for 2002–2007 ($p = 0.021$; see Appendix A Table A4) suggesting the importance of factors beyond just population density and metropolitan designation are driving market dynamics.

The total number of 'Chain community pharmacies' was inversely related to 'Independent community pharmacies' displaying an increase between 2002–2007 (530 to 718), a decline between 2007–2012 (718 to 707), followed by growth again in 2012–2017 (707 to 807) resulting in a net increase of 277 'Chain community pharmacies' over 15 years (see Table 2). Population density retained a statistically significant relationship with market dynamics of 'Chain community pharmacies' throughout each five year interval of the study (p-values: 0.014, 0.009, 0.022; see Appendix A Tables A1–A3), while metropolitan designation was significant only for the five year interval between 2012–2017 ($p = 0.013$; see Appendix A Table A6). This again suggests that other factors beyond metropolitan designation would be useful for data interpretation.

When analyzed as a whole, the results do not yield a consistent relationship between the study's independent variables and the market dynamic patterns that carry throughout the analyzed time periods. This finding differs from the conclusions of previous work by Schommer et al. that suggested the best opportunities for growth in the number of pharmacies occurred where population density was increasing and adequate infrastructure, logistics, resources, and markets, represented by a metropolitan area designation, existed [9]. This suggests that different or additional factors beyond the traditional market dynamic predictors were at play in each 5 year intervals of this study. We propose that the traditional dichotomy of independent and chain community pharmacy groupings no longer provide an optimal characterization for the market dynamics of pharmacies today. Each of these possibilities is better evaluated as a part of this study's second objective.

The second objective was to describe the number and proportion of community pharmacies for each county in the state of Minnesota every five years over a 15 year period (i.e., 2002–2017) by (1) 'Business Organization Structure' and (2) 'Pharmacy Type'.

In 2002, 'Single entity'—'Independent community pharmacies' represented the highest number and proportion of business organization structures for community pharmacies in the state of Minnesota (See Table 2). By 2007, these totals plummeted from 35% (N = 346) to 21% (N = 227), with gains by 'State/regional chains' and 'National chains' surpassing the overall difference (see Figure 8). Previous research has suggested this result as being the consequence of the latter outcompeting and acquiring the former in conveniently dispensing medications to patients utilizing a product-oriented, fee for service reimbursement systems [9]. These conditions combined with a strong economy may have also led to overall increases in 'State/regional chain' and 'National chain' community pharmacies between 2002–2007 that surpassed what would be expected based on population densities and metropolitan designation (See Table 2). Community pharmacy types between 2002–2007 remained fairly stable with the most notable changes being a four-point decline in 'Health and personal care' community pharmacies and a four-point rise in 'Mass merchandiser' pharmacies. The decrease in the former reflects losses of independent 'Single entity' community pharmacies explained at the beginning of the paragraph which was offset by gains of 'State/regional chains' in this category. The four-point rise of 'Mass merchandiser' community pharmacies also was accounted for by the growth of 'National chains' and reflected the expansion of big box stores like Walmart nationwide during this time period.

The interval between 2007–2012 saw a relative reversal of the business organization structure trends from the preceding five years, although not at the same magnitude as 2002–2007. 'Single entity'—'Independent community pharmacies' grew in number (227 to 260) and proportion (21% to 24%), while 'State/regional chains' declined and 'National chains' held steady (see Figure 8). This significant change in market dynamic trends points to macro forces at play such as the near economic collapse of 2008 and passage of the Affordable Care Act of 2010 (ACA). It may be that these events created an uncertain and altered business environment difficult for larger healthcare entities to deftly navigate, which created niche opportunities for the more nimble 'Independent community pharmacies' to fill. In some cases, pharmacists who left chain positions may have utilized their experiential knowledge to start new businesses in areas such as compounding, home infusion, and other specialty services that were historically not thought of or classified as independent community pharmacies. Additionally, the ACA was a major piece of healthcare legislation that may represent a watershed moment for community pharmacy practice and market dynamics by increasing the business viability of pharmacies as healthcare access points with the capacity to provide and be reimbursed for patient care and public health services like medication therapy management, immunizations, and more. Community pharmacy types between 2007–2012 continued to remain fairly stable with small declines in 'Health and personal care' pharmacies and 'Mass merchandiser' community pharmacies with the difference made up by small increases in 'Specialty' community pharmacies.

The market dynamic trends of business organization structure changed again between 2012–2017, as 'Single entity'—independent community pharmacies saw a return of sharp declines in their number and proportion (see Figure 8 and Table 2) and large rises in 'State/regional chains' and 'National chains'. These findings suggest that these larger community pharmacy entities adjusted to the new healthcare law and were bolstered by a stronger economy to once again outpace the growth of 'Single entity' and 'Small chain' community pharmacies through by beginning to providing patient care services along with its convenient dispensing. This time period also saw chain pharmacies grow or attempt to grow via mergers and acquisitions for the purposes of horizontal integration (e.g., CVS acquiring Target pharmacies, Walgreens acquiring Rite Aid) to increase customer access and vertical integration (e.g., CVS-Aetna, Walgreens-AmerisourceBergen, Walmart-Humana) to contain customers within comprehensive service networks. This is particularly evidenced by the type of community pharmacies that showed the most growth during this time period. 'Clinic/medical center' community pharmacies showed the greatest increase in number and proportion, indicating their natural advantage over other pharmacy types in integrating advanced pharmacist services and patient information into comprehensive and quality healthcare services. The time periods between 2012–2017 also showed a rise in 'Health and personal care' community pharmacies like CVS, Thrifty White, and Walgreens which also began offering patient care services. The largest decline during this time period was 'Mass merchandiser' community pharmacies, which reflected a reduction in the number of box stores nationwide due to a general shift in consumer preferences for online retail providers like Amazon [25].

Another interesting note pertaining to market dynamics is the limited growth of 'Specialty' community pharmacies in comparison to the proportional growth of healthcare dollars on specialty drugs over the 15 year period of the study. In fact, even the small fluctuations in 'Specialty' pharmacies may be due to methodological variation from how the category was defined/coded at the time of this study (2007 and 2017 data) and the previous work by Schommer et al. that this study drew from (2002 and 2012 data).

Study Limitations

The limitations of this study should be considered when interpreting the findings. First, these analyses were performed for only 87 counties making up a single state and therefore did not account for the outside influences or characteristics of border counties that could impact affect market dynamics, making multivariate statistical analysis impractical. Another factor that was not accounted for was the impact of insurance mandates for prescription mail order services or changes to third party payment contracts, particularly for independent/small chain pharmacies. Furthermore, the limited number of counties prevented the use of multivariate statistical analysis. Another limitation of the study is that only licensed community pharmacies were considered, rather than all locations where pharmacist services are provided such as in managed care organizations and medical centers. The inclusion of these entities would be outside the scope of this paper, but future research focusing on the type and quality of pharmacist services rather than the business structure and location of pharmacies. Finally, there may be other characteristics pertaining to pharmacy organizations and the demographics they serve which can explain the market dynamics in this study.

5. Conclusions

The findings showed that community pharmacy distribution in Minnesota's 87 counties may have shifted between 2002 and 2017 from traditional retail models to emerging healthcare models based on population health needs. This signals the need for not only a new approach for tracking community pharmacy market dynamics but also adjustments by community pharmacies to remain relevant in a new environment of patient care services.

Author Contributions: A.W.O. wrote the manuscript. J.C.S. and R.S.H. contributed to the design of the study, provided comments for each step of the study, and reviewed the manuscript. All authors approved the submitted version for publication.

Acknowledgments: The authors would like to thank Akeem Yusuf, Reshmi Singh, and Richard Cline for their previous work on this topic which served as an inspiration for this work.

Appendix A

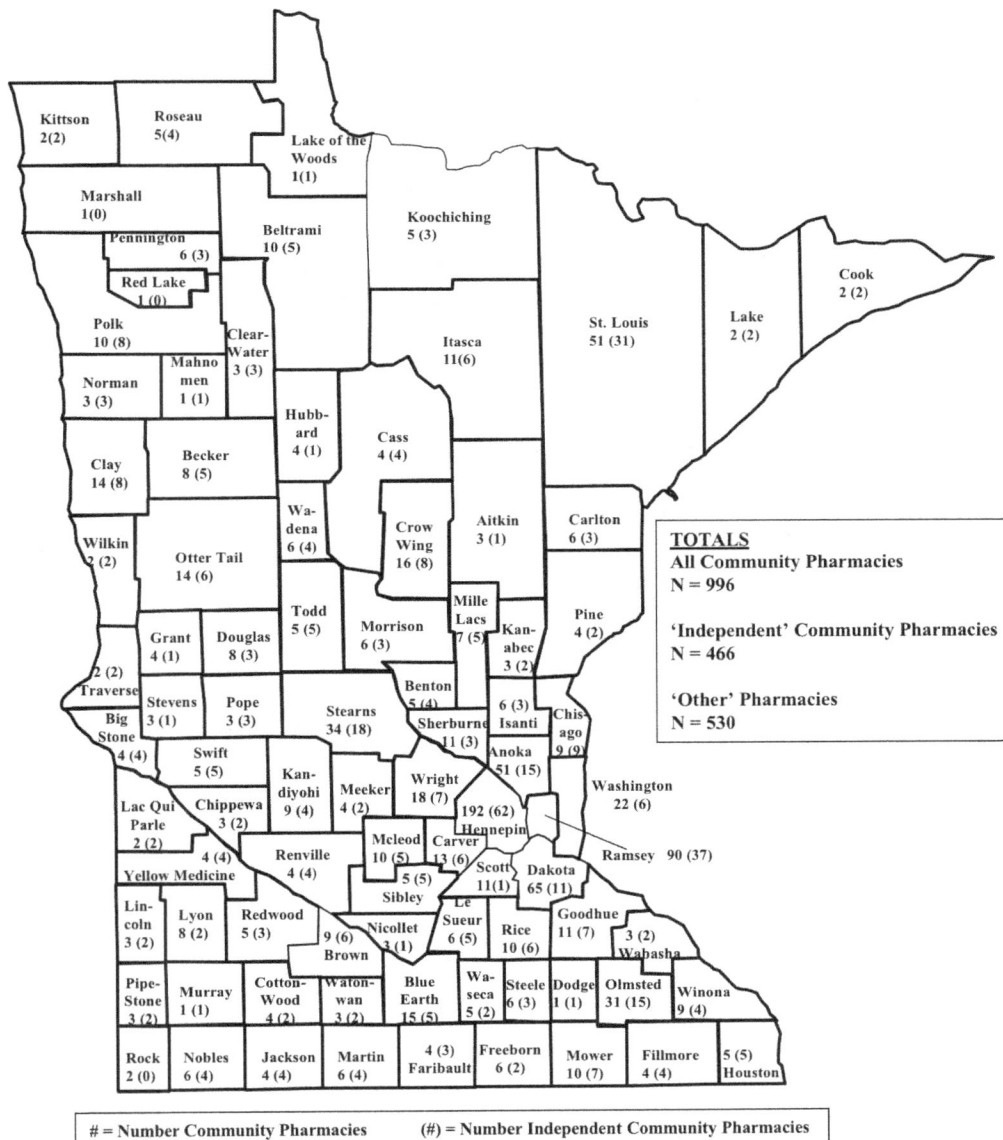

Figure A1. Community pharmacies in Minnesota counties (2002) [9].

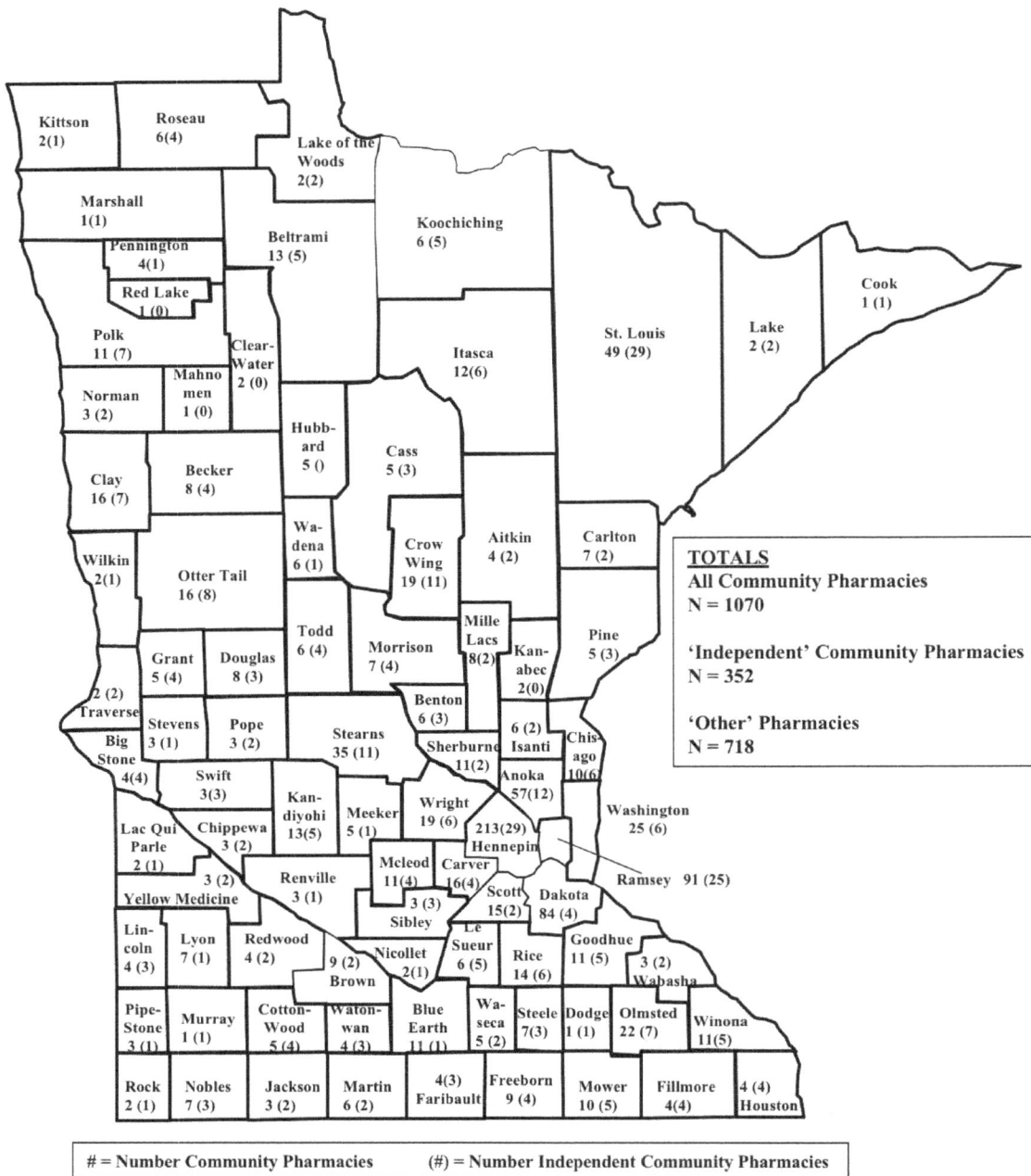

Figure A2. Community pharmacies in Minnesota counties (2007).

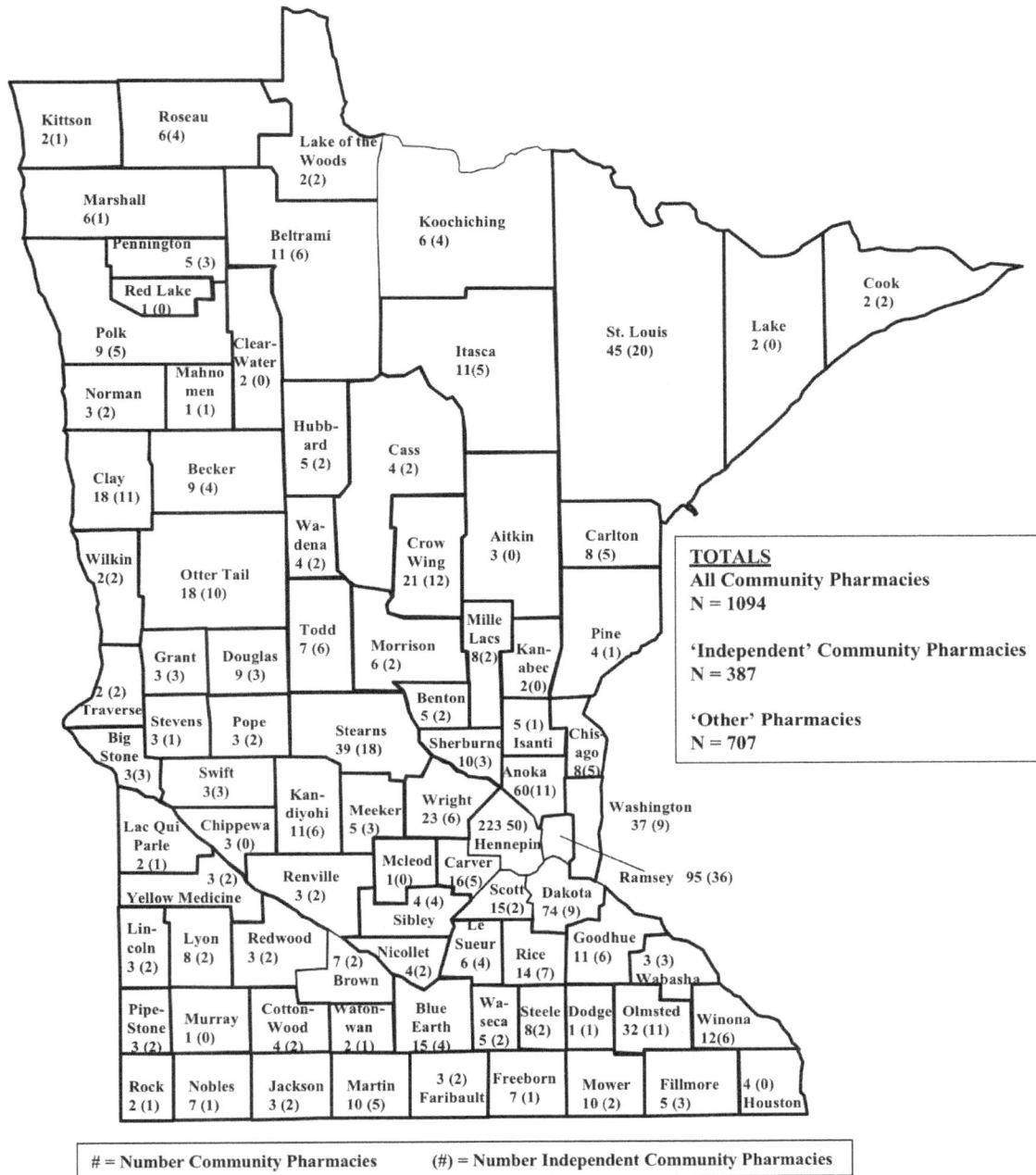

Kittson 2(1)
Roseau 6(4)
Lake of the Woods 2(2)
Koochiching 6 (4)
Cook 2 (2)
Marshall 6(1)
Pennington 5 (3)
Beltrami 11 (6)
Red Lake 1 (0)
St. Louis 45 (20)
Lake 2 (0)
Polk 9 (5)
Clear-Water 2 (0)
Itasca 11(5)
Norman 3 (2)
Mahnomen 1 (1)
Hubbard 5 (2)
Cass 4 (2)
Clay 18 (11)
Becker 9 (4)
Wadena 4 (2)
Crow Wing 21 (12)
Aitkin 3 (0)
Carlton 8 (5)
Wilkin 2(2)
Otter Tail 18 (10)
Todd 7 (6)
Morrison 6 (2)
Mille Lacs 8(2)
Pine 4 (1)
Kanabec 2(0)

TOTALS
All Community Pharmacies
N = 1094

'Independent' Community Pharmacies
N = 387

'Other' Pharmacies
N = 707

Grant 3 (3)
Douglas 9 (3)
Benton 5 (2)
Traverse 2 (2)
Stevens 3 (1)
Pope 3 (2)
Stearns 39 (18)
Sherburne 10(3)
Isanti 5 (1)
Chisago 8(5)
Big Stone 3(3)
Swift 3(3)
Kandiyohi 11(6)
Meeker 5 (3)
Wright 23 (6)
Anoka 60(11)
Washington 37 (9)
Lac Qui Parle 2 (1)
Chippewa 3 (0)
Renville 3 (2)
Mcleod 1(0)
Carver 16(5)
223 50) Hennepin
Ramsey 95 (36)
Yellow Medicine 3 (2)
Sibley 4 (4)
Scott 15(2)
Dakota 74 (9)
Lincoln 3 (2)
Lyon 8 (2)
Redwood 3 (2)
Nicollet 7 (2)
Le Sueur 6 (4)
Brown 4(2)
Rice 14 (7)
Goodhue 11 (6)
Wabasha 3 (3)
Pipe-Stone 3 (2)
Murray 1 (0)
Cotton-Wood 4 (2)
Waton-wan 2 (1)
Blue Earth 15 (4)
Waseca 5 (2)
Steele 8(2)
Dodge 1 (1)
Olmsted 32 (11)
Winona 12(6)
Rock 2 (1)
Nobles 7 (1)
Jackson 3 (2)
Martin 10 (5)
Faribault 3 (2)
Freeborn 7 (1)
Mower 10 (2)
Fillmore 5 (3)
Houston 4 (0)

= Number Community Pharmacies   (#) = Number Independent Community Pharmacies

Figure A3. Community pharmacies in Minnesota counties (2012) [9].

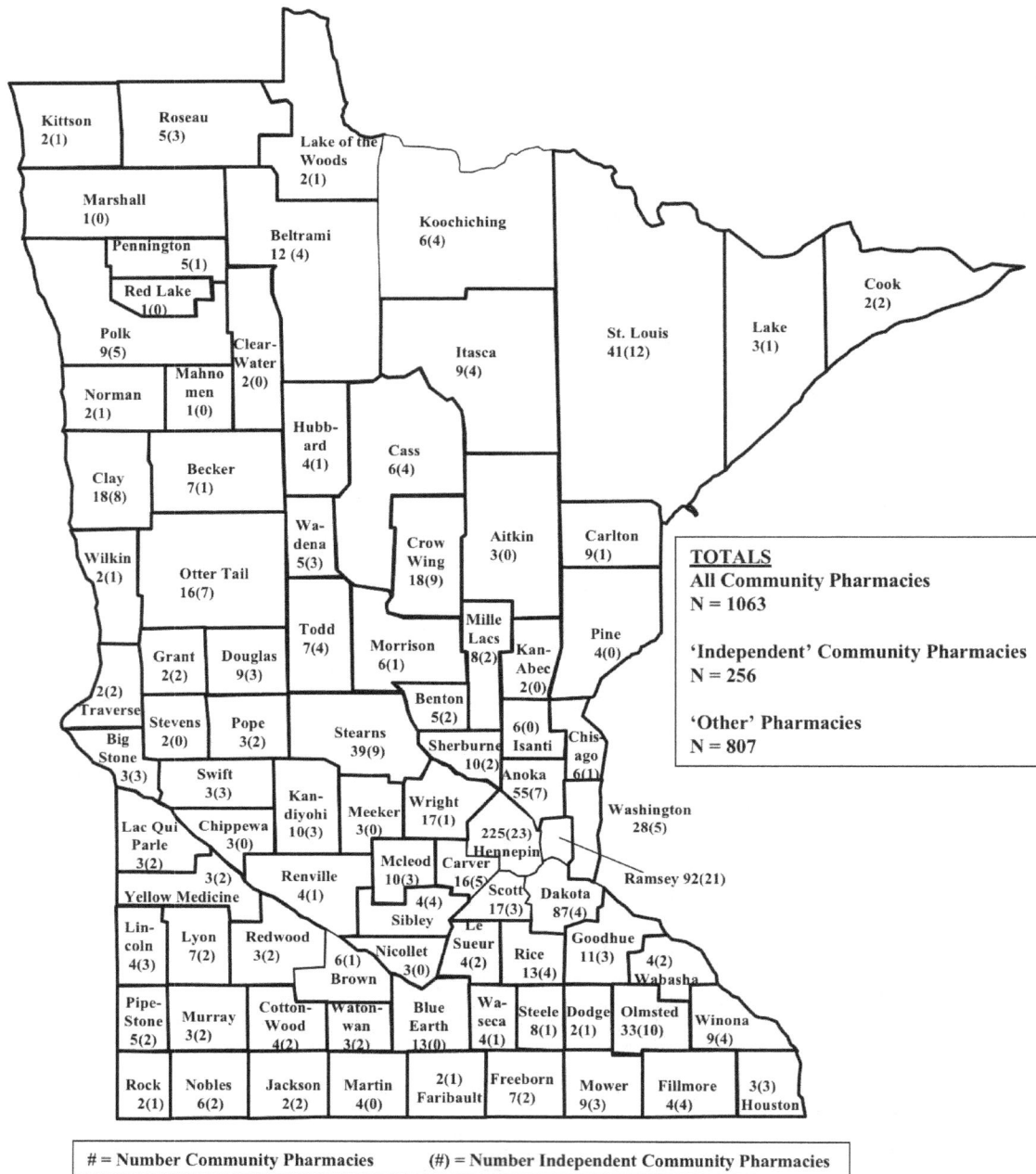

Figure A4. Community pharmacies in Minnesota counties (2017).

Table A1. The relationship between change in population density (p/mi^2) and market dynamics for community pharmacies in Minnesota counties between 2002 and 2007 (N = 87).

Pharmacy Category Market Dynamic	Counties with <0 p/mi^2 Change	Counties with 0–5 p/mi^2 Change	Counties with >5 p/mi^2 Change	Overall
	N = 43	N = 29	N = 15	N = 87
All community pharmacies				
Lost pharmacies	23%	17%	7%	18%
Stayed the same	51%	24%	13%	36%
Gained pharmacies	26%	59%	80%	46%
$p = 0.002$				

Table A1. *Cont.*

Pharmacy Category Market Dynamic	Counties with <0 p/mi² Change	Counties with 0–5 p/mi² Change	Counties with >5 p/mi² Change	Overall
	N = 43	N = 29	N = 15	N = 87
Independent pharmacies				
Lost pharmacies	56%	41%	80%	55%
Stayed the same	23%	35%	13%	25%
Gained pharmacies	21%	24%	7%	20%
p = 0.185				
Chain pharmacies				
Lost pharmacies	12%	3%	7%	8%
Stayed the same	42%	45%	0%	36%
Gained pharmacies	47%	52%	93%	56%
p = 0.014				

Notes: p/mi^2 = persons per square mile; percentages may not total 100% due to rounding.

Table A2. The relationship between change in population density (p/mi^2) and market dynamics for community pharmacies in Minnesota counties between 2007 and 2012 (N = 87).

Pharmacy CategoryMarket Dynamic	Counties with <0 p/mi² Change	Counties with 0–5 p/mi² Change	Counties with >5 p/mi² Change	Overall
	N = 44	N = 31	N = 12	N = 87
All community pharmacies				
Lost pharmacies	30%	26%	33%	29%
Stayed the same	55%	36%	17%	43%
Gained pharmacies	16%	39%	50%	29%
p = 0.052				
Independent pharmacies				
Lost pharmacies	43%	23%	25%	33%
Stayed the same	39%	19%	17%	29%
Gained pharmacies	18%	58%	58%	38%
p = 0.005				
Chain pharmacies				
Lost pharmacies	18%	45%	42%	31%
Stayed the same	54%	26%	8%	38%
Gained pharmacies	27%	29%	50%	31%
p = 0.009				

Notes: p/mi^2 = persons per square mile; percentages may not total 100% due to rounding.

Table A3. The relationship between change in population density (p/mi^2) and market dynamics for community pharmacies in Minnesota counties between 2012 and 2017 (N = 87).

Pharmacy CategoryMarket Dynamic	Counties with <0 p/mi² Change	Counties with 0–5 p/mi² Change	Counties with >5 p/mi² Change	Overall
	N = 44	N = 33	N = 10	N = 87
All community pharmacies				
Lost pharmacies	32%	46%	40%	38%
Stayed the same	48%	36%	20%	40%
Gained pharmacies	21%	18%	40%	22%
p = 0.349				

Table A3. *Cont.*

Pharmacy CategoryMarket Dynamic	Counties with <0 p/mi² Change	Counties with 0–5 p/mi² Change	Counties with >5 p/mi² Change	Overall
	N = 44	N = 33	N = 10	N = 87
Independent pharmacies				
Lost pharmacies	43%	61%	80%	54%
Stayed the same	36%	27%	10%	30%
Gained pharmacies	21%	12%	10%	16%
p = 0.234				
Chain pharmacies				
Lost pharmacies	16%	12%	30%	16%
Stayed the same	59%	36%	10%	45%
Gained pharmacies	25%	52%	60%	39%
p = 0.022				

Notes: p/mi² = persons per square mile; percentages may not total 100% due to rounding.

Table A4. The relationship between Metropolitan Designation and market dynamics for community pharmacies in Minnesota counties between 2002 and 2007 (N = 87).

Pharmacy CategoryMarket Dynamic	Metropolitan Counties	Non-Metropolitan Counties	Overall
	N = 21	N = 66	N = 87
All community pharmacies			
Lost pharmacies	14%	19%	18%
Stayed the same	19%	41%	36%
Gained pharmacies	67%	39%	46%
p = 0.083			
Independent pharmacies			
Lost pharmacies	81%	47%	55%
Stayed the same	14%	29%	25%
Gained pharmacies	5%	24%	20%
p = 0.021			
Chain pharmacies			
Lost pharmacies	5%	9%	8%
Stayed the same	19%	41%	36%
Gained pharmacies	76%	50%	56%
p = 0.108			

Notes: percentages may not total 100% due to rounding.

Table A5. The relationship between Metropolitan Designation and market dynamics for community pharmacies in Minnesota counties between 2007 and 2012 (N = 87).

Pharmacy CategoryMarket Dynamic	Metropolitan Counties	Non-Metropolitan Counties	Overall
	N = 21	N = 66	N = 87
All community pharmacies			
Lost pharmacies	33%	27%	29%
Stayed the same	24%	49%	43%
Gained pharmacies	43%	24%	29%
p = 0.111			
Independent pharmacies			
Lost pharmacies	33%	33%	33%
Stayed the same	14%	33%	29%
Gained pharmacies	52%	33%	38%
p = 0.171			

Table A5. *Cont.*

Pharmacy CategoryMarket Dynamic	Metropolitan Counties	Non-Metropolitan Counties	Overall
	N = 21	N = 66	N = 87
Chain pharmacies			
Lost pharmacies	48%	26%	31%
Stayed the same	24%	42%	38%
Gained pharmacies	29%	32%	31%
p = 0.138			

Notes: percentages may not total 100% due to rounding.

Table A6. The relationship between Metropolitan Designation and market dynamics for community pharmacies in Minnesota counties between 2012 and 2017 (N = 87).

Pharmacy CategoryMarket Dynamic	Metropolitan Counties	Non-Metropolitan Counties	Overall
	N = 27	N = 60	N = 87
All community pharmacies			
Lost pharmacies	41%	37%	38%
Stayed the same	30%	45%	40%
Gained pharmacies	30%	18%	22%
p = 0.323			
Independent pharmacies			
Lost pharmacies	67%	48%	54%
Stayed the same	22%	33%	30%
Gained pharmacies	11%	18%	16%
p = 0.282			
Chain pharmacies			
Lost pharmacies	19%	15%	16%
Stayed the same	22%	55%	45%
Gained pharmacies	59%	30%	39%
p = 0.013			

Notes: percentages may not total 100% due to rounding.

References

1. Gaither, C.A.; Schommer, J.C.; Doucette, W.R.; Kreling, D.H.; Mott, D.A. *Final Report of the 2014 National Sample Survey of the Pharmacist Workforce to Determine Contemporary Demographic Practice Characteristics and Quality of Work-Life*; American Association of Colleges of Pharmacy: Arlington, VA, USA, 2015; Available online: https://www.aacp.org/sites/default/files/finalreportofthenationalpharmacistworkforcestudy2014.pdf (accessed on 7 May 2018).

2. Bureau of Labor and Statistics. Occupational Employment and Wages, May 2017: 29-1051 Pharmacists. *Occup. Employ. Stat.* **2017**, *9*. Available online: https://www.bls.gov/oes/current/oes291051.htm (accessed on 7 May 2018).

3. Cranor, C.W.; Christensen, D.B. The Asheville Project: Short-term outcomes of a community pharmacy diabetes care program. *J. Am. Pharm. Assoc.* **2003**, *43*, 149–159. Available online: http://www.ncbi.nlm.nih.gov/pubmed/12688433 (accessed on 8 May 2018). [CrossRef]

4. Isetts, B.J.; Schondelmeyer, S.W.; Artz, M.B.; Lenarz, L.A.; Heaton, A.H.; Wadd, W.B.; Brown, L.M.; Cipolle, R.J. Clinical and economic outcomes of medication therapy management services: The Minnesota experience. *J. Am. Pharm. Assoc.* **2003**, *48*, 203–211. [CrossRef] [PubMed]

5. Bacci, J.L.; McGrath, S.H.; Pringle, J.L.; Maguire, M.A.; McGivney, M.S. Implementation of targeted medication adherence interventions within a community chain pharmacy practice: The Pennsylvania Project. *J. Am. Pharm. Assoc.* **2014**, *54*, 584–593. [CrossRef] [PubMed]

6.   Qato, D.M.; Daviglus, M.L.; Wilder, J.; Lee, T.; Qato, D.; Lambert, B. "Pharmacy Deserts" Are Prevalent In Chicago's Predominantly Minority Communities, Raising Medication Access Concerns. *Health Aff.* **2014**, *33*, 1958–1965. [CrossRef] [PubMed]

7.   Qato, D.M.; Zenk, S.; Wilder, J.; Harrington, R.; Gaskin, D.; Alexander, G.C. The availability of pharmacies in the United States: 2007–2015. van Wouwe JP, ed. *PLoS ONE* **2017**, *12*, e0183172. [CrossRef] [PubMed]

8.   Schommer, J.C.; Singh, R.L.; Cline, R.R.; Hadsall, R.S. Market dynamics of community pharmacies in Minnesota. *Res. Soc. Adm. Pharm.* **2006**, *2*, 347–358. [CrossRef] [PubMed]

9.   Schommer, J.C.; Yusuf, A.A.; Hadsall, R.S. Market dynamics of community pharmacies in Minnesota, U.S. from 1992 through 2012. *Res. Soc. Adm. Pharm.* **2014**, *10*, 217–231. [CrossRef] [PubMed]

10.   Minnesota Board of Pharmacy. *Pharmacy Immunization Practice in Minnesota*; Minnesota Board of Pharmacy: Minneapolis, MN, USA, 2016; Volume 2, Available online: www.health.state.mn.us/divs/idepc/immunize/ hcp/protocols/ (accessed on 8 May 2018).

11.   Baroy, J.; Chung, D.; Frisch, R.; Apgar, D.; Slack, M.K. The impact of pharmacist immunization programs on adult immunization rates: A systematic review and meta-analysis. *J. Am. Pharm. Assoc.* **2016**, *56*, 418–426. [CrossRef] [PubMed]

12.   Salazar, D. Turning the Tide: Community Pharmacy Grapples with the Opioid Epidemic. *Drug Store News* **2018**, *1*. Available online: https://www.pharmacist.com/article/turning-tide-community-pharmacy- grapples-opioid-epidemic (accessed on 8 May 2018).

13.   National Association of Boards of Pharmacy. *NABP Issues Policy Statement Supporting the Pharmacist's Role in Increasing Access to Opioid Overdose Reversal Drug*; National Association of Boards of Pharmacy: Mount Prospect, IL, USA, 2014; Available online: http://www.nabp.net/news/nabp-issues-policy-statement- supporting-the-pharmacist-s-role-in-increasing-access-to-opioid-overdose-reversal-drug (accessed on 8 May 2018).

14.   Smolen, A. Role of the Pharmacist in Proper Medication Disposal. *US Pharm.* **2011**, *36*, 52–55.

15.   Rickles, N.M.; Skelton, J.B.; Davis, J.; Hopson, J. Cognitive memory screening and referral program in community pharmacies in the United States. *Int. J. Clin. Pharm.* **2014**, *36*, 360–367. [CrossRef] [PubMed]

16.   Staudt, A.M.; Amtower, J.E.; George, J.; Daniels, N.C.; Allou, J.N.; Laswell, E.; Ballentine, J. The Correlation of Free Health Screenings at Community Pharmacies on Diabetes. *Innov. Pharm.* **2017**, *8*. [CrossRef]

17.   DeLoach, L.A.; Leonard, C.E.; Galdo, J.A. Specialty Pharmacy: What's the Impact on Community Practice? *US Pharm.* **2016**, *41*, 35–40. Available online: https://www.uspharmacist.com/article/specialty-pharmacy- whats-the-impact-on-community-practice (accessed on 8 May 2018).

18.   Carrion, A.; Martin, T.S. The Affordable Care Act and the Pharmacist. *US Pharm.* **2015**, *40*, 33–38.

19.   Melody, K.; McCartney, E.; Sen, S.; Duenas, G. Optimizing care transitions: The role of the community pharmacist. *Integr. Pharm. Res. Pract.* **2016**, *5*, 43–51. [CrossRef] [PubMed]

20.   Pringle, J.L.; Rucker, N.L.; Domann, D.; Chan, C.; Tice, B.; Burns, A.L. Value-Based Incentives in Community Pharmacy. *Am. J. Pharm. Benefits* **2016**, *8*, 22–29.

21.   Minnesota Department of Health. Minnesota Board of Pharmacy. 2018. Available online: https://mn.gov/ boards/pharmacy/ (accessed on 8 May 2018).

22.   US Census Bureau. *Statistical Abstract of the United States*; United States Department of Commerce: Washington, DC, USA. Available online: https://www.census.gov/history/www/reference/publications/ statistical_abstracts.html (accessed on 7 May 2018).

23.   Minnesota State Demographic Center (SDC). Available online: https://mn.gov/admin/demography/ (accessed on 8 May 2018).

24.   The Office of the Revisor of Statutes. *Minnesota Administrative Rules*; Part 6800.0100; Minnesota Legislature: St. Paul, MN, USA, 2011; Volume 3. Available online: https://www.revisor.mn.gov/rules/?id=6800.0100 (accessed on 8 May 2018).

25.   Welch, D.; Burritt, C.; Coleman-Lochner, L. Retail's Big Box Era at an End. *Financ. Post* **2012**, *6*. Available online: http://business.financialpost.com/news/retail-marketing/retails-big-box-era-at-an-end (accessed on 8 May 2018).

18

Pharmacy Technicians' Willingness to Perform Emerging Tasks in Community Practice

William R. Doucette [1],* and Jon C. Schommer [2]

[1] College of Pharmacy, University of Iowa, 115 S. Grand Avenue, S518 PHAR, Iowa City, IA 52242, USA
[2] College of Pharmacy, University of Minnesota, 308 Harvard Street, S.E., Minneapolis, MN 55455, USA; schom010@umn.edu
* Correspondence: william-doucette@uiowa.edu

Abstract: New tasks are being developed for pharmacy technicians in community practice. The objectives of this study were to (1) assess the willingness of community pharmacy technicians to perform new tasks, and (2) to identify factors affecting technicians in assuming new tasks in community pharmacy practice. An online survey asked about the respondent characteristics, involvement in pharmacy technician tasks, willingness to perform emerging pharmacy technician tasks, and influences on pharmacy technicians' performance of emerging tasks. Descriptive statistics were calculated for all items. A total of 639 usable surveys from community pharmacy technicians were used in the analyses. The respondents reported a mean of 11.5 years working as a pharmacy technician, with 79.2% working full time. Technicians reported high willingness to perform four emerging tasks, moderate willingness for six tasks, and low willingness to perform two tasks. The low willingness tasks were administering a vaccination and drawing a blood sample with a finger stick. Four workplace influences on willingness to perform emerging tasks were insufficient staffing, insufficient time to complete additional tasks, employers not classifying technicians based on specialized skills, and usually feeling stress at work. It appears likely that pharmacy technicians will be willing to perform the new tasks needed to support the emerging patient care services in community pharmacies.

Keywords: pharmacy technician; community pharmacy; willingness; services

1. Introduction

Community pharmacy practice continues to evolve as payers seek higher quality care for limited payment, providers pursue improved coordination of care, healthcare systems strive for collaborative care models, and chronically ill patients prefer care from a pharmacist they know [1–3]. As new community pharmacy services are expanded and developed, typically there are changes in workflow and staffing within the pharmacies. While pharmacists are being called upon to provide greater patient care through collaborative and other innovative healthcare models, pharmacy technicians are also undertaking new roles in community pharmacy practice. New roles for pharmacy technicians are derived from new services, such as medication management [4,5], technician prescription validation (i.e., tech-check-tech) [6], medication reconciliation [7], medication synchronization [8], and immunizations [9–11]. Although some growth has occurred with these services, as pharmacy payment and care models also evolve, it is likely that these services, and others, will continue to become a part of community pharmacy practice [12,13]. To succeed in this environment, community pharmacies will need a strong supply of well-trained and motivated pharmacy technicians. Such technicians can free up pharmacists to deliver additional patient care services, while performing new tasks themselves.

The purpose of this study was to evaluate the willingness of pharmacy technicians to perform new tasks as community pharmacy practice changes in the future.

The specific objectives of this study were as follows:

(1) Assess the willingness of pharmacy technicians to perform new tasks in community pharmacy practice;

(2) Identify factors that can affect pharmacy technicians in assuming new roles in community pharmacy practice.

2. Materials and Methods

This study was an online survey sent to 29,084 certified pharmacy technicians. The sample was obtained through the Pharmacy Technician Certification Board (PTCB) and the National Health-Career Association (NHA). The sample frames did not support a priori screening to identify technicians working in community pharmacies, so such screening was done in the survey itself. A Qualtrics online survey was prepared by the research team, and links to it were sent out via email by PTCB and NHA. Three email contacts containing a survey link were sent to the sample about 10 days apart from each other. The survey was open for 40 days overall.

The survey asked about four primary topics: respondent characteristics, involvement in pharmacy technician tasks, willingness to perform emerging pharmacy technician tasks, and potential influences on pharmacy technicians' performance of emerging tasks. See the supplementary material for the formatted survey questions. The respondent characteristics included several demographics (e.g., age, gender), as well as practice-related variables (e.g., practice experience). Technician involvement in 12 emerging pharmacy technician tasks was rated with a 3-point scale (1 = not at all involved, 2 = somewhat involved, 3 = regularly involved). Respondents also rated their willingness to perform the 12 emerging pharmacy technician tasks using a 4-point scale (1 = unwilling, 2 = slightly willing, 3 = moderately willing, 4 = very willing). Finally, the survey respondents used a 7-point Likert scale (1 = strongly disagree, 2 = disagree, 3 = somewhat disagree, 4 = neither agree nor disagree, 5 = somewhat agree, 6 = agree, 7 = strongly agree) to rate workplace variables. The list of emerging technician tasks was developed from the literature and with input from community pharmacy informants. Based on the willingness ratings of respondents, the emerging tasks were categorized as high willingness (at least 60% very willing), moderate willingness (25–59% very willing) and low willingness (less than 25% very willing). Descriptive statistics (e.g., mean, median, frequencies) were calculated for all items, using data from respondents who reported current employment as a pharmacy technician in a community pharmacy setting. This study was approved by the University of Iowa Human Subjects Office.

3. Results

A total of 1257 survey responses were received. Of these, 639 were usable surveys from people working as community pharmacy technicians which were used in the analyses described in this article. The overall response rate was 4.3 percent. All of these respondents reported being a certified pharmacy technician. The most common setting type was large chain community pharmacy (36.2%), followed by mass merchandiser (28.8%), independent (15.2%), supermarket (10.6%) and other (9.3%). The regions the respondents came from were the Midwest (39.1%), South (37.6%), West (15.4%) and Northeast (7.9%). The respondents reported a mean of 11.5 (S.D. = 8.7) years working as a pharmacy technician. A majority (79.2%) of respondents reported full-time employment (>30 h a week). Similarly, a large percentage (87.5%) of respondents were female. The mean age of the community pharmacy technician respondents was 42.5 (S.D. = 12.4) years. Over half (54.3%) of the respondents reported their primary method of training to work as a pharmacy technician was unaccredited on-the-job training from their employer. Other reported training methods included unaccredited structured training program from their employer (11.3%), accredited standalone training program (10.6%), accredited structured training program from their employer (10.2%) and other (13.5%).

At least half of the community pharmacy technician respondents reported regular involvement with only two of the emerging tasks (Table 1): calling a prescriber for clarification of a prescription order (56.2%) and collecting patient medication history from a patient (51.3%). Less than 20% of respondents reported regular involvement with eight of the emerging tasks. This last set of activities has historically been performed by pharmacists, often due to legal restrictions preventing technicians from performing them. Three of these activities are related to dispensing: performing final prescription verification, taking a prescription order over the telephone, and transferring a prescription to another pharmacy. The three least commonly performed tasks were part of relatively new services, and perhaps were beyond the traditional scope of pharmacy technician roles: obtaining patient vital signs, administering a vaccination, and drawing a blood sample with a finger stick.

The respondents also reported their willingness to perform the 12 emerging technician tasks. For four of these tasks, at least 60% of the respondents stated that they would be very willing to perform them, while less than 8% said they were unwilling to do them (Table 1). These "high willingness" tasks were calling a prescriber to clarify a prescription order, collecting patient medication history, documenting patient care, and calling patients prior to medication synchronization filling. Another set of six tasks had lesser willingness, being rated as very willing to perform by 37–53% of respondents, and showing greater unwillingness (17–29%).

Table 1. Involvement [A] and willingness [B] to perform emerging technician tasks.

Emerging Technician Tasks	Not at All Involved n, (%)	Regularly Involved n, (%)	Unwilling n, (%)	Very Willing n, (%)
• Call prescriber for clarification of electronic or written prescription order	95, (14.9)	359, (56.2)	34, (5.3)	482, (75.4)
• Collect patient medication history from patient	111, (17.4)	328, (51.3)	40, (6.3)	418, (65.4)
• Document pharmacy care in patient records	220, (34.4)	204, (31.9)	41, (6.4)	403, (63.1)
• Call patient prior to medication synchronization to clarify medications to be filled	188, (29.4)	236, (36.9)	49, (7.7)	389, (60.9)
• Prepare vaccination for administration by pharmacist	392, (61.3)	121, (18.9)	144, (22.5)	337, (52.7)
• Take prescription order from physician over the telephone	457, (71.5)	90, (14.1)	137, (21.4)	320, (50.1)
• Transfer a prescription to another pharmacy	437, (68.4)	71, (11.1)	117, (18.3)	314, (49.1)
• Conduct medication reconciliation after patient is discharged from hospital	443, (69.3)	58, (9.1)	111, (17.4)	284, (44.4)
• Obtain patient vital signs (blood pressure, heart rate, temperature)	594, (93.0)	13, (2.0)	186, (29.1)	279, (43.7)
• Perform final prescription verification during dispensing	423, (66.2)	125, (19.6)	157, (24.6)	240, (37.6)
• Administer a vaccination to a patient	599, (93.7)	11, (1.7)	301, (47.1)	156, (24.4)
• Draw a blood sample from a patient (finger stick)	617, (96.6)	6, (0.9)	311, (48.7)	151, (23.6)

[A] Involvement rated with a 3-point scale: 1 = not at all involved, 2 = somewhat involved, 3 = regularly involved.
[B] Willingness rated with a 4-point scale: 1 = unwilling, 2 = slightly willing, 3 = moderately willing, 4 = very willing.

Two final "low willingness" tasks were rated as very willing to perform by less than 25% of respondents, and unwilling to perform by at least 47% of respondents: administering a vaccination, and drawing a blood sample with a finger stick.

The final section of the survey asked respondents about 11 workplace variables that could affect their willingness to perform emerging pharmacy technician tasks. For reporting, the number and percentage of respondents who rated any level of agreement (i.e., somewhat agree, agree, strongly agree) were calculated for each variable, as well as the scale mean and standard deviation. Seven variables expected to support pharmacy technician willingness to perform emerging tasks had agreement from at least 59% of respondents (Table 2). The remaining four variables showed less likelihood to support technicians' performance of new tasks, having strong agreement with a negative factor (1 item) or having low agreement with a positive factor (3 items). These four variables were that current staffing may not support technicians assuming new tasks (negative item), having enough time to complete additional tasks, employers classifying technicians based on specialized skills, and not usually feeling stress at work.

Table 2. Work environment variables.

Rate your level of agreement with each of the following statements in regard to pharmacy technicians working in your pharmacy.	Agreement n, (%)	Mean (SD)
• At my workplace the technicians work well with the pharmacists.	583 (91.5%)	6.12 (1.22)
• If I had to learn to do new tasks for my job, I feel confident that I could do so readily.	580 (91.2%)	6.14 (1.16)
• Performing new tasks in my workplace helps keep my work interesting.	552 (86.7%)	5.91 (1.33)
• I would be excited to have a new opportunity if we implemented a new service at my pharmacy.	515 (80.8%)	5.69 (1.51)
• At my workplace the managers would be supportive when technicians are performing new tasks.	472 (74.1%)	5.31 (1.57)
• When implementing a new service, technicians at my workplace may receive training to perform the tasks.	457 (71.7%)	5.05 (1.66)
• Current staffing levels at my pharmacy may not support technicians assuming additional tasks.	427 (67.0%)	4.98 (1.85)
• My fellow pharmacy staff would be supportive of implementing a new service in the pharmacy.	375 (59.0%)	4.78 (1.67)
• There is enough time in my current workday to complete additional tasks and responsibilities.	233 (36.6%)	3.43 (2.01)
• My employer classifies technicians based on specialized skills.	225 (35.4%)	3.78 (1.89)
• I don't usually feel stress when working at my job.	224 (35.2%)	3.43 (1.97)

Agreement was rated on a 7-point scale: 1 = strongly disagree, 2 = disagree, 3 = somewhat disagree, 4 = neither agree nor disagree, 5 = somewhat agree, 6 = agree, 7 = strongly agree. Agreement variable = sum of somewhat agree, agree and strongly agree. Note: Unshaded variables are expected to support technician willingness to perform new tasks, while shaded variables are not.

4. Discussion

There were four emerging tasks with moderate involvement ratings. Three of these moderate involvement tasks were related to communication: two with patients (i.e., collecting patient medication history and calling prior to medication synchronization filling) and one with providers (i.e., calling a prescriber for clarification of a prescription order). These tasks show the importance of communication skills in expanding the roles of community pharmacy technicians. Technicians that regularly interact with patients need to be effective in gathering information from them, as well as in giving pertinent details to them. The other task categorized in the moderate involvement sector was documenting patient care. This task would typically be outside of dispensing, for which documentation occurs automatically through the dispensing software. Rather, this task likely relates to non-dispensing services, such as documentation of immunizations in state registries and of medication management services. Lengel et al. reported low participation by trained pharmacy technicians in documenting medication therapy management (MTM) services [5].

Based on reported technician involvement, eight tasks were categorized as low involvement. These tasks may not be performed by technicians in many community pharmacies due to legal or regulatory restrictions. For example, many states do not currently allow technicians to perform the final prescription verification in community pharmacies. Desselle and Holmes also reported technician verification of other technicians' work as having low involvement from community pharmacy technicians [14]. Similarly, transferring a prescription to another pharmacy and taking a prescription order over the telephone are restricted to pharmacists in some states. Until state laws address these tasks, it is likely they will not be shifted largely to technicians. Conducting medication reconciliation after discharge from a hospital was reported as being done regularly by almost 10% of respondents in this study. Given the strong interest in smooth care transitions, this could be a task that becomes more common as more community pharmacies deliver such a service. Three tasks had no more than 2% of respondents rate that they are regularly involved in them: obtaining patient vital signs, administering a vaccination, and drawing a blood sample with a finger stick. These tasks are not widely performed in community pharmacies by technicians. Thus, it is likely that community pharmacy technicians have little or no opportunity to perform these tasks at this time. Desselle et al. also reported very low involvement by pharmacy technicians in administering immunizations [15].

The respondents' involvement ratings indicate that most of these emerging tasks are not widespread in community pharmacy practice. Considering the involvement and willingness to perform ratings together, it can be seen that respondents tended to be less willing to perform tasks with which they had lower involvement. That is, some of the unwillingness to perform might simply derive from a lack of familiarity with the low-rated tasks. Another characteristic of the two tasks with the lowest willingness ratings is they involve needles. It could be that some of the respondents are not comfortable with such activities, which may be outside of their technician training.

Over half (54.3%) of respondents stated they used unaccredited on-the-job training from their employer, while the next most frequent method was unaccredited structured training program from their employer (11.3%). In addition, another 10.2 percent of respondents reported using an accredited structured training program from their employer. Thus, about three-fourths (75.8%) of the respondents completed technician training through their employer. Accredited technician training programs accounted for just over 20%, between accredited standalone (10.6%) and accredited employer (10.2%) programs. It is clear that employer-led training programs are currently, and will likely continue to be, a key factor in training pharmacy technicians for emerging roles. As new standards are developed for training pharmacy technicians, their employers are likely to influence the future content and delivery of such training.

Based on technician ratings, seven of the work environment variables very likely would support new technician tasks, while four would be less supportive or even unsupportive. Four of the more supportive workplace characteristics represented organizational factors: technicians working well with pharmacists, managerial support for technicians performing new tasks, technicians receiving training to perform new tasks, and support of fellow pharmacy staff to implement a new service. As new activities are introduced into a workplace, the support of the employees at all levels is needed for the activities to be performed properly. These findings point to the need for technicians to be supported by their managers and fellow pharmacy staff when taking on new pharmacy technician duties. The other three more supportive variables were characteristics of individuals: confidence to learn new tasks, belief that new tasks keep work interesting, and being excited about implementing a new service. These individual characteristics could be considered at the time of hiring technicians. In addition, confidence relates to self-efficacy, which can be increased by education, mastery experience and social modeling [16].

The four workplace characteristics that were expected to be less supportive of technicians performing new tasks included current staffing being unable to support new tasks, insufficient time in the current workday to support new tasks, feeling stress at work, and the employer not classifying technicians based on specialized skills. Any workplace that introduces new tasks will need to be aware of how the new tasks affect employee time and workload. Pharmacies that utilize technicians in new roles to implement new services will need to manage the workload of their technicians. It is expected that new tasks would add to technicians' stress level, which likely could be managed by training and experience. As technicians begin to perform new tasks, some of them will need specialized skills and training. Training and some type of credentialing could be used to support technicians obtaining advanced knowledge and skills.

This study has several limitations. The low response rate limits its generalizability to the population of community pharmacy technicians. Thus, the findings should be interpreted conservatively. Another limitation is that many of the questions had not been used in previous studies. To try to assure clear understanding by respondents, the items were evaluated and improved through a cognitive testing process in which pharmacy technicians read the items aloud and provided feedback on vague language. Also, content experts read the survey and provided feedback prior to the main survey. It is possible that pharmacy technicians' willingness to perform emerging tasks varies by state due to differences in state law. Although this was a national sample, over half of the states had less than ten responses. Future research could be done to examine the effects of state laws and regulations on technicians' willingness to perform new tasks. Finally, the limited detail collected in the survey about technician training did not allow study of the extent to which these emerging topics are being taught during technician training. Again, future research is recommended to investigate this issue.

5. Conclusions

Overall, community pharmacy technicians reported being willing to perform almost all of the emerging tasks that were rated in this study. It is likely that technicians will be able to increase their roles where community pharmacy practice offers expanded and new patient care services and where permitted by law. As pharmacies work to integrate into collaborative care and other innovative care models, it appears likely that pharmacy technicians will be willing to perform the new tasks needed to support the evolution and advancement of patient care services delivered in the community pharmacy setting.

Author Contributions: Conceptualization—W.R.D., methodology—shared, software—shared, validation—shared, formal analyses—shared, investigation—shared, resources—W.R.D., data curation—W.R.D., writing original draft—shared, writing review & editing—shared, visualization—shared, supervision—W.R.D., project administration—W.R.D., funding acquisition—W.R.D.

Funding: This research was funded by National Association of Chain Drug Stores.

Acknowledgments: The authors would like to acknowledge Emily Schommer, CPhT for her assistance with reviewing early drafts of the survey. Also, we acknowledge Alina Cernasav, PharmD, for her assistance with coding and analyzing.

References

1. Easter, J.C.; DeWalt, D.A. The medication optimization value proposition: Aligning teams and education to improve care. *NCJM* **2017**, *78*, 168–172. [CrossRef] [PubMed]

2. Trygstad, T. Payment reform meets pharmacy practice and education transformation. *NCJM* **2017**, *78*, 173–176. [CrossRef] [PubMed]

3. Urick, B.Y.; Prown, P.; Easter, J.C. Achieving better quality and lower costs in Medicaid through enhanced pharmacy services. *NCJM* **2017**, *78*, 188–189. [CrossRef] [PubMed]

4. Powers, M.F.; Bright, D.R. Pharmacy technicians and medication therapy management. *J. Pharm. Technol.* **2008**, *24*, 336–339. [CrossRef]

5. Lengel, M.; Kuhn, C.H.; Worley, M.; Wehr, A.M.; McAuley, J.W. Pharmacy technician involvement in community pharmacy medication therapy management. *J. Am. Pharm. Assoc.* **2018**, *58*, 179–185. [CrossRef] [PubMed]

6. Adams, A.J.; martin, S.J.; Stolpe, S.F. "Tech-check-tech": A review of the evidence on its safety and benefits. *Am. J. Health-Syst. Pharm.* **2011**, *68*, 1824–1833. [CrossRef] [PubMed]

7. Kraus, S.K.; Sen, S.; Murphy, M.; Pontiggia, L. Impact of a pharmacy technician-centered medication reconciliation program on medication discrepancies and implementation of recommendations. *Pharm. Pract.* **2017**, *15*, 1–4. [CrossRef] [PubMed]

8. America's Pharmacist. *All Aboard the Synchronization Train*; America's Pharmacist: Alexandria, VA, USA, September 2013.

9. Powers, M.F.; Hohmeier, K. Pharmacy technicians and immunizations. *J. Pharm. Technol.* **2011**, *27*, 111–116. [CrossRef]

10. Bright, D.; Adams, A.J. Pharmacy Technician-Administered Vaccines in Idaho (letter). *Am. J. Health-Syst. Pharm.* **2017**, *74*, 2033–2034. [CrossRef] [PubMed]

11. McKeirnan, K.C.; Frazier, K.R.; Nguyen, M.; MacLean, L.G. Training pharmacy technicians to administer immunizations. *J. Am. Pharm. Assoc.* **2018**, *58*, 174–178. [CrossRef] [PubMed]

12. Bryan, K.; Mattingly, T.J.I.I.; Gernant, S.A. Optimizing the Role of Pharmacy Technicians in Patient Care Settings. *J. Am. Pharm. Assoc.* **2018**, *58*, 7–11. [CrossRef] [PubMed]
13. Mattingly, A.N.; Mattingly, T.J., II. Advancing the Role of the Pharmacy Technician: A Systematic Review. *J. Am. Pharm. Assoc.* **2018**, *58*, 94–108. [CrossRef] [PubMed]
14. Desselle, S.P.; Holmes, E.R. Results of the 2015 National Certified Pharmacy Technician Workforce Survey. *Am. J. Health-Syst. Pharm.* **2017**, *74*, e295–e305. [CrossRef] [PubMed]
15. Desselle, S.P.; Hoh, R.; Holmes, E.R.; Gill, A.; Zamora, L. Pharmacy technician self-efficacies: Insight to aid future education, staff development, and workforce planning. *Res. Soc. Adm. Pharm.* **2018**, *14*, 581–588. [CrossRef] [PubMed]
16. Bandura, A. Health promotion by social cognitive means. *Health Educ. Behav.* **2004**, *31*, 143–164. [CrossRef] [PubMed]

19

Impact of Pharmacy Based Travel Medicine with the Evolution of Pharmacy Practice

Derek Evans [iD]

FRPharmS, FRGS, MFTM RCPS, Independent Prescriber, 58 The Nurseries, Langstone, Wales NP18 2NT, UK; d.p.evans@btinternet.com

Abstract: Background: Pharmacy has utilised the changes in legislation since 2000 to increase the range and supply function of services such as travel health to travellers. With the number of travellers leaving the UK and trying new destinations there is an increasing need for more travel health provision. Working models: The models of supply of a travel health service vary according to the size of the corporate body. The large multiples can offer assessment via a specialist nurse or doctor service and then supply through the pharmacy. Others will undertake an onsite risk assessment and supply through the pharmacist. The sole Internet suppliers of medication have been reviewed and the assessment standards questioned following survey and inspection. Education: There is no dedicated pharmacist-training programme in advanced level travel health. As a consequence one academic institution allows pharmacists to train on a multidisciplinary course to obtain an academic membership. With training for travel health not being mandatory for any travel health supply function the concern is raised with standards of care. Future: There is a consultation paper on the removal of travel vaccines from NHS supply due to be decided in the future. If these vaccines are removed then they will provide a greater demand on pharmacy services. Discussion: The starting of a travel health service can be made without any additional training and remains unregulated, giving cause for concern to the supply made to the traveller. Conclusions: Pharmacies in the UK offer a range of options for supplying travel health services; however these need to be with improved mandatory training and supply.

Keywords: travel medicine; health; pharmacist; pharmacy; vaccinations; prescribing and education

1. Introduction

This is a review of the development of the practice of pharmacy in the UK developing from the legal changes that occurred in the 2000s to include modern working models and specialist eduction that is available to pharmacists.

In the UK, prior to 2000 the role of the pharmacist was that of the traditional supply function against the supply of a prescription and the sale of over the counter products (OTC). Within the UK the legislation is defined in 3 legal categories of medicines, prescription only (POM)—only supplied against a doctors or dentists prescription (private and National Health Service (NHS)); pharmacy only medicines (PM)—only supplied from a licensed pharmacy in the presence of a pharmacist and OTC products. At this time there was no legislation that allowed pharmacists to provide routine or travel vaccinations or to supply POMs without a relevant prescription.

With changes to both the legal supply of POMs and the increasing requirement to use pharmacist's clinical skills then evolvement of influenza vaccination was introduced. This led onto the consideration of travel health health services from a pharmacy, by a pharmacist, to become established.

The changes to a nationally funded travel health service remain under scrutiny and with increasing numbers of patients travelling abroad annually (+5%) and +27% intending to to travel a country they have never visited before [1] the NHS is reviewing the current funding of these services.

2. Legislative Changes

In 1998 the NHS reviewed the medicines that where be allowed to be supplied on a prescription. This review included the removal of chloroquine for malaria prophylaxis and the change to PM status allowing it to be purchased from pharmacies, (Figure 1). The NHS continues to supply free of charge to all travellers' vaccines against hepatitis A, typhoid, diphtheria/tetanus/polio and cholera from surgery that is contracted to provide vaccinations. All other vaccinations remained on a private supply along with the antimalarials.

In 2000 following lobbying from the Royal College of Nurses (RCN) for group protocols to supply national immunisation services, the law was changed to allow the supply of medication by healthcare professionals using Patient Group Directions [2].

At the same time-work was underway to allow a new category of prescribers to be formed. This became known as supplementary prescribing, which was originally given to practice and district nurses working alongside a doctor to reduce the workload [3]. A supplementary prescriber was a healthcare professional who had the authority to supply a range of previously agreed drugs according to an agreed clinical management plan.

With the increase in clinical knowledge and skills being taught and applied to other healthcare professions the role of independent prescriber was created in 2006, which included pharmacists [4]. This role allowed a pharmacist, with a formal qualification in independent prescribing to be able to write diagnose, treat and write prescriptions. The ethical area of competence is unregulated and such prescribers a can legally write a prescription that may include schedule 2 Controlled Drugs [5].

A major change in the law occurred in 2012 with the introduction of the Human Medicines Regulations [6]. This allowed the widening of the range of medication that could be supplied under a PGD allowing more services to be created. Additional NHS regulations introduced at the same time allowed the concept of a new style of pharmacy, that of the at distance or "postal service" pharmacies, where a pharmacy could make an online sale or supply of a prescription without face to face contact with the patient. Alongside these regulations came the new standards of pharmacy premises which included the minimum design standards for every pharmacy to have a their own consultation room to provide services.

With the UK Government reviewing the impact of annual influenza absences and the pressure for new roles to be allowed to pharmacy the first pharmacy flu vaccination services were introduced in 2007 as a private service utilising PGDs. This continued until 2015 when it was extended and included as a pharmacy NHS funded service.

Alongside the provision of seasonal influenza vaccinations other vaccination services supplied by PGDs and Pharmacist Independent Prescriber (PIPs) evolved such as travel vaccinations and the supply of antimalarials for prophylaxis. With the austerity measures imposed on public spending private clinical services were considered as a part solution to maintaining financial solvency.

In late 2017 the PHE was tasked with a consultation between professionals to consider if the total withdrawal of all vaccines for pre-travel should be removed from the NHS [7] and made private supply only.

The significance of the changes to practice working at a faster rate than legislative changes has led to the introduction of support networks for pharmacists providing travel health service using telemedicine or at distance triage services completed by a nurse or doctor [8].

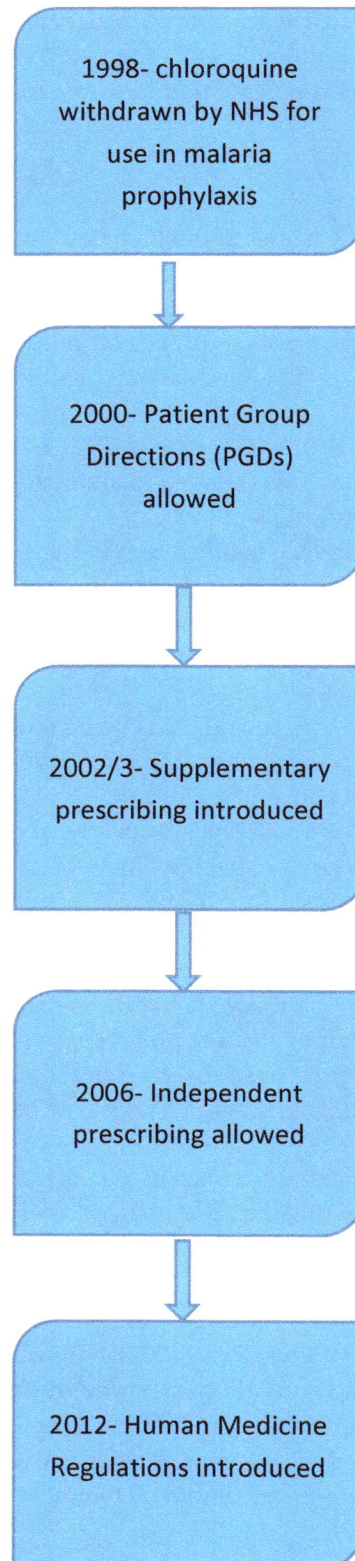

Figure 1. Key legislative changes allowing pharmacists to practice travel medicine.

3. Models of Working Practices

Within the pharmacy population in the UK, 49.2% of pharmacies are owned by groups and termed large multiples. Examples of these include Boots, Lloyds, Well, Rowlands and the supermarket groups of Asda, Morrisons and Tesco. Other smaller independents provide 12.4% and the remainder is made up small chains (<3 outlets) and independents 38.4% of the market [9].

Access to travel health or medicine services is varied and one type of model includes a risk assessment being completed externally by a doctor, nurse or pharmacist and then the vaccination or anti-malarial supply being authorised by either a private prescription or directed to a pharmacist through a Patient Specific Direction (PSD). (A PSD is a formal arrangement, which allows a doctor or independent prescriber to direct the supply of vaccination through another healthcare professional to a patient).

Other pharmacies, allow an online booking service to be made with one of its selected stores (not all stores are included) for a risk assessment lasting up to 40 min. The clinical support and backup is provided by a nurse led service to which the pharmacist can refer. The pharmacist can administer the vaccinations and supply the medication at the appointment.

The UK legislation differs at this point regarding the regulation of the standards of practice between solely organised pharmacist clinics and those by other healthcare professions. The regulating body in England, the Care Quality Commission (CQC) [10] regulates the standards to be applied in nurse or doctor led clinics; whilst the General Pharmaceutical Council (GPhC) regulates the standards in pharmacies. In 2017 the joint regulators investigated online prescribing to patients. The report highlighted significant areas of failure between some online prescribers and those in a patient-facing scenario [11]. A previous study evaluating the supply of atovaquone/proguanil through online prescribing highlighted that potential questions were no addressed such as previous ADR to the drugs (59%) or the length of stay in the malarial area (50%) [12].

A small independent survey study in 2018 concluded that a pharmacy travel health service was well accepted by patients and met their needs, providing a value for money service [13].

4. Travel Health Education

With the supply of POM medication made by pharmacists either under a PGD or as an Independent Prescriber the professional expectation is that the standard of training to use these preparations should be of the a similar standard at an advanced level. Within the UK there is no legal requirement to have received any formal advanced level training before using a PGD and whilst an Independent Prescriber qualifies in a defined area of competence, they are legally allowed to prescribe any medicinal product outside of their competence, including controlled drugs.

To ensure that basic immunisation is practiced correctly the GPhC in alliance with the Royal College of Nursing and Public Health England have published a document that lists the national minimum standards and core curriculum for immunisation training for registered healthcare practitioners [14].

For those pharmacists who do elect to undertake extended training there are ranges of courses in travel health that are shared with other professions allowing an equality between practitioners. Examples of this can be found at the centres of excellence of in London, Liverpool and Glasgow. Details of the courses available to pharmacists are seen in Table 1, an overview suggests that pharmacy professional courses are of a basic level and many of the advanced level courses are restricted to registered doctors and nurses only.

Table 1. Travel health training and education available to pharmacists in UK.

Institution	Travel Medicine Post-Graduate Course Available to Pharmacist	Formal Professional Accreditation
Faculty of Travel Medicine (FTM) of the Royal College of Physicians and Surgeons (Glasgow)	Diploma in Travel Medicine (12–15 months)	Membership of Faculty of Travel Medicine of RCPS
	Foundation in Travel Medicine (6 months) https://rcpsg.ac.uk/travel-medicine/education	None
London School of Hygiene and Tropical Medicine	None-professional diplomas only available to physicians based in London and nurses/midwives (3–12 months) https://www.lshtm.ac.uk/study/courses/professional-development/professional-diplomas	None
	Pharmacists can have access to a short course (4 days) https://www.lshtm.ac.uk/study/courses/short-courses/travel-medicine	None
Liverpool School of Tropical Medicine	Travel Vaccination- Principles and Practice (5 weeks)	None
	Malaria prevention in Travel Health (3 weeks) http://www.lstmed.ac.uk/study/courses	None
Centre for Pharmacy Postgraduate Education	Travel health- understanding and supporting travellers' wellbeing https://www.cppe.ac.uk/programmes/l/travel-e-02/	Evidence for Royal Pharmaceutical Society Faculty framework https://www.rpharms.com/professional-development/faculty/about-the-faculty
National Pharmacy Association	Travel PGDs https://www.npa.co.uk/training/patient-group-directions/travel-pgd/	None
British Global Travel Health Association (BGTHA)	ABC of travel health https://www.abcoftravelhealth.com	None
National Travel Health Network and Centre (NaTHNaC)	Yellow training and clinic registration https://nathnacyfzone.org.uk	Accreditation to provide Yellow Fever vaccination and registration of clinic

Additionally an external representative body, the British Global Travel Health Association (BGTHA) has produced its own e-learning programme that is currently awaiting accreditation.

5. Future

The Association of British Travel Agents travel trends report [1] indicates that there is a growth in early bookings for 2018 holidays and people are travelling to destinations not visited before. In the summer of 2017 the UK government announced a review of cost controls throughout areas of the NHS. Amongst this was a proposal to remove all vaccines currently provided free of charge for travel (hepatitis A, typhoid, combined tetanus/diphtheria/polio, and cholera) from NHS supply. The NHS has since requested a feasibility study to be completed by Public Health England [7] on the complete removal of these vaccines and the subsequent impact on public health services. The findings are awaiting publication.

6. Discussion

Within the UK the changes in national legislation have provided wider and more extensive powers for pharmacists to supply POM medication. The term travel health is undefined and yet to be recognised by the General Medical Council as a medical speciality. The consequence is that a pharmacist can initiate a travel health service and the levels of service being offered can vary from the supply of antimalarial medication to specialists who have completed an extensive level of training. To become competent in travel health, pharmacist practitioners should consider the need to complete an independent prescribers course, a recognised formal qualification in travel health and membership to a medical Royal College. This has been accomplished by a small number of pharmacist practitioners, however the practice of travel health without all of the additional skill sets, relies on the pharmacist to understand the limits of their competency when assessing and providing a clinical service.

As highlighted before, the supply function of POMs can be made using a PGD, however no mandatory training on the use is required to use these. The other supply function is using an independent prescriber that trains in a specific area of competency but are legally allowed to prescribe any POM. A consequence of this is that pharmacist independent prescribers can supply travel health medication without being specifically trained in the specialist clinical area.

The professional guidelines advise that independent prescribers should only practice within their competency and that PGDs are only used following specific training. Due to the complex nature of travel health a review is required of the supply provision and training and that should include arrangements for referral of complex patient cases to specialist pharmacists. The need of specialist, mandatory training is supported by the Faculty of Travel Medicine who have published a statement indicating that there is no licensing or checks on the level of care and that travellers are at risk [15].

By comparison in Alberta, Canada pharmacist provided travel health services are supplied by suitably trained pharmacists with basic life support skills and prescribing skills. The additional requirement is the completion of a formally recognised qualification in travel health, such as the Certificate of Knowledge of the International Society of Travel Medicine [16].

7. Conclusions

Travel health provision through UK community pharmacies is well advanced due to changes in national legislation. The supply of POM medications using PGD and independent prescriber services allows any pharmacist to privately supply travel health medication; however the minimum skill base to provide these services remains undefined and not legally required. To ensure the ongoing safety of travellers then the UK licensing authorities need to consider working with the specialist education providers to define minimum standards of competence for pharmacists. The formal training of advanced level services available to pharmacists is supplied through a single awarding institution, with other institutions selectively offering to medical practitioners and nurses only. To match the demand of pharmacist level travel health services more formally certified post-graduate courses in travel medicine would need to be made available. The future would indicate that with more people travelling there would be an increased demand on travel health services in the UK.

References

1. Association of British Travel Agents (ABTA). Travel Trends Report. 2018. Available online: https://abta.com/assets/uploads/general/ABTA_Travel_Trends_Report_2018.pdf (accessed on 12 March 2018).
2. Department of Health. *Health Service Circular 2000/026*; National Health Service Executive: London, UK, 2000.
3. Cook, R. A brief guide to the new supplementary prescribing. *Nurs. Times* **2002**, *98*, 26. [PubMed]
4. Department of Health. A Guide to Implementing Nurse and Pharmacist Independent Prescribing within the NHS in England. 2006. Available online: http://webarchive.nationalarchives.gov.uk/20130124072757/http://www.dh.gov.uk/prod_consum_dh/groups/dh_digitalassets/@dh/@en/documents/digitalasset/dh_4133747.pdf (accessed on 12 March 2018).
5. NICE Pathways. Non-Medical Prescribing. 2018. Available online: https://bnf.nice.org.uk/guidance/non-medical-prescribing.html (accessed on 12 March 2018).
6. Statutory Instruments. *The Human Medicines Regulations*; No 1916; U.K. Government Statutory Instruments: London, UK, 2012.
7. Public Health England. Public Health England to consider removing travel vaccinations from NHS prescriptions. *Pharm. J.* **2017**, *299*, 7906. [CrossRef]
8. Valneva in Partnership (VIP). 2018. Available online: https://vip.valnevauk.com/home/?confirmedhcp=1 (accessed on 20 June 2018).

9.   Sukkar, E. Community Pharmacy in Great Britain 2016: A Fragmented Market. 2016. Available online: https://www.pharmaceutical-journal.com/news-and-analysis/infographics/community-pharmacy-in-great-britain-2016-a-fragmented-market/20201210.article (accessed on 12 March 2018).

10. Care Quality Commission. Healthcare Clinic. 2018. Available online: http://www.cqc.org.uk/what-we-do/services-we-regulate/find-healthcare-clinic (accessed on 19 March 2018).

11. Care Quality Commission. Regulating Digital Healthcare Providers in Primary Care. 2017. Available online: http://www.cqc.org.uk/sites/default/files/20170303_pms-digital-healthcare_regulatory-uidance.pdf (accessed on 19 March 2018).

12. Goodyer, L.; Devgi, V. A survey of Travel related medicines available through e-prescribing services in the UK. *J. BGTHA* **2014**, *24*, 53–55.

13. Hind, C.; Bond, C.; Lee, A.; van Teijlingen, E. Travel medicine services from a community pharmacy: Evaluation of a pilot service. *Pharm. J.* **2008**, *281*, 625–632.

14. Public Health England. National Minimum Standards and Core Curriculum for Immunisation Training for Registered Healthcare Practitioners. 2018. Available online: https://www.gov.uk/government/uploads/system/uploads/attachment_data/file/679824/Training_standards_and_core_curriculum_immunisation.pdf (accessed on 21 March 2018).

15. Royal College of Physicians and Surgeons. Protecting the Health of Travellers from the UK and Ireland. 2015. Available online: https://rcpsg.ac.uk/documents/agm-and-elections/ftm/255-health-of-travellers/file (accessed on 26 June 2018).

16. Houle, S.; Bascom, C.; Rosenthal, M. Clinical outcomes and satisfaction with a pharmacist—Managed travel clinic in Alberta, Canada. *Travel Med. Infect. Dis.* **2018**, *23*, 21–26. [CrossRef] [PubMed]

20

Pharmacists Becoming Physicians: For Better or Worse?

Eugene Y. H. Yeung [1,2] (iD)

1   Education Centre, Royal Lancaster Infirmary, Lancaster LA1 4RP, UK; eugeney@doctors.org.uk

2   Department of Medical Microbiology, The Ottawa Hospital General Campus, The University of Ottawa, Ottawa, ON K1H 8L6, Canada

Abstract: Physicians and pharmacists nowadays are often described as adversaries rather than members of the same team. Some pharmacists apply to medical school later in their careers, and experience obstacles during the transition process. This article details interviews with two physician–pharmacists, who each have a past pharmacist license and current physician license. The respondents described the limitations of pharmacists' scope of practice as their main reasons to pursue a medical career. However, the respondents enjoy applying their pharmacy knowledge and experience to improve their medical practice. They do not feel pharmacy seniors and medical recruiters are supportive towards their chase for medical careers. The respondents noted the importance of peer-reviewed articles to promote pharmacist involvement in patient care and collaboration between physicians and pharmacists. Conflicts between physicians and pharmacists tend to happen because of their different focuses on patient care. The respondents do not see themselves having an edge over other medical school applicants, and noted that recruiters could negatively view their pharmacy experience. The respondents believe that physician–pharmacists are catalysts to foster collaboration between physicians and pharmacists, because they clearly understand the role of each profession. Nevertheless, the respondents feel that physicians and pharmacists are generally lukewarm towards pharmacists transitioning into physicians.

Keywords: collaboration; pharmacist; physician; pharmacy education; medical education; interprofessional; multidisciplinary; conflict; interview

1. Introduction

Prior to the Edict of Frederich II, which officially created the profession of pharmacy from medicine in the Western World, the roles of "prescriber" and "dispenser" were virtually identical [1]. One might expect pharmacy to inherit the cultural norms from medicine. However, physicians and pharmacists nowadays are often described as "adversaries rather than members of the same team" [2]. Some pharmacists apply to medical school later in their careers, and experience "culture shocks" during the process of becoming physicians [1]. The culture of "physician–pharmacists" (professionals with past pharmacist licenses and current physician licenses) is unique [1], but peer-reviewed literature in this area is very limited. The lack of literature could be due to pharmacists recognizing the adversarial relationship between pharmacy and medicine, and thus being secretive about their intention to pursue medical careers. Some may fear being accused of using pharmacy education as a stepping stone to medicine. For instance, the pharmacy director of Mount Sinai Hospital, Canada, questioned whether pharmacists are "MD wannabees" for performing physical assessment [3].

Perhaps the best people to comment on physician–pharmacist collaboration would be those who completed the undergraduate training and understand the hardship in both professions. The current commentary adapted the self-interview style of a published qualitative study [4], in which pharmacists shared how they integrated experience into practice, managed challenges, and advised for pharmacists wishing to do the same. The aim of the interview was to explore details about physician–pharmacists' culture and suggestions on how to improve interprofessional collaboration between the two professions. As a disclaimer, the two physician–pharmacists' responses do not represent the views of all pharmacists and physicians, and are meant to be starting points for future research.

2. Materials and Methods

The semistructured interviews were undertaken with two ex-pharmacists who are now physicians, and follow the methods adapted from two previous studies [1,4]. As an inclusion criterion, each participant must have a past pharmacist license and current physician license. No specific exclusion criteria were used. The author administered the questions through key informant interviews, asked for elaboration of answers, and compiled and edited the manuscript. The interview consisted of open questions about the participants' background, experience as pharmacists and physicians, motivation to study medicine, and their opinions on how to improve collaboration between pharmacy and medicine. All respondents provided informed consents and received no monetary compensation for their participation.

3. Results

Question 1: Describe your pharmacy experience and motivation to study medicine.

Response: I worked as a pharmacist in both community and hospital settings for years. I also completed a research degree in pharmacy to explore my scope of practice. However, I was not satisfied with my jobs at that time. For example, when working in community, I had no access to patients' clinical and laboratory findings, and thus found it difficult to monitor patients' drug effectiveness and adverse effects. When I asked physicians to provide patients' clinical details and management plans, I did not always feel welcomed. Similarly, when I asked patients to provide more details about their illness, some questioned my intention and simply said their physicians alone are sufficient to manage their health. Not every pharmacy employer appreciates your research experience; some can see you as being a "non-clinical" person. These experiences make me want to take a more comprehensive role in health care and pursue a medical career.

Response: Before going to medical school, I worked as a community pharmacist, which I very much enjoyed. However, I also like hands-on experience with patients, which I experienced during my volunteer work in a labor and delivery unit in a developing country. I realized I could practice surgeries and clinical procedures as a physician, but probably not as much as a pharmacist. However, I still appreciate the training I received in pharmacy, which is applicable to my current medical practice, especially when managing patients with multiple morbidities.

Question 2: What have been some of the most satisfying experiences that you had using your pharmacy knowledge?

Response: I taught medical students on how to dose vancomycin and gentamicin, and apply pharmacokinetics in clinical settings, because medical students have limited exposure in these areas. I shared my clinical pharmacology knowledge to improve the antimicrobial stewardship program in a teaching hospital [5]. In other projects, I used my pharmacy experience to advocate for better medication reconciliation [6], adverse drug reaction documentations [7], and collaboration between physicians and pharmacists [8]. Pharmacists can improve public perception by publications and word of mouth, especially from physician–pharmacists. For example, I suggested modifications of pharmacy training to improve their physical examination skills [9]. Since becoming a physician, I still actively contribute to pharmacology research and have published the findings in medical journals [10–12].

Response: Pharmacology knowledge is especially useful in clinics, where we prescribe for patients with menopause, infertility, and abnormal uterine bleeding. It is also useful in gyne-oncology, antepartum, and postpartum wards, where we encounter various medications beyond the usual scope of practice of obstetricians and gynecologists. Although our specialty physicians are very familiar with medications commonly used in our field, we need additional help managing patients' multiple morbidities—that is when general knowledge on medications could help. For example, I helped patients to differentiate some over-the-counter medications, and advised them to check with their community pharmacists. I feel I empower my pharmacy colleagues, and facilitate seamless care and interprofessional collaboration.

Question 3: What barriers have you faced when applying to medical schools?

Response: Not all pharmacy seniors are supportive. When I asked for reference letters, one replied, "If you want career counselling, my door is always open. I have seen this movie many times." That comment did not discourage me, but motivated me to persevere in my application.

Response: Contrary to popular belief, I do not see obvious advantages of being a pharmacist. Some medical recruiters may think you are having a good life even without becoming a physician. Why should they not give the medical school positions to candidates who sacrifice all their lives to become physicians? Other candidates also have their own skill sets that make them favorable in medical school admissions.

Question 4: What are ongoing challenges in encouraging pharmacist involvement in medical settings?

Response: During a presentation, a medical colleague said research studies conducted by physicians are more clinically relevant than ones conducted by other healthcare professionals, which are sometimes self-glorifying their own practices. I cannot completely disagree—I often see articles about the benefit of pharmacy services in pharmacy journals; in contrast, physicians tend to be well-regarded in the public eye, and do not need as much validation of their services. There are peer-reviewed articles that question the benefits of pharmacists in multidisciplinary care [13,14], that led me to write letters to editors to express my concerns [15,16]. I understand that peer-reviewed articles can improve the image of the pharmacy profession, but believe the focus should now be shifted towards how collaboration with physicians improves patients' clinical outcomes. However, when submitting articles about physician–pharmacist collaboration to pharmacy journals, my collaborators and I received responses like "pharmacists do not want to become physicians." Journal reviewers and editors denied our topic being relevant to pharmacy practice, and questioned our insight and knowledge about pharmacy.

Response: It is not easy for pharmacists to meet all physicians' expectations. Physicians' clinics tend to run late and overtime [17,18], so they may not want pharmacists to interrupt for trivial issues. But some other physicians complain about pharmacists changing medications without informing physicians beforehand. Some physicians dislike the long waiting time in pharmacy and cost of dispensing fees. But many physicians' clinics also have long waiting times and charge the government consultation fees. There are still prejudices towards pharmacists and double-standards on both professions.

Question 5: Why do you think conflicts happen between physicians and pharmacists?

Response: Physicians and pharmacists have different priorities. The most important drug-related problem is not always the most important medical issue. Hospital physicians, for example, tend to focus on patients' main reasons for admissions, whereas pharmacists want to take care of all drug-related issues. Once, a pharmacist urged to restart a myocardial infarcted patient's vitamin tablets; my medical colleagues questioned whether the situation was urgent. Another reason for conflicts is that physicians do not want to work beyond their usual competency level, as recommended by their regulatory bodies, but pharmacists tend to feel competent in any drug-related issues. For instance, a pharmacist asked a general pediatric staff physician to change a psychiatric medication started by a community psychiatrist; the pediatrician had to pass the issue to the patient's general practitioner because that is out of her area of expertise; the general practitioner might have to hand over the issue to the psychiatrist, due to worries of changing the psychiatrist's management plan. Physicians have prescribing power, but are not allowed to freely prescribe anything they want. When their suggestions are denied, pharmacists could interpret that as their service being undervalued.

Response: In pharmacy school, I was taught to actively look for drug-related problems and ask the prescribers to make changes. It seems like a sign of professional achievement when pharmacists successfully intervene in patients' medical therapies. I heard of a pharmacist wanting to start a patient on metformin despite the patient's poor prognosis after a cardiac arrest. On the contrary, physicians like to keep patients' management plans status quo. Physicians' goals of care are usually bringing a patient's clinical status back to baseline, safely discharging the patient home, and monitoring in community settings. As the Hippocratic Oath states, first do no harm. Making unnecessary therapeutic changes could put a patient at a higher risk of experiencing adverse effects, and delay one's discharge date. Another common area of conflicts is when to order an investigation. Many hospital pharmacists are knowledgeable about the tests available, and tend to promptly recommend a test to rule in a diagnosis. I heard of a pharmacist suggesting a d-dimer test to rule in thromboembolism in a septic shock patient. However, physicians are trained to ensure the clinical presentations and examination findings fit with the working diagnosis, and avoid ordering tests when the clinical situations show low predictive values [19]. Physicians are taught the art of reassurance to avoid unnecessary testing, which wastes healthcare funding and causes health anxiety for patients [20].

Question 6: What is your opinion on pharmacists wanting to become physicians?

Response: Physicians and pharmacists alike need to be open-minded. Yes, you lose a pharmacist to medical school, but then you have a physician who truly understands the benefits of physician–pharmacist collaboration to health care. As an ex-pharmacist, I tend to be interested in anything drug-related, including research and clinical work in any specialties. This curiosity could come back to haunt me. In an interview, I was criticized for lack of focus in one specialty, and questioned about my intent to apply for the job position. I jokingly rebutted, "Well, I played a lot of sports too. It does not mean I want to be a professional athlete." None of interviewers even smiled. Apparently, we did not share the same sense of humor.

Response: Many physicians applied more than once to medical school. After years of medical school, one needs to complete years of postgraduate training. Family and financial factors play big roles in your decision-making—you should not become physicians simply because of the perceived stable income. You should be humble and not see yourselves as having an edge over other applicants.

4. Discussion

We identified similar perspectives of physician–pharmacists who integrate their pharmacy experience into medical practices. They have faced barriers in applying to medical schools, which stemmed from the adversarial relationship between pharmacy and medicine. They advocated collaboration between physicians and pharmacists, but are aware of its difficulty. A major barrier is the different priorities between physicians and pharmacists, which were also noted in a survey conducted on pharmacists and physicians [21]. The study showed that physicians want pharmacists to help with insurance approvals and medication counselling, whereas pharmacists want to manage patients' drug-related problems.

One possible solution for interprofessional strain is collaborative teaching to medical and pharmacy students, which can be used as a bridge to understand each other's role and minimize unnecessary conflicts in practice [8]. The University of British Columbia (Canada) has long developed elective interprofessional modules for students in various health disciplines [22]. However, studies on interprofessional education tend to show aversion towards teaching delivered by the other healthcare professional [5,23]. Interprofessional education requires further honing to improve physicians' and pharmacists' acceptance towards each other.

The respondents illustrated how their use of pharmacy knowledge results in more comprehensive care. They understand the limitation of their involvement if they were not physicians, and described the double standard on physicians and pharmacists. The findings are consistent with a previous qualitative study on physician–pharmacists, which described the physician–pharmacist relationship like the Canada–US (or New Zealand–Australia) effect: physicians are like Americans who were born through liberty and revolution, whereas pharmacists are like Canadians who compromise and negotiate [1]. Similarly, a semistructured interview with 11 pharmacists and 8 physicians concluded that pharmacists confer trust based on ones' title, degree, and status, whereas physicians build trust based on ones' competency and performance [24]. Like physicians and pharmacists, other professions also experience intra- and interprofessional strains on status and prestige [25].

The respondents described the importance of peer-reviewed publications to better define pharmacists' roles and debunk myths. These perspectives illustrated how physician–pharmacists are catalysts to foster collaboration between physicians and pharmacists, because they clearly understand the role of each profession. Nevertheless, pharmacists may face obstacles in applying to medical schools, as both physicians and pharmacists are reportedly lukewarm towards how pharmacists transition into physicians.

The findings of the current article add to the limited peer-reviewed literature on the unique culture of physician–pharmacists [1]. Although there are online forums and Youtube videos on how pharmacists transition into physicians, these are not peer-reviewed and are thus omitted in the current article. Limitations of this article include a small sample size, which makes broad generalizations of the findings difficult. It is difficult to recruit licensed physicians who had pharmacist licenses and are willing to participate in an interview with no monetary compensation, and, thus, selection bias might have occurred. It is understandable that some interview questions, such as commenting on why conflicts happen between the professions, are controversial and involve critique on how each profession practices. That makes the recruitment process even more difficult. It is noted that the responses from the two physician–pharmacists could be opinions but not facts. The respondents do not represent all pharmacists, especially those who work in other countries and experience different educational systems. These limitations are common among qualitative studies, especially the ones on innovative ideas. Qualitative studies on how pharmacists perform physical examinations and contribute to general practice recruited only 3 and 16 respondents, respectively [4,26]. A hypothesis was generated in the current article that encourages researchers to conduct future research on the culture and struggles of physician–pharmacists. With more studies, we would collectively increase the sample size and make the findings more generalizable.

5. Conclusions

From the perspective of the two interview respondents, physician–pharmacists understand the culture of each profession, and are good liaisons to promote interprofessional collaboration. They believe they can integrate their pharmacy knowledge to aid their practice in medicine. Nevertheless, the respondents feel that physicians and pharmacists are generally lukewarm towards pharmacists transitioning into physicians. The current article has a sample size of only two physician–pharmacists, but their responses are good starting points for future research. We require more peer-reviewed articles and research to explore the unique culture of physician–pharmacists, and their contribution towards the healthcare system.

Funding: This interview received no external funding.

References

1. Austin, Z.; Gregory, P.A.M.; Martin, J.C. Negotiation of interprofessional culture shock: The experiences of pharmacists who become physicians. *J. Interprof. Care* **2007**, *21*, 83–93. [CrossRef] [PubMed]

2. Ma, C.S.J.; Holuby, R.S.; Bucci, L.L. Physician and pharmacist collaboration: The University of Hawai'i at Hilo College of Pharmacy—JABSOM experience. *Hawaii Med. J.* **2010**, *69*, 42–44. [PubMed]

3. Simpson, S.H.; Wilson, B. Should pharmacists perform physical assessments? *Can. J. Hosp. Pharm.* **2007**, *60*, 271–273. [CrossRef]

4. Chua, D.; Ladha, F.; Pammett, R.T.; Turgeon, R.D. Pharmacist performance of physical assessment: Perspectives of clinical pharmacists working in different practice settings. *Can. J. Hosp. Pharm.* **2017**, *70*, 305–308. [CrossRef] [PubMed]

5. Yeung, E.Y.H.; Alexander, M. Use of junior doctor-led peer education to improve antibiotic stewardship. *Br. J. Clin. Pharmacol.* **2017**, *83*, 2831–2832. [CrossRef] [PubMed]

6. Yeung, E.Y.H. Are We Legitimately Stopping Medications? Use of Pharmacist and Junior Doctor Teaching to Improve Medication Reconciliation. Available online: http://bjgp.org/content/are-we-legitimately-stopping-medications-use-pharmacist-and-junior-doctor-teaching-improve (accessed on 11 November 2016).

7. Yeung, E.Y.H. Adverse drug reactions: A potential role for pharmacists. *Br. J. Gen. Pract.* **2015**, *65*, 511. [CrossRef] [PubMed]

8. Yeung, E.Y.H. Collaborative Interprofessional Healthcare Education. Available online: http://bjgp.org/content/collaborative-interprofessional-healthcare-education (accessed on 3 June 2018).

9. Mohammed, R.S.D.; Yeung, E.Y.H. Physical examinations by pharmacists: Practising the right thing makes perfect. *Can. J. Hosp. Pharm.* **2017**, *70*, 468–469. [CrossRef] [PubMed]

10. Yeung, E.Y.; Comben, E.; McGarry, C.; Warrington, R. STI testing in emergency contraceptive consultations. *Br. J. Gen. Pract.* **2015**, *65*, 63–64. [CrossRef] [PubMed]

11. Yeung, E.Y.H.; Chun, S.; Douglass, A.; Lau, T.E. Effect of atypical antipsychotics on body weight in geriatric psychiatric inpatients. *SAGE Open Med.* **2017**, *5*. [CrossRef] [PubMed]

12. Yeung, E.Y.H.; Buhagiar, K. Correlation of age and metabolic adverse effects of antipsychotics. *Clin. Drug Investig.* **2017**, *38*, 381–384. [CrossRef] [PubMed]

13. Lynes, S. Multidisciplinary care. *Br. J. Gen. Pract.* **2017**, *67*, 348. [CrossRef] [PubMed]

14. Avery, A.J. Pharmacists working in general practice: Can they help tackle the current workload crisis? *Br. J. Gen. Pract.* **2017**, *67*, 390–391. [CrossRef] [PubMed]

15. Yeung, E.Y.H. Explaining the role of pharmacists in multidisciplinary care. *Br. J. Gen. Pract.* **2017**, *67*, 447–448. [CrossRef] [PubMed]

16. Yeung, E.Y.H. Pharmacists are not physician assistants. *Br. J. Gen. Pract.* **2017**, *67*, 548. [CrossRef] [PubMed]

17. McCartney, M. Margaret McCartney: Why GPs are always running late. *BMJ* **2017**, *358*, j3955. [CrossRef] [PubMed]

18. Irving, G.; Holden, J. Calling time on the 10-minute consultation. *Br. J. Gen. Pract.* **2012**, *62*, 238–239. [CrossRef] [PubMed]

19. Malhotra, A.; Maughan, D.; Ansell, J.; Lehman, R.; Henderson, A.; Gray, M.; Stephenson, T.; Bailey, S. Choosing Wisely in the UK: The Academy of Medical Royal Colleges' initiative to reduce the harms of too much medicine. *BMJ* **2015**, *350*, h2308. [CrossRef] [PubMed]

20. Tomlinson, J. Beyond patient reassurance. *Br. J. Gen. Pract.* **2015**, *65*, 656–657. [CrossRef] [PubMed]

21. Kelly, D.V.; Bishop, L.; Young, S.; Hawboldt, J.; Phillips, L.; Keough, T.M. Pharmacist and physician views on collaborative practice: Findings from the community pharmaceutical care project. *Can. Pharm. J.* **2013**, *146*, 218–226. [CrossRef] [PubMed]

22. The University of British Columbia Interprofessional Health & Human Service Electives. Available online: https://socialwork.ubc.ca/current-students/bsw-undergrad-program-info/ihhs-courses/ (accessed on 1 June 2018).

23. Van Winkle, L.J.; Bjork, B.C.; Chandar, N.; Cornell, S.; Fjortoft, N.; Green, J.M.; La Salle, S.; Lynch, S.M.; Viselli, S.M.; Burdick, P. Interprofessional workshop to improve mutual understanding between pharmacy and medical students. *Am. J. Pharm. Educ.* **2012**, *76*, 150. [CrossRef] [PubMed]

24. Gregory, P.A.; Austin, Z. Trust in interprofessional collaboration: Perspectives of pharmacists and physicians. *Can. Pharm. J.* **2016**, *149*, 236–245. [CrossRef] [PubMed]

25. Abbott, A. Status and status strain in the professions. *Am. J. Sociol.* **1981**, *86*, 819–835. [CrossRef]

26. Butterworth, J.; Sansom, A.; Sims, L.; Healey, M.; Kingsland, E.; Campbell, J. Pharmacists' perceptions of their emerging general practice roles in UK primary care: A qualitative interview study. *Br. J. Gen. Pract.* **2017**, *67*, e650–e658. [CrossRef] [PubMed]

21

Young Muslim Women Living with Asthma in Denmark: A Link between Religion and Self-Efficacy

Louise C. Druedahl [1,*] 🆔, **Duaa Yaqub** [1], **Lotte Stig Nørgaard** [1], **Maria Kristiansen** [2] 🆔 and **Lourdes Cantarero-Arévalo** [1]

[1]   Social and Clinical Pharmacy Group, Department of Pharmacy, Faculty of Health and Medical Sciences, University of Copenhagen, Universitetsparken 2, DK-2100 Copenhagen, Denmark; iwear_aps@hotmail.com (D.Y.); lotte.norgaard@sund.ku.dk (L.S.N.); lou.cantarero@sund.ku.dk (L.C.-A.)

[2]   Department of Public Health, Faculty of Health and Medical Sciences, University of Copenhagen, Øster Farimagsgade 5, DK-1014 Copenhagen, Denmark; makk@sund.ku.dk

*   Correspondence: louise.druedahl@sund.ku.dk

Abstract: Asthma is a chronic respiratory disease that can be controlled with appropriate medicinal treatment. Adherence to pharmacological treatment is therefore critical. Self-efficacy plays a key role in adherence to medicine in chronic diseases, including asthma. Additionally, ethnic minorities have poor adherence to medicines. However, the impact of religion on self-efficacy and adherence is understudied. Therefore, the aim of this study was to explore the role of self-efficacy in adherence to asthma medicine treatment and the influence of religion on self-efficacy among young, Muslim minority women. A focus group and individual interviews with 10 Muslim minority women (14–24 years of age) living in Denmark were conducted. Data analysis was deductive using Bandura's theory of self-efficacy and modes of agency. Overall, religion was shown to affect self-efficacy. The women reported changes in self-perceived self-efficacy during the holy month of Ramadan. In addition, praying was used as an alternative to medicine for controlling asthma symptoms. However, the women did not perceive religion and treating asthma with medicine as mutually exclusive, but rather as coexisting for the shared goal of controlling asthma symptoms. It is important for healthcare professionals (HCPs) to be aware of the link between self-efficacy, religion and adherence to asthma medicine treatment. This awareness can aid HCPs in giving advice regarding adherence to asthma treatment, and when monitoring treatment to improve the quality of asthma care for young Muslim minority women.

Keywords: adherence; asthma; Bandura; Denmark; ethnic minority; self-efficacy; young adults; women

---

1. Introduction

Asthma is a chronic inflammatory airway disease that affects people irrespective of their gender, age and country of birth [1–3]. Asthma is the most common chronic disease affecting the lower respiratory tract in children [3]. More boys than girls are affected by asthma, although by young adulthood, this pattern either cannot be detected or has reversed [2,4]. Hormonal changes are thought to contribute to the shift in gender-dependent disease patterns [4,5]. In 2017, the World Health Organization estimated that about 235 million people worldwide have asthma [6], and that the prevalence is increasing [7].

Minimising the health impact of asthma requires individuals to have the necessary skills to manage their disease. Most patients can manage the symptoms successfully using pharmacotherapy, patient education, symptom monitoring and/or by avoiding triggers [3]. Treatment includes long-term control and fast-acting relief medicine, the former to prevent symptoms and the latter for acute symptom relief [3,8,9]. Correct use of controller medicine such as inhaled corticosteroids (ICS) can control asthma symptoms and reduce the risk of exacerbation [8]. However, adherence to ICS treatment is low: 49–73% for children and less than 50% for adolescents and adults [10]. One reason for the low medicine adherence of adolescents could be that healthcare professionals (HCPs) do not provide sufficient preparation or support to parents and/or affected children for the transition in responsibility for medicine [11]. Parents or caregivers are responsible for managing asthma in children, including redeeming prescriptions, communicating with HCPs and administering medicine [11]. For the future adult to take on this responsibility, the transfer must be successfully made starting in the early stages of adolescence [11]. One relevant aspect for this is self-efficacy, which is an individual's belief in his/her own ability to perform a specific action to manage a particular situation [12,13]. Furthermore, self-efficacy is essential for managing asthma [14–16] and for medication adherence in general [17].

Ethnicity is a complex concept that describes the group to which persons belong/are perceived to belong on basis of shared characteristics such as geographical, language and cultural traditions, but may also include facets of religion [18]. Some ethnic minority patients have a higher disease burden of asthma than ethnic majority patients, illustrated by their increased rate of hospital admissions compared with the majority population [19,20]. In Scotland, the highest hospital admission rate was seen among Pakistanis [20]. Ethnic minority also seems relevant for adherence to controller asthma medicine. Studies in the Netherlands and USA, respectively, have found that ethnic minority children and adolescents have the same [21] or lower [22] adherence to controller asthma medicine than the majority population. A study in UK found children of parents from Pakistan to more often have wheezing the last 12 months, but also physician's diagnosis of asthma and medicine usage compared to British background [23]. Although asthma morbidity and mortality have been found disproportionately high in ethnic minority children, cultural tailoring of treatment is rarely incorporated into treatment regimens [24]. A Danish study comparing Danish ethnicity to Turkish, Lebanese and Iraqi ethnicity found that ethnic inequalities in asthma treatment were not caused by differences in household income, but may result from a lack of parental knowledge about the Danish healthcare system [25]. Other factors affecting ethnic inequalities in asthma include poor health literacy, religious and health beliefs and challenges in cross-cultural communication [26]. One example hereof is that Muslims may prefer to avoid using medicine during Ramadan [27]. However, overall, supported self-management from HCPs can possibly improve quality of life for ethnic minority patients with asthma [28].

In Denmark, asthma prevalence is higher among boys than girls, but with a shift in proportion in adolescents and young adults [29]. In addition, women with asthma (above 16 years of age) have more emergency department visits and a higher societal disease burden compared with men [29]. Therefore, the aim of this study was to explore self-efficacy to adhere to asthma medicine treatment to assess the influence of religion on self-efficacy and adherence among young, ethnic minority women ages 14–24.

1.1. The Setting

In Denmark in 2015, non-Danish origin comprised 11.7% of the population [30]. Most of these were first generation immigrants (8.9%), and the remainder were their descendants (second generation 2.8%) [30]. The largest groups originated from non-Western countries: Turkey, Iraq, Pakistan, Bosnia-Herzegovina, Iran and Lebanon [30]. The definitions of 'immigrant' and 'descendant' are based on definitions of Statistics Denmark [30]. According to these, 'immigrants' are born outside of Denmark and none of the parents are both born in Denmark and a Danish citizen. Furthermore, 'descendants' are born in Denmark, but none of the parents are both born in Denmark and a Danish citizen. In addition, 'Danish origin' is if one of the parents is both born in Denmark and is a Danish citizen [30].

Ethnic minority is in Denmark defined by the country of origin of the parents. Middle Eastern countries comprise five out of six of the largest non-Western groups in Denmark and all where Islam is the official religion, and therefore interviewees with Middle Eastern origin practicing Islam was the focus of the study.

1.2. Theory of Self-Efficacy

As previously mentioned, Albert Bandura's theory of self-efficacy describes an individual's belief in his/her own ability to perform a specific action to manage a particular situation [12,13]. The theory relates to behavioural choices, which may or may not have adverse effects [12]. Therefore, self-efficacy can be used for the health-related behaviour of taking asthma medicine.

Self-efficacy is linked to the individual's expectations to reach a certain outcome. Achieving the outcome is influenced by the individual's expectation about (i) his/her ability to behave in a certain way, and (ii) the behaviour resulting in the desired outcome [12]. A person with high self-efficacy will increase his/her efforts when faced with difficulties. In contrast, a person with low self-efficacy may behave ineffectively despite knowing what to do [13].

Although the theory of self-efficacy does not address religion [12], Bandura briefly links religion to self-efficacy via the concept of agency [31]. Three modes of agency are relevant to religious practice: personal agency, proxy agency and collective agency [31]. For example, personal agency increases if religious teachings inspire an individual to believe that he/she can exert control over his/her own actions and surroundings [32]. Active proxy agency relates to the belief that a divine or supreme being (usually referred to as God) can exercise power over events [31]. The effect of divine proxy agency can be either to increase self-efficacy, if God is perceived as a collaborating partner, or to cause passivity (i.e., reduce self-efficacy), if God is being depended on to solve problems experienced [31]. Prayers are a way of invoking proxy agency, which individuals often use in times of distress due to physical or emotional problems [31]. Collective agency refers to the pooling of knowledge, resources and skills, and builds on the perception of people as social (not isolated) creatures [31]. Religious beliefs can provide both psychological support and a model for behaviour [31].

Lower self-efficacy may be associated with an ethnic minority background [33], and with more emergency department visits and hospital admissions [34]. Patients with asthma who have high self-efficacy link to a higher quality of life [35], fewer asthma symptom days [33] and higher adherence to controller medicine [36]. Moreover, high adherence to asthma controller medicine use links with positive outcome expectations, which influences self-efficacy [36]. A recent study found that self-efficacy was more important to asthma outcome than knowledge about asthma, attitudes towards asthma management and perceived barriers to care [34]. Thus, improvement in self-efficacy among asthma patients may lead to better self-management and disease control [14,37,38].

2. Materials and Methods

A qualitative approach was used. Data were collected between May and July 2016, via a focus group and individual interviews with young, Muslim minority women. The data were collected in the capital region of Denmark.

2.1. Recruitment

Convenience sampling via Facebook was used to recruit 14–24-year-old Muslim minority women who had asthma and treated asthma with medicine. Other inclusion criteria include Middle Eastern origin (see Section 1.1) and practicing Islam. The presence of asthma was self-reported by interviewees. The first 10 eligible interviewees were selected. The recruitment included posting several calls for interviewees in 11 Facebook groups or pages for ethnic minority groups in Denmark. The language of the calls was Danish. The calls were posted by the second author, a young, bilingual Danish-Arabic female pharmacist who shares ethnic and religious background with the interviewees.

2.2. Conducting Interviews

The study sample comprised 10 interviewees, all of whom participated in an individual interview and were invited to participate in a focus group. All 10 individual interviews and the single-focus group interview of three interviewees were semi-structured. The second author constructed the interview guides, which were informed by a systematic review of literature in the PubMed and Embase databases on ethnic and minority groups, self-efficacy and anti-asthmatic agents. The interview guide used for individual interviews was designed to encourage interviewees to describe their experience of everyday life with asthma medicine, including their use of opinions and attitudes about asthma medicines, as well as coping strategies for handling exacerbations. Thematic content in the interview guide for individual interviews was asthma history, medication compliance, social aspects of having asthma, ethnicity, religion, limitations due to asthma and self-efficacy. Themes for the focus group were medication compliance, ethnicity and the Muslim holy month of Ramadan. See the interview guides in Supplementary Material. To explore the influence of religion on medication adherence, questions addressing the influence of faith and religious practice on the course of the disease and medicine use were included in both of the interview guides.

The second author conducted and moderated all interviews in Danish. Individual interviews were carried out either in person or by online video call, according to the interviewee's preference. The focus group interview was conducted in person at the University of Copenhagen. Each interviewee was given one gift certificate of 100 DKK (~13 EUR or ~16 USD) for participating. All interviews were audio-recorded and transcribed verbatim. Quoted text from interview transcripts was translated from Danish to English by the first author. The interview guides were translated from Danish to English by the first and third authors.

2.3. Data Analysis

The data were deductively analysed using Bandura's theory of self-efficacy [12,13,31,39] and three types of agency relevant to religion [31] to explore the experiences of young, Muslim minority women with self-efficacy and adherence to asthma medicine treatment.

De-identified interview transcripts were analysed by extracting all text with behavioural, emotional or belief-related content on relevant themes. The themes were classified into low and high categories as part of the process. The themes were:

• Outcome expectations (high/low)

Expectations were labelled high outcome, if the interviewee indicated that using medicine would provide higher control of asthma symptoms. Similarly, expectations were labelled low outcome, if the interviewee described using medicine as inadequate to improve control of asthma symptoms.

• Self-perceived self-efficacy to use asthma medicine (high/low)

Self-perceived self-efficacy was the interviewee's perception of her ability to use asthma medicine. If this was not described, the interviewee's general self-efficacy was assessed instead based on general statements about asthma-related experiences and whether the interviewee described having a more positive or more negative attitude (corresponding to high or low general self-efficacy, respectively).

• Adherence to asthma medicine treatment (high/low)

Adherence (to asthma medicine) was assessed based on the interviewee's statements about actual medicine use

Interview transcripts were de-identified prior to analysis by the second author. Data were analysed by the first author, who is also a pharmacist, but does not share a cultural or religious background with the interviewees. All co-authors discussed the analysis to ensure rigor and that the analysis reflected the data as a whole.

2.4. Ethics

According to Danish [Order no. 410 of 09/05/2012] [40], ethics approval is not necessary when personal data are handled as part of a master's thesis research project, as long as the interviewee provides explicit consent. According to the Danish Data Protection Agency, these personal data include data obtained from interviews. The interview data in this study were handled as part of the second author's master's thesis research project. Written informed consent to participate in the study was obtained from all interviewees or parents of minors (age < 18 years) on behalf of their child.

3. Results

The study sample comprised 10 interviewees with self-reported asthma, who identified themselves as Muslims. Interviewees were 14–24 years old and had had asthma for 2–18 years. All interviewees used inhaler asthma medicine. All interviewees participated in individual interviews and three (IP3, IP6 and IP8) also participated in a focus group interview held after the individual interviews. Individual interviews varied in length from 30 min to one hour, and the focus group interview lasted for one hour. Demographics of the interviewees can be seen in Table 1.

Table 1. Demographics of interviewees.

Pseudonym	Age	Years with Asthma	Medicine Prescribed [1] (Current Use)	Immigrant Status [2] (Country of Origin)
IP1	15	5	Reliever & controller (reliever only)	Descendant (Iraq)
IP2	14	2	Reliever & controller (both)	Descendant (Iraq)
IP3	19	16	Reliever & two types of controller (only reliever)	Immigrant (Iraq)
IP4	22	2	Reliever & controller (both)	Descendant (Palestine)
IP5	14	14	Reliever & controller (both)	Descendant (Palestine)
IP6	21	12	Reliever & controller (only reliever)	Descendant (Lebanon)
IP7	18	18	Reliever & controller (primarily reliever)	Descendant (Lebanon)
IP8	15	10	Reliever & two types of controller (all)	Descendant (Pakistan)
IP9	24	4	Reliever & controller (primarily reliever)	Descendant (Turkey)
IP10	20	10	Reliever & controller (both)	Descendant (Turkey)

[1] Information about medicine use was obtained during interviews. [2] Descendant (born in Denmark) or immigrant was self-reported, and evaluated based on the definitions of Statistics Denmark [30].

3.1. Perceptions of Asthma and the Experience of Having Asthma

All interviewees said that they tried to live a normal life despite their asthma and its treatment. They stated that they spend a lot of time with their friends and using asthma medicine is not an issue with their friends, and that they do not feel stigmatised by having the disease. Even so, the experience of using asthma medicine varied among interviewees. For example, IP1 (15 years old) described an episode in which she experienced relief after using fast-acting reliever medicine to control her asthma symptoms. However, IP6 (21 years old) described a contrasting episode in which she took reliever medicine just prior to her annual or semi-annual hospitalisations, but did not achieve the expected symptom relief: *"If I usually use [terbutaline, relief medicine] and it doesn't help, it gets even worse" (IP6).* Observing relatives with asthma using asthma medicine seemed to reassure the interviewees by helping them to contextualise their situation as normal and manageable. However, the way the interviewees thought about their illness differed profoundly: five saw asthma as unproblematic or not chronic, while others did perceive asthma as a problem and believed it would continue to be so throughout their lifetime. For example, IP10 stated that she can remain calm when having an exacerbation and that she can get rid of asthma, whereas IP9 said she is nervous about having to live with asthma for the rest of her life. Remaining calm or nervous during an asthma attack were unrelated to the interviewees' age or age of onset of asthma.

Focus group interviewees distinguished their ethnicity and described their feelings of being ethnic minority patients due to traditions, culture and religion. A re-occurring theme in both individual and focus group interviews was that ethnicity and religion influence self-efficacy, which will be elaborated on in the following paragraphs.

While some interviewees claimed high self-efficacy in their approach to asthma medicine, their self-described behaviour mainly comprised examples of not using the medicine (i.e., low self-efficacy; Table 2, see e.g., IP7). Please see Table 2 for an overview of the adherence of each interviewee with regard to her medicine use, her expectations of how medicines will affect her asthma symptoms and her assessed level of self-efficacy.

Table 2. Overview of interviewees, their opinions, and the assessment of their self-perceived self-efficacy with regard to medicine use and their adherence to asthma medicine.

Pseudonym	Outcome Expectations (High/Low)	Self-Efficacy—General or in Relation to Medicine (High/Low)	Adherence to Asthma Medicine (High/Low)
IP1	High for reliever "I use it [the medicine] and then I get tremors and after half an hour it works. And I begin to feel the effect" Low for controller [2nd author: "Do you think the controller medicine would help you not experience these asthma exacerbations?"] "No, it doesn't matter"	High (in general) "[I am] an energetic young woman who fights for good results in life that can benefit me in my future"	Low (for medicine) "I tell her [the physician] that I don't use my medicine"
IP2	High "Now I can feel when I need to use it/ . . . /you don't get better by not using it [the medicine]"	High (for medicine) "The blue [reliever] I always carry with me when I am not home, but I don't use it that often. It is mostly the brown one [controller] that I use morning and evening every day"	High (for medicine) "In gym class when I felt ill, my teacher came and said that I should sit down / . . . /and use my medicine / . . . /But now I can feel when I need to use it"
IP3	Low "Because the medicine does not give you an immediate effect. You still feel bad even after [using] the medicine. Actually it takes a long time before the medicine works"	High (for medicine) [2nd author: "Where are you on a scale from 1–10 about remembering to use the medicine, where 1 is bad and 10 is good?"] "I actually think I am about 7–8"	Low (for medicine) "Sometimes I take it [medicine] twice a day. It depends on how I feel . . . I actually think [my asthma] has improved over time, therefore I am thinking about quitting [using medicine]"
IP4	High for reliever, low for controller "I don't think I see a difference in the one [controller] that I use morning and evening. But more to a higher degree with the one I use when necessary; its effect I feel right away"	High (for medicine) "[I] just put it by my bed so that I remember to use it both morning and evening. And the blue one [reliever] I always have with me in the car"	High (for medicine) "And right during my workout, I felt I needed air, but I did not get enough / . . . /I took my medicine right away"
IP5	High for reliever, low for controller: "I use the blue [reliever] one [mostly], that is probably the strongest [medicine]"	High (in general) "I am probably very positive. I am always lively. I always have energy"	High (for medicine) "I had started coughing/ . . . /so I went home and took my medicine and then I went back to the party"
IP6	High "[Terbutaline, reliever]. That is [used] when I feel worst/ . . . /if I don't use the brown one [controller] for a period, then there can come a time where I get an exacerbation and am hospitalised"	Low (for medicine) "I am irresponsible regarding my own medicine. But I always remember my mom's"	Low (for medicine) "With asthma, it is first when I start to feel ill that I remember to use it. Once, two months passed where I didn't use my medicine. Not one single [time]"
IP7	Low "If I use my medicine, I will probably get better, but I probably won't be completely asthma-free"	High (in general) "I am very strong-willed and occasionally stubborn, but at the same time I see myself as a responsible, mature and sensible young woman"	Low (for medicine) "Would say I am pretty bad at using the one I need daily. So when I feel ill, I get motivated to use it"

Table 2. *Cont.*

Pseudonym	Outcome Expectations (High/Low)	Self-Efficacy—General or in Relation to Medicine (High/Low)	Adherence to Asthma Medicine (High/Low)
IP8	High *"Sometimes the two don't help, the brown and the red [controllers]. Then, it is only the blue [reliever] that helps, because it works faster than the other two"*	High (for medicine) [2nd author: *"Where are you on a scale from 1–10 about remembering to use the medicine, where 1 is bad and 10 is good?]* *"Maybe 8"*	High (for medicine) *"I use my medicine morning and evening"*
IP9	Low *"I was told that it would go away when I used my inhaler daily for a while, but I haven't seen the effect yet. When I don't use it for 3–4 days, I get a severe cough and breathing difficulties"*	High (in general) *"I am very outgoing, helpful, and can be aggressive but also friendly"*	Low (for medicine) *"I don't need to do anything [to remember the medicine]. When I don't use it my cough reminds me right away"*
IP10	High *"I can really feel how the medicine helps"*	High (for medicine) *"I use the brown one [controller] morning and evening, and the blue [reliever] when needed. The blue I also use before exercising"*	High (for medicine) *"I set the alarm so I remember to use my medicine"*

3.2. Expectations about Medicine to Control Asthma Symptoms

Interviewees used other ways to control their asthma symptoms besides asthma medicine, which relates to Bandura's different modes of agency related to religion.

Despite technical competency in using inhalers, interviewees indicated a lack of knowledge about the outcome from using asthma medicine (especially long-term controllers). For example, IP9 did not consider it necessary to remind herself to take her medicine, because she knew her cough would remind her, which means that she failed to effectively adhere to controllers to prevent asthma symptoms: *"I don't have to do anything [to remember to use medicine]. When I don't use it, my coughing reminds me right away" (IP9).* Therefore, not all interviewees linked the action of using medicine to the outcome of controlling asthma symptoms. In addition, a few interviewees said that they became better at remembering to use the controller medicine when they experienced more frequent asthma symptoms.

Some interviewees had low expectations about the controller medicine as a means to prevent asthma symptoms. For example, IP1, IP3, IP4, IP5, IP7 and IP9 stated that long-term control medicine was unable to improve their sense of well-being because it lacked an immediate effect (unlike fast-acting reliever medicine). For this reason, controller medicine was believed to have less effect than reliever medicine (IP6, IP7 and IP9). However, some interviewees indicated that the controller medicine had an effect. For example, IP6 said that she knew the controller medicine helped without having a perceptive effect: *"The brown [controller medicine]/ . . . / does not [seem to] help, but it helps without my feeling it" (IP6).*

3.3. Influence of Religion, Modes of Agency and Ramadan on Self-Efficacy and Asthma Medicine Adherence

Religion was crucial to the interviewees in managing their asthma. All interviewees described religious practices such as praying or fasting during Ramadan. Interviewees described religion as influencing their feelings about having and managing asthma. For IP9, this meant that the effect of reading a religious text, a hadith, helped her to feel more positive and strengthened her belief in her abilities to manage her asthma. *"Without my religion, I don't think I would have seen any good sides of the illness/ . . . /It [asthma] heavily affects my everyday life/ . . . /but according to my religion, Allah Teala [God] gives an illness to someone to cleanse their sins/ . . . /I see it [asthma] as an opportunity to cleanse my sins/ . . . /He [God] loves me so much that he wants me in Paradise, so I have been blessed with an illness/ . . . /and hadith [religious text]/ . . . /has motivated me and given me a positive approach" (IP9).* This example related to active proxy agency as well as personal agency, but it was the only example of personal agency described by an interviewee.

The most frequently expressed mode of agency was active proxy agency: most interviewees (seven out of 10) described the supreme being (referred to as God or Allah) as an active proxy agent. This was illustrated, for example, by praying for help from Allah to be cured of asthma or to increase self-efficacy to use asthma medicine. *"I ask Allah if he could please make my asthma better"* (IP8). Some interviewees considered an improvement in asthma symptoms to be an answer to prayers or a reason to be thankful to Allah (IP4, IP6, IP7 and IP8). The interviewees described Allah as exercising power over events and said that Allah ensured control of their asthma symptoms. Overall, achieving control of asthma symptoms was described as the result of using medicine as well as the answer to prayers.

However, praying was also described as a collective agency; for example, IP8's mother also prayed for improvement of her daughter's asthma: *"And my mom, she also always asks Allah to make me healthy in her prayers"* (IP8).

The interviewees described fasting during the holy month of Ramadan as an essential part of their religious practices. Opinions among the interviewees appear to differ about whether or not taking medicine means breaking the fast. IP3 stated that it was acceptable not to fast when having an illness even though she did not want to take medicine when fasting, whereas IP7 and IP9 expressed the opinion that taking medicine does not break the fast. However, IP5 was not sure whether it was *haram* (sinful) to use medicine during Ramadan if she felt ill from asthma, and IP3 was determined not to break her fast despite experiencing asthma symptoms that previously had led to a two-day hospitalisation. Interviewees sought information about whether or not it was considered appropriate to use medicine during Ramadan from their families, the Internet and religious texts. Interviewees differed as to whether they included physicians in their decision-making about using asthma medicine during Ramadan. IP2 and IP8 said that they discussed the new treatment regimen with their physicians, whereas IP6 and IP9 made decisions without their physician's advice.

All interviewees wanted to fast, but their abilities to do so differed. IP8 fasted for a couple of days even though her physician told her not to, so that she could take her medicine, whereas IP6 stated that she was unable to fast for seven days because of her asthma. The focus group interviewees indicated that they were unaffected by verbal attempts at persuasion from parents, husbands and physicians to abstain from fasting.

All interviewees explained that they perceived to combine fasting with using medicine. Although some interviewees mentioned altering the dosage regimen, this was perceived by them as combining fasting with medicine use. Thus, fasting affected the self-perceived self-efficacy to use medicine. Most interviewees described aligning the intake of controller medicine with sunrise and sunset, for example: *"I will use it at suhoor [morning before sunrise] and at iftar [after sunset]"* (IP5). In contrast, IP3 and IP6 stated that using reliever medicine regularly as a safety precaution during Ramadan made them feel better psychologically even though they did not have an asthma attack when using it. The medicine regimen differed during Ramadan compared to other months of the year, although focus group interviewees emphasised that both fasting and asthma medicine use are important:

IP3: *"You should prioritise both [fasting and using medicine.]"*

IP6: *" . . . if you are only using the medicine once in the morning, then you shift it to somewhere in the evening. In that way, you are both fasting and complying with the medicine and thereby prioritising [them] equally high."*

IP3: *"That way one still gets the same effect of the medicine . . . "*

2nd author: *"But is that something you also carry out? Rotating the time of using medicine depending on sunrise and sunset?"*

All interviewees: *"Yes"* (focus group interview)

Religion and religious practice played a large part in self-efficacy related to asthma health behaviour, including using medicine. According to the interviewees, using medicine and carrying out religious practices do not need to be mutually exclusive: the two can co-exist.

4. Discussion

The main finding of this study is that religion and religious practice influence self-efficacy to adhere to asthma medicine treatment.

The adherence to medicine treatment differed among these young, Muslim minority women. A reason for this might be found in their varying descriptions about the effect of their medicine. In particular, it was observed in this sample that low outcome expectations for controller medicine link to low adherence. This might be a part of the explanation for the reported lower redemption of prescriptions for asthma controller medicine compared to reliever medicine among Muslim minorities in Denmark [25]. This is supported by a study showing that adherence to asthma controller medicine links with positive outcome expectations [36]. Self-efficacy is a concept relevant for investigating asthma adherence [33,35,36]. Thus, it should be investigated whether low outcome expectations in general contribute to low adherence via its influence on self-efficacy.

4.1. Religion and Religious Practice Influence Self-Efficacy

Medicine adherence for these young, Muslim minority women shifts during Ramadan, often to either once a day or twice a day, at both *suhoor* and *iftar*. Individuals with asthma have previously reported this pattern [27,41]. A review of the health impact of fasting during Ramadan recommended that individuals with asthma avoid fasting to prevent possible worsening of bronchoconstriction [42]. Similar to the findings by Azizi [42], this study reports that different traditions of Islam appear to provide different beliefs about whether inhaler use nullifies the fast, leading to inter-individual differences in adherence to asthma treatment during Ramadan compared with other months of the year.

All interviewees demonstrated religious commitment by their strong intention to fast despite their illness, which has also been reported for Turkish adults with asthma [41]. However, the interviewees generally expressed the opinion that they would break the fast if they felt ill, similar to Pakistanis with type 2 diabetes [43]. The self-efficacy to fast appears to be strong, despite verbal persuasion against fasting and the experience of worsening asthma symptoms as a consequence of fasting. This can be considered a counteractive influence on the self-efficacy to use asthma medicine.

Therefore, Bandura's theory of self-efficacy [12,13,31,39] and modes of agency relevant to religion [31] cannot explain how religion shapes self-efficacy as revealed in this study.

The findings show that these young Muslim minority women with asthma perceive religion as offering an alternative (to using medicine) to obtain the desired outcome of controlling asthma symptoms. The interviewees used praying as part of religious practice to invoke the supreme being to exercise influence as an active proxy agent. A Danish study previously found that non-Western immigrants in Denmark may think their efforts to improve health are not important, which the authors report could be related to self-efficacy [44]. These results by Molin et al. [44] might be explained by the findings of this study connected with Bandura's modes of agency. Bandura [35] states that passivity can develop due to a belief that God will help solve personal issues, and, in this present study, God was considered to be an active proxy agent in controlling asthma symptoms. Ahmedani et al. [45] reported that participants who believed that God determines health and health outcomes had lower ICS adherence compared to participants with other beliefs, although they did not explore the effects of a specific religion. A distinction can be made between a belief in God and a belief that God is an active proxy agent, and only the latter seems to influence asthma health behaviour. However, praying was also reported to heighten self-efficacy for using medicine, which is predicted to result in higher medicine adherence.

It is important for HCPs to be aware of the link between self-efficacy, religion and adherence to asthma medicine treatment. An understanding of how these can interact can help both prescribers and pharmacy staff provide better counselling to young, Muslim minority women and aid the monitoring of treatment for this subgroup of patients. In turn, this could improve the quality of asthma care for young, Muslim minority women.

4.2. Strengths and Limitations of the Study

The interviewer's shared gender and religious background with the interviewees might have added to better interactions during the interview [46]. This also could have lead to muted opinions if thought to differ from the interviewer's, but it was not the impression to be the case. Data saturation may not have been reached in this study due to the relatively small group of interviewees. Using the quality criteria of Lincoln and Guba [47], the authors sought to ensure the trustworthiness and transferability of data by transparency in data collection, data analysis and result reporting. The transferability is limited due to the small convenience sample, but may give an indication of possible opinions hold by young, Muslim women. One study strength was the reflexive discussion of data analysis among co-authors because this greatly strengthens the trustworthiness of results.

The self-assessment of adherence can be a limitation of the study because other means were not used to ensure the validity of the assessment.

The recruitment strategy was successful in using social media, consistent with a previously conducted qualitative study that recruited participants in a comparable age range [48]. A potential issue is that this sampling approach does not target eligible participants not using Facebook. This might favour recruitment of interviewees who share the same views or beliefs, thus limiting data completeness. As it was not possible to discover why some potential recruits chose not to respond to the call for participation, it cannot be determined how responders differ from non-responders. However, the study did not aim to generalise the findings to a wider population, but instead aimed to gain insight into the experiences of young, Muslim minority women in Denmark using asthma medicine.

The theory of self-efficacy proved applicable for analysing adherence to asthma medicine treatment. However, it is important to be aware that dichotomisations, such as classifications of low and high self-efficacy levels in the present analysis, should be used with some caution. The insights into the lives of young, Muslim minority women obtained via the interviews are based on only a single time point in their lives; therefore, the self-perceived self-efficacy level might have shifted from low to high or vice versa if interviewees had chosen to tell other life stories. However, despite this limitation, it is of interest to understand the adherence and asthma health behaviour of this subgroup of patients.

4.3. Future Perspectives

More knowledge is needed about how to help Muslims combine fasting with adherence to asthma medicine treatment. A possible approach would be to explore the effect of providing health and medicine treatment information at mosques and by other means, as previously suggested for cancer treatment adherence in England [49]. In addition, there is a need for more research to update the theory of self-efficacy to conceptualise the impact of religion on self-efficacy.

5. Conclusions

Self-efficacy to adhere to asthma medicine treatment is linked to religion and religious practice. During the holy month of Ramadan, changes in self-perceived self-efficacy were reported by interviewees. In addition, praying was used as an alternative to medicine for controlling asthma symptoms. Feelings of improvement in asthma symptoms were considered as either an answer to prayers or a reason to be thankful to Allah. This was because the outcome of controlling asthma symptoms was perceived to be achieved by Allah. However, the use of medicine and religion was not perceived to be mutually exclusive, but rather to coexist with the shared goal of controlling asthma symptoms.

It is important for HCPs to be aware of the link between self-efficacy, religion and adherence to asthma medicine treatment. The understanding of how these can interact can help both prescribers and pharmacy staff to provide better counselling to young Muslim women and aid the monitoring of treatment for this subgroup of patients. In turn, this could improve the quality of asthma care for young Muslim women.

39. Justitsministeriet. Bekendtgørelse om ændring af bekendtgørelse om undtagelse fra pligten til anmeldelse af visse behandlinger, som foretages for en privat dataansvarlig: BEK nr. 410 af 09/05/2012 [Decree Amending the Decree on Exemption from the Obligation to Ceclare Certain Procedures Which Are Made for a Private Data Controller: Order No. 410 of 09/05/2012]. 2012. Available online: https://www.retsinformation.dk/Forms/R0710.aspx?id=141758 (accessed on 14 May 2018).

40. Aydin, Ö.; Celik, G.E.; Önen, Z.P.; Yilmaz, I.; Özdemir, S.K.; Yildiz, Ö.; Mungan, D.; Demirel, Y.S. How do patients with asthma and COPD behave during fasting? *Allergol. Immunopathol.* **2014**, *42*, 115–119. [CrossRef] [PubMed]

41. Car, J.; Sheikh, A. Fasting and asthma: An opportunity for building patient-doctor partnership. *Prim. Care Respir. J.* **2004**, *13*, 133–135. [CrossRef] [PubMed]

42. Azizi, F. Islamic fasting and health. *Ann. Nutr. Metab.* **2010**, *56*, 273–282. [CrossRef] [PubMed]

43. Mygind, A.; Kristiansen, M.; Wittrup, I.; Nørgaard, L.S. Patient perspectives on type 2 diabetes and medicine use during Ramadan among Pakistanis in Denmark. *Int. J. Clin. Pharm.* **2013**, *35*, 281–288. [CrossRef] [PubMed]

44. Molin, K.R.; Mygind, A.; Nørgaard, L.S. Perceptions of disease aetiology and the effect of own behavior on health among poly-pharmacy patients with non-Western backgrounds in Denmark. *Int. J. Pharm. Pract.* **2013**, *21*, 386–392. [CrossRef] [PubMed]

45. Ahmedani, B.K.; Peterson, E.L.; Wells, K.E.; Rand, C.S.; Williams, L.K. Asthma medication adherence: The role of God and other health locus of control factors. *Ann. Allergy Asthma Immunol.* **2013**, *110*, 75–79. [CrossRef] [PubMed]

46. Richards, H.; Emslie, C. The 'doctor' or the 'girl from the University'? Considering the influence of professional roles on qualitative interviewing. *Fam. Pract.* **2000**, *17*, 71–75. [CrossRef] [PubMed]

47. Lincoln, Y.S.; Guba, E.G. But is it rigorous? Trustworthiness and authenticity in naturalistic evaluation. In *Naturalistic Evaluation*; Williams, D.D., Ed.; Jossey-Bass: San Francisco, CA, USA, 1986; pp. 73–81.

48. Fergie, G.; Hunt, K.; Hilton, S. Social media as a space for support: Young adults' perspectives on producing and consuming user-generated content about diabetes and mental health. *Soc. Sci. Med.* **2016**, *170*, 46–54. [CrossRef] [PubMed]

49. Whyte, A. Ready for Ramadan. *Nurs. Stand.* **2010**, *24*, 18–19. [CrossRef] [PubMed]

Permissions

All chapters in this book were first published in PHARMACY, by MDPI; hereby published with permission under the Creative Commons Attribution License or equivalent. Every chapter published in this book has been scrutinized by our experts. Their significance has been extensively debated. The topics covered herein carry significant findings which will fuel the growth of the discipline. They may even be implemented as practical applications or may be referred to as a beginning point for another development.

The contributors of this book come from diverse backgrounds, making this book a truly international effort. This book will bring forth new frontiers with its revolutionizing research information and detailed analysis of the nascent developments around the world.

We would like to thank all the contributing authors for lending their expertise to make the book truly unique.

They have played a crucial role in the development of this book. Without their invaluable contributions this book wouldn't have been possible. They have made vital efforts to compile up to date information on the varied aspects of this subject to make this book a valuable addition to the collection of many professionals and students.

This book was conceptualized with the vision of imparting up-to-date information and advanced data in this field. To ensure the same, a matchless editorial board was set up. Every individual on the board went through rigorous rounds of assessment to prove their worth. After which they invested a large part of their time researching and compiling the most relevant data for our readers.

The editorial board has been involved in producing this book since its inception. They have spent rigorous hours researching and exploring the diverse topics which have resulted in the successful publishing of this book. They have passed on their knowledge of decades through this book. To expedite this challenging task, the publisher supported the team at every step. A small team of assistant editors was also appointed to further simplify the editing procedure and attain best results for the readers.

Apart from the editorial board, the designing team has also invested a significant amount of their time in understanding the subject and creating the most relevant covers. They scrutinized every image to scout for the most suitable representation of the subject and create an appropriate cover for the book.

The publishing team has been an ardent support to the editorial, designing and production team. Their endless efforts to recruit the best for this project, has resulted in the accomplishment of this book. They are a veteran in the field of academics and their pool of knowledge is as vast as their experience in printing. Their expertise and guidance has proved useful at every step. Their uncompromising quality standards have made this book an exceptional effort. Their encouragement from time to time has been an inspiration for everyone.

The publisher and the editorial board hope that this book will prove to be a valuable piece of knowledge for researchers, students, practitioners and scholars across the globe.

List of Contributors

Antonio Sánchez-Pozo
Department of Biochemistry, Faculty of Pharmacy, University of Granada, Campus Cartuja s/n, Granada 18071, Spain

Roxana Sandulovici
Faculty of Pharmacy, Titu Maiorescu University, 22, Dâmbovnicului, Sector 4, 040441 Bucharest, Romania

Constantin Mircioiu and Cristina Rais
Faculty of Pharmacy, University of Medicine and Pharmacy "Carol Davila", 6th Traian Vuia, Sector 2, 020956 Bucharest, Romania

Jeffrey Atkinson
Pharmacolor Consultants Nancy, 12 rue de Versigny, 54600 Villers, France

Sawsan Abdullah Alamri and Mastour Safer Al Ghamdi
College of Clinical Pharmacy, Imam Abdulrahman Bin Faisal University (University of Dammam), Dammam 31441, Saudi Arabia

Raniah Ali Al Jaizani and Atta Abbas Naqvi
Department of Pharmacy Practice, College of Clinical Pharmacy, Imam Abdulrahman Bin Faisal University (University of Dammam), Dammam 31441, Saudi Arabia

Morag C. E. McFadyen and Lesley Diack
School of Pharmacy and Life sciences, Robert Gordon University, Riverside East, Garthdee Road, Aberdeen AB10 7GJ, UK

Minji Sohn and Mohamed Bazzi
College of Pharmacy, Ferris State University, 220 Ferris Drive, Big Rapids, MI 49307, USA

Meghan Burgess
College of Health Professions, Ferris State University, 200 Ferris Drive, Big Rapids, MI 49307, USA

Constantin Mircioiu
Pharmacy Faculty, University of Medicine and Pharmacy "Carol Davila" Bucharest, Dionisie Lupu 37, Bucharest 020021, Romania

Jeffrey Atkinson
Pharmacolor Consultants Nancy, 12 rue de Versigny, Villers 54600, France

Gennaro A. Paolella
Naval Medical Center San Diego, United States Navy, San Diego, CA 92101, USA

Andrew D. Boyd
Department of Biomedical and Health Information Sciences, University of Illinois at Chicago, Chicago, IL 60612, USA

Scott M. Wirth and Sandra Cuellar
Department of Pharmacy Practice, Ambulatory Pharmacy Services, University of Illinois at Chicago, Chicago, IL 60612, USA

Neeta K. Venepalli
Department of Medicine, Hematology/Oncology, University of Illinois at Chicago, Chicago, IL 60612, USA

Stephanie Y. Crawford
Department of Pharmacy Systems, Outcomes and Policy, University of Illinois at Chicago, Chicago, IL 60612, USA

Urszula Religioni
Department of Public Health, Medical University of Warsaw, Banacha 1a, 02-097 Warsaw, Poland

Damian Swieczkowski, Natalia Cwalina and Miłosz J. Jaguszewski
First Department of Cardiology, Medical University in Gdansk, Dębinki 7, 80-952 Gdánsk, Poland

Anna Gawrónska
Institute of Logistics and Warehousing, Ewarysta Estkowskiego 6, 61-755 Poznán, Poland

Anna Kowalczuk
National Medicines Institute, Chełmska 30/34, 00-725 Warsaw, Poland

Mariola Drozd
Department of Applied Pharmacy, Medical University of Lublin, Chodźki 1, 20-093 Lublin, Poland

Mikołaj Zerhau
Hospital Pharmacy, Mazowiecki Szpitala Specjalistyczny w Ostrołęce, Al. Jana Pawła II 120 A, 07-410 Ostrołęka, Poland

Dariusz Smolínski
Community Pharmacy, Poland

Stanisław Radomínski
Quizit Sp. z. o. o., Unit Dose, Sprinterów 2/6, 94-022 Łódź, Poland

David Brindley
Department of Paediatrics, University of Oxford, Level 2, Children's Hospital, John Radcliffe, Headington, Oxford OX3 9DU, UK
The Oxford—UCL Centre for the Advancement of Sustainable Medical Innovation (CASMI), The University of Oxford, Tavistock Square, London WC1H 9JP, UK
Centre for Behavioural Medicine, UCL School of Pharmacy, University College London, BMA House, Tavistock Square, London WC1H 9JP, UK
Harvard Stem Cell Institute, Cambridge, MA 02138, USA
USCF-Stanford Centre of Excellence in Regulatory Science and Innovation (CERSI), San Francisco, CA 94158, USA

Piotr Merks
Department of Pharmaceutical Technology, Faculty of Pharmacy Collegium Medicum in Bydgoszcz, Nicolaus Copernicus University in Torun, 85-089 Bydgoszcz, Poland

Meagen M. Rosenthal and Erin R. Holmes
Department of Pharmacy Administration, School of Pharmacy, University of Mississippi, 223 Faser Hall, University, MS 38677-1848, USA

Tessa J. Hastings, Lindsey A. Hohmann and Salisa C. Westrick
Health Outcomes Research and Policy, Harrison School of Pharmacy Auburn University, 020 James E. Foy Hall, Auburn, AL 36849, USA

Stuart J. Mc Farland
College of Medicine, University of South Alabama, 307 N University Blvd, Mobile, AL 36688, USA

Benjamin S. Teeter
Department of Pharmacy Practice, College of Pharmacy, University of Arkansas for Medical Sciences, 4301W Markham St, Little Rock, AR 72205, USA

Agnieszka Skowron, Justyna Dymek, Anna Gołda and Wioletta Polak
Faculty of Pharmacy, Jagiellonian University Medical College, Krakow 30-699, Poland

Vanessa Marvin and Emily Ward
Department of Pharmacy, Chelsea and Westminster Hospital NHS Foundation Trust, London SW10 9NH, UK

Medicines Optimisation, NIHR CLAHRC NW London, London SW10 9NH, UK

Barry Jubraj
Medicines Optimisation, NIHR CLAHRC NW London, London SW10 9NH, UK
Institute of Pharmaceutical Science, King's College London, London SE1 9NH, UK

Mark Bower
Department of Oncology, Chelsea and Westminster Hospital NHS Foundation Trust, London SW10 9NH, UK

Iñaki Bovill
Department of Elderly Medicine, Chelsea and Westminster Hospital NHS Foundation Trust, London SW10 9NH, UK

Fatimah Ali Albusalih
College of Clinical Pharmacy, Imam Abdulrahman Bin Faisal University (University of Dammam), Dammam 31441, Saudi Arabia

Atta Abbas Naqvi
Department of Pharmacy Practice, College of Clinical Pharmacy, Imam Abdulrahman Bin Faisal University (University of Dammam), Dammam 31441, Saudi Arabia

Rizwan Ahmad
Natural Products and Alternative Medicines, College of Clinical Pharmacy, Imam Abdulrahman Bin Faisal University (University of Dammam), Dammam 31441, Saudi Arabia

Niyaz Ahmad
Department of Pharmaceutics, College of Clinical Pharmacy, Imam Abdulrahman Bin Faisal University (University of Dammam), Dammam 31441, Saudi Arabia

Jeffrey Atkinson
Pharmacolor Consultants Nancy, Villers 54600, France

Whitney J. Kiel
Bronson Methodist Hospital, 601 John St. Suite M-020, Kalamazoo, MI 49007, USA

Shaun W. Phillips
Clinical and Pharmacy Services, Bronson Healthcare Group, 300 North Avenue, Battle Creek, MI 49017, USA

Valentina Petkova
Faculty of Pharmacy, Medical University-Sofia, 2-Dunav Street, 1000 Sofia, Bulgaria

Jeffrey Atkinson
Pharmacolor Consultants Nancy, 12 rue de Versigny, 54600 Villers, France

Anthony W. Olson, Jon C. Schommer and Ronald S. Hadsall
College of Pharmacy, University of Minnesota, 308 Harvard Street, S.E., Minneapolis, MN 55455, USA

William R. Doucette
College of Pharmacy, University of Iowa, 115 S. Grand Avenue, S518 PHAR, Iowa City, IA 52242, USA

Jon C. Schommer
College of Pharmacy, University of Minnesota, 308 Harvard Street, S.E., Minneapolis, MN 55455, USA

Derek Evans
FRPharmS, FRGS, MFTM RCPS, Independent Prescriber, 58 The Nurseries, Langstone, Wales NP18 2NT, UK

Eugene Y. H. Yeung
Education Centre, Royal Lancaster Infirmary, Lancaster LA1 4RP, UK
Department of Medical Microbiology, The Ottawa Hospital General Campus, The University of Ottawa, Ottawa, ON K1H 8L6, Canada

Louise C. Druedahl, Duaa Yaqub, Lotte Stig Nørgaard and Lourdes Cantarero-Arévalo
Social and Clinical Pharmacy Group, Department of Pharmacy, Faculty of Health and Medical Sciences, University of Copenhagen, Universitetsparken 2, DK-2100 Copenhagen, Denmark

Maria Kristiansen
Department of Public Health, Faculty of Health and Medical Sciences, University of Copenhagen, Øster Farimagsgade 5, DK-1014 Copenhagen, Denmark

Index